D0744619

Fetal Surgery

Guest Editor

HANMIN LEE, MD

CLINICS IN PERINATOLOGY

www.perinatology.theclinics.com

June 2009 • Volume 36 • Number 2

SAUNDERS an imprint of ELSEVIER, Inc.

W.B. SAUNDERS COMPANY
A Division of Elsevier Inc.

Elsevier, Inc. • 1600 John F. Kennedy Blvd. • Suite 1800 • Philadelphia, PA 19103-2899

http://www.theclinics.com

CLINICS IN PERINATOLOGY Volume 36, Number 2
June 2009 ISSN 0095-5108, ISBN-10: 1-4377-0521-9, ISBN-13: 978-1-4377-0521-8

Editor: Carla Holloway
Developmental Editor: Donald Mumford

© 2009 Elsevier ■ **All rights reserved.**

This journal and the individual contributions contained in it are protected under copyright by Elsevier, and the following terms and conditions apply to their use:

Photocopying
Single photocopies of single articles may be made for personal use as allowed by national copyright laws. Permission of the Publisher and payment of a fee is required for all other photocopying, including multiple or systematic copying, copying for advertising or promotional purposes, resale, and all forms of document delivery. Special rates are available for educational institutions that wish to make photocopies for non-profit educational classroom use. For information on how to seek permission visit www.elsevier.com/permissions or call: (+44) 1865 843830 (UK)/(+1) 215 239 3804 (USA).

Derivative Works
Subscribers may reproduce tables of contents or prepare lists of articles including abstracts for internal circulation within their institutions. Permission of the Publisher is required for resale or distribution outside the institution. Permission of the Publisher is required for all other derivative works, including compilations and translations (please consult www.elsevier.com/permissions).

Electronic Storage or Usage
Permission of the Publisher is required to store or use electronically any material contained in this journal, including any article or part of an article (please consult www.elsevier.com/permissions). Except as outlined above, no part of this publication may be reproduced, stored in a retrieval system or transmitted in any form or by any means, electronic, mechanical, photocopying, recording or otherwise, without prior written permission of the Publisher.

Notice
No responsibility is assumed by the Publisher for any injury and/or damage to persons or property as a matter of products liability, negligence or otherwise, or from any use or operation of any methods, products, instructions or ideas contained in the material herein. Because of rapid advances in the medical sciences, in particular, independent verification of diagnoses and drug dosages should be made. Although all advertising material is expected to conform to ethical (medical) standards, inclusion in this publication does not constitute a guarantee or endorsement of the quality or value of such product or of the claims made of it by its manufacturer.

Clinics in Perinatology (ISSN 0095-5108) is published in quarterly by Elsevier Inc., 360 Park Avenue South, New York, NY 10010-1710. Months of issue are March, June, September, and December. Business and Editorial offices: 1600 John F. Kennedy Blvd., Suite 1800, Philadelphia, PA 19103-2899. Customer Service Office: 6277 Sea Harbor Drive, Orlando, FL 32887-4800. Periodicals postage paid at New York, NY and additional mailing offices. Subscription prices are $217.00 per year (US individuals), $321.00 per year (US institutions), $255.00 per year (Canadian individuals), $408.00 per year (Canadian institutions), $314.00 per year (foreign individuals), $408.00 per year (foreign institutions) $105.00 per year (US students), and $153.00 per year (Canadian and foreign students). Foreign air speed delivery is included in all Clinics subscription prices. All prices are subject to change without notice. **POSTMASTER:** Send address changes to *Clinics in Perinatology*; Elsevier Periodicals Customer Service, 11830 Westline Industrial Drive, St. Louis, MO 63146. Customer Service (orders, claims, online, change of address): Elsevier Periodicals Customer Service, 11830 Westline Industrial Drive, St. Louis, MO 63146. Tel: 1-800-654-2452 (U.S. and Canada); 314-453-7041 (outside U.S. and Canada). Fax: 314-453-5170. E-mail: journalscustomerservice-usa@elsevier.com (for print support); journalsonlinesupport-usa@elsevier.com (for online support).

Reprints. For copies of 100 or more, of articles in this publication, please contact the Commercial Reprints Department, Elsevier Inc., 360 Park Avenue South, New York, NY 10010-1710. Tel. (212) 633-3812; Fax: (212) 482-1935; email: reprints@elsevier.com.

Clinics in Perinatology is also pubilshed in Spanish by McGraw-Hill Interamericana Editores S.A., P.O. Box 5-237, 06500 Mexico D.F., Mexico.

Clinics in Perinatology is covered in *MEDLINE/PubMed (Index Medicus) Current Contents, Excepta Medica, BIOSIS* and *ISI/BIOMED.*

Printed in the United States of America.

Contributors

GUEST EDITOR

HANMIN LEE, MD
Associate Professor of Surgery, Pediatrics, and Obstetrics/Gynecology; Reproductive Health Sciences Director, Fetal Treatment Center, University of California, San Francisco, San Francisco, California

AUTHORS

N. SCOTT ADZICK, MD
Director, Center for Fetal Diagnosis and Treatment; Surgeon-in-Chief, Children's Hospital of Philadelphia; C.Everett Koop Professor of Pediatric Surgery, University of Pennsylvania School of Medicine, Philadelphia, Pennsylvania

KAREL ALLEGAERT, MD, PhD
Woman and Child Division, Fetal Medicine Unit, University Hospital Gasthuisberg, Leuven, Belgium

ROBERT H. BALL, MD
Director, HCA Fetal Therapy Initiative, Maternal-Fetal Services of Utah, St Mark's Hospital, Salt Lake City, Utah

FRANK A. CHERVENAK, MD
Given Foundation Professor and Chair, Department of Obstetrics and Gynecology, New York Weill Cornell Medical Center, New York Presbyterian Hospital, New York, New York

FILIP CLAUS, MD, PhD
Professor, Division of Medical Imaging, University Hospital Gasthuisberg, Leuven, Belgium

FERGUS V. COAKLEY, MD
Department of Radiology, University of California, San Francisco, San Francisco, California

TIMOTHY CROMBLEHOLME, MD
Fetal Care Center of Cincinnati; Division of Pediatric General, Thoracic and Fetal Surgery, Cincinnati Children's Hospital; University of Cincinnati, College of Medicine, Cincinnati, Ohio

ANNE DEBEER, MD
Woman and Child Division, Fetal Medicine Unit, University Hospital Gasthuisberg, Leuven, Belgium

JAN A. DEPREST, MD, PhD
Professor, Woman and Child Division, Fetal Medicine Unit, University Hospital Gasthuisberg, Leuven, Belgium

ELISE DONE, MD
Woman and Child Division, Fetal Medicine Unit, University Hospital Gasthuisberg, Leuven, Belgium

DIANA L. FARMER, MD
Division of Pediatric Surgery, Department of Surgery, Fetal Treatment Center, University of California, San Francisco, San Francisco, California

DARIO O. FAUZA, MD
Associate, Department of Surgery, Children's Hospital Boston; Associate Professor of Surgery, Harvard Medical School, Boston, Massachusetts

VICKIE A. FELDSTEIN, MD
Professor of Clinical Radiology, Department of Radiology, University of California, San Francisco, San Francisco, California

ALAN W. FLAKE, MD
Professor of Surgery, Department of Surgery; Director, Children's Center for Fetal Research, Children's Hospital of Philadelphia, University of Pennsylvania School of Medicine, Philadelphia, Pennsylvania

ORIT A. GLENN, MD
Department of Radiology, University of California, San Francisco, San Francisco, California

EDUARDO GRATACOS, MD, PhD
Professor and Chair, Department of Obstetrics, Hospital Clinic, Barcelona, Spain

LEONARDO GUCCIARDO, MD
Woman and Child Division, Fetal Medicine Unit, University Hospital Gasthuisberg, Leuven, Belgium

MOUNIRA HABLI, MD
Fetal Care Center of Cincinnati; Division of Pediatric General, Thoracic and Fetal Surgery, Cincinnati Children's Hospital; Maternal Fetal Medicine, University of Cincinnati, College of Medicine, Cincinnati, Ohio

R. WHIT HALL, MD
Professor of Pediatrics, Division of Neonatology, University of Arkansas for Medical Sciences, Little Rock, Arkansas

MICHAEL R. HARRISON, MD
Professor Emeritus, Division of Pediatric Surgery, Department of Surgery, Fetal Treatment Center, University of California, San Francisco, San Francisco, California

SHINJIRO HIROSE, MD
Division of Pediatric Surgery, Department of Surgery, Fetal Treatment Center, University of California, San Francisco, San Francisco, California

LINDA M. HOPKINS, MD
Assistant Professor, Division of Perinatal Medicine and Genetics, University of California, San Francisco, San Francisco, California

LISA K. HORNBERGER, MD
Department of Pediatrics, Division of Cardiology, Fetal and Neonatal Cardiology Program;
Professor of Pediatrics and Obstetrics and Gynecology, Department of Obstetrics and
Gynecology, University of Alberta, Edmonton, Alberta, Canada

TIM JANCELEWICZ, MD
Division of Pediatric Surgery, Department of Surgery, Fetal Treatment Center, University
of California, San Francisco, San Francisco, California

ERIC JELIN, MD
Division of Pediatric Surgery, Department of Surgery, Fetal Treatment Center, University
of California, San Francisco, San Francisco, California

RUSSELL W. JENNINGS, MD
Associate Professor, Department of Surgery, Harvard Medical School; Director,
Advanced Fetal Care Center, Department of Surgery, Children's Hospital Boston, Boston,
Massachusetts

MARK PAUL JOHNSON, MD
Associate Professor, Department of Obstetrics and Gynecology; Associate Professor,
Department of Surgery; Associate Professor, Department of Pediatrics, University of
Pennsylvania School of Medicine, The Center for Fetal Diagnosis and Treatment,
The Children's Hospital of Philadelphia, Philadelphia, Pennsylvania

HANMIN LEE, MD
Associate Professor of Surgery, Pediatrics, and Obstetrics/Gynecology; Reproductive
Health Sciences Director, Fetal Treatment Center, University of California, San Francisco,
San Francisco, California

FOONG YEN LIM, MD
The Fetal Care Center of Cincinnati; Division of Pediatric General, Thoracic and Fetal
Surgery, Cincinnati Children's Hospital; University of Cincinnati, College of Medicine,
Cincinnati, Ohio

LAURENCE B. McCULLOUGH, PhD
Dalton Tomlin Chair, Center for Medical Ethics and Health Policy, Baylor College
of Medicine, Houston, Texas

KYPROS NICOLAIDES, MD, PhD
Professor, Harris Birthright Center for Fetal Medicine, King's College Hospital, London,
United Kingdom

LARRY RAND, MD
Director of Perinatal Services, Fetal Treatment Center; Assistant Professor, Department
of Obstetrics, Gynecology, and Reproductive Sciences, University of California,
San Francisco, San Francisco, California

IRWIN REISS, MD, PhD
Neonatal Intensive Care, Departments of Intensive Care and Pediatric Surgery, Erasmus
Medical Centre, Sophia Kinderziekenhuis, Rotterdam, The Netherlands

JESSICA L. ROYBAL, MD
Research Fellow, Department of Surgery, Children's Center for Fetal Research, Children's
Hospital of Philadelphia, University of Pennsylvania School of Medicine, Philadelphia,
Pennsylvania

MATTHEW T. SANTORE, MD
Research Fellow, Department of Surgery, Children's Center for Fetal Research, Children's Hospital of Philadelphia, University of Pennsylvania School of Medicine, Philadelphia, Pennsylvania

PRIYA SEKAR, MD, MPH
Clinical Research Fellow, Department of Pediatrics, Division of Cardiology, Fetal and Neonatal Cardiology Program, Stollery Children's Hospital, Edmonton, Alberta, Canada

ROLLA M. SHBAROU, MD
Assistant Professor of Pediatrics, Division of Neurology, University of Arkansas for Medical Sciences, Arkansas Children's Hospital, Little Rock, Arkansas

DICK TIBBOEL, MD, PhD
Professor and Chair, Intensive Care Department of Pediatric Surgery, Erasmus Medical Centre, Sophia Kinderziekenhuis, Rotterdam, The Netherlands

CHRISTOPHER G.B. TURNER, MD
Research Fellow, Department of Surgery, Children's Hospital Boston, Boston, Massachusetts

WAYNE TWORETZKY, MD
Assistant Professor, Department of Pediatrics, Harvard Medical School; Director, Fetal Cardiology Program, Children's Hospital Boston, Boston, Massachusetts

TIM VAN MIEGHEM, MD
Woman and Child Division, Fetal Medicine Unit, University Hospital Gasthuisberg, Leuven, Belgium

LOUISE E. WILKINS-HAUG, MD, PhD
Associate Professor Harvard Medical School; Division Director, Maternal Fetal Medicine and Reproductive Genetics, Department of Maternal Fetal Medicine, Brigham and Women's Hospital, Boston, Massachusetts

DANNY WU, MD
Assistant Professor of Obstetrics, Gynecology, and Reproductive Sciences, University of California, San Francisco, San Francisco, California

SERENA WU, MD
Fellow, General Surgery, The Center for Fetal Diagnosis and Treatment, The Children's Hospital of Philadelphia, Philadelphia, Pennsylvania

Contents

R. Whit Hall and Rolla M. Shbarou

> Painful procedures in the neonatal ICU are common, undertreated, and
> lead to adverse consequences. The drugs most commonly used to treat
> neonatal pain include the opiates, benzodiazepines, barbiturates, ket-
> amine, propofol, acetaminophen, and local and topical anesthetics. This
> article discusses the indications for and advantages and disadvantages
> of the commonly used analgesic drugs. Guidance and references for drugs
> and dosing for specific neonatal procedures are provided.

Fetal Surgery

Overview

Tim Jancelewicz and Michael R. Harrison

> Over the past 3 decades, fetal surgery for congenital disease has evolved
> from merely a fanciful concept to a medical field in its own right. Tech-
> niques for open hysterotomy, minimal-access hysteroscopy, and image-
> guided percutaneous fetal access have become well established, first in
> animal models and subsequently in humans. At the same time, major
> advances in fetal imaging and diagnosis, anesthesia, and tocolysis have
> allowed fetal intervention to become a vital tool for subsets of patients
> who would otherwise endure significant morbidity and mortality. This
> article offers a concise overview of the history of fetal surgery, from its
> tumultuous early days to its current status as an important means for the
> early treatment of potentially devastating congenital anomalies.

Frank A. Chervenak and Laurence B. McCullough

> This article provides a comprehensive approach to the ethics of clinical
> investigation of fetal surgery. Investigators should address the initiation
> and assessment of clinical trials to determine whether they establish a stan-
> dard of care and use an appropriate informed consent process to recruit
> and enroll subjects, consider whether selection criteria should include the
> abortion preferences of the pregnant woman, and consider whether

In this review, the authors explore the role of noninvasive and invasive fetal interventions in fetal cardiovascular disease guided by observations at fetal echocardiography. They first review fetal cardiac lesions that may be ameliorated by fetal intervention and then review noncardiac fetal pathologic findings for which fetal echocardiography can provide important insight into the pathophysiology and aid in patient selection for and timing of intervention and postintervention surveillance.

Specific Diseases

Congenital diaphragmatic hernia (CDH) should be diagnosed in the prenatal period and prompt referral to a tertiary referral center for imaging, genetic testing, and multidisciplinary counseling. Individual prediction of prognosis is based on the absence of additional anomalies, lung size, and liver herniation. In severe cases, a prenatal endotracheal balloon procedure is currently being offered at specialized centers. Fetal intervention is now also offered to milder cases within a trial, hypothesizing that this may reduce the occurrence of bronchopulmonary dysplasia in survivors. Postnatal management has been standardized by European high-volume centers for the purpose of this and other trials.

Congenital diaphragmatic hernia (CDH) is characterized by a defect in the diaphragm that permits abdominal viscera to herniate into the chest. These herniated viscera are thought to compress the growing lung and cause lung parenchymal and vascular hypoplasia. The genetic defects that cause the diaphragmatic defect may also contribute primarily to lung hypoplasia. Postnatal reduction of the herniated abdominal viscera and correction of the diaphragmatic defect are easily achievable, but the lung hypoplasia persists, often leading to persistent fetal circulation and respiratory failure. This article reviews the experimental basis of fetal therapy for CDH and the US clinical experience with tracheal occlusion.

of patients referred for suspected TTTS have a different underlying patho-logic condition, however, and differentiating the subcategories of MC path-ophysiologic conditions may change treatment course and outcome. The key to understanding complicated MC pregnancies lies in the placental an-gioarchitecture and intertwin vascular communications between the fetuses.

Fetal intervention for myelomeningocele (MMC) may improve hydroceph-alus and hindbrain herniation associated with the Arnold-Chiari II malfor-mation and may reduce the need for ventriculoperitoneal shunting. As of now, there is little evidence that prenatal repair of MMC improves neuro-logic function. MMC is the first nonlethal disease under consideration and study for fetal surgery. As a result, potential improvements in outcome must be balanced with maternal safety and well-being, in addition to that of the unborn patient.

Congenital heart disease (CHD) is an attractive target for fetal therapy. With the development of successful neonatal repair for many types of CHD over the last 20 years, fetal therapy has become the next frontier. Concurrent advances in interventional catheterization and fetal imaging provided a foundation for the novel field of fetal cardiac intervention. This article focuses on the current status of in utero catheter interventions for CHD with particular interest in therapy for defects characterized by pro-gressive stenosis or atresia of the semilunar valves, the aortic and pulmo-nary, with development of subsequent ventricular hypoplasia.

Research/Future Directions

At the present time, the most likely and eminent application of stem cell therapy to the fetus is in utero hematopoietic stem cell transplantation (IUHCT), and this stem cell type will be discussed as a paradigm for all pre-natal stem cell therapy. The authors feel that the most likely initial applica-tion of IUHCT will use adult HSC derived from bone marrow (BM) or peripheral blood (PB), and will focus this article on this specific approach. The article also reviews the experimental data that support the capacity of IUHCT to induce donor-specific tolerance.

Christopher G.B. Turner and Dario O. Fauza

Attempts at harnessing the prospective benefits of the therapeutic use of fetal cells or tissues date many decades before the modern era of transplantation. The first reported transplantation of human fetal tissue took place in 1922. Fetal cells or tissues also have been used as helpful investigational tools since the 1930s. Still, it was only in the last three decades that fetal tissue transplantation in people has started to lead to favorable outcomes, yet by and large anecdotally. This article offers an outlook on a relatively new dimension in fetal cell-based therapies, namely the engineering of tissues in the laboratory, along with its prospective applications.

GOAL STATEMENT

The goal of *Clinics in Perinatology* is to keep practicing neonatologists and maternal-fetal medicine specialists up to date with current clinical practice in perinatology by providing timely articles reviewing the state of the art in patient care.

ACCREDITATION

The *Clinics in perinatology* is planned and implemented in accordance with the Essential Areas and Policies of the Accreditation Council for Continuing Medical Education (ACCME) through the joint sponsorship of the University of Virginia School of Medicine and Elsevier. The University of Virginia School of Medicine is accredited by the ACCME to provide continuing medical education for physicians.

The University of Virginia School of Medicine designates this educational activity for a maximum of 15 *AMA PRA Category 1 Credits*™ for each issue, 60 credits per year. Physicians should only claim credit commensurate with the extent of their participation in the activity.

The American Medical Association has determined that physicians not licensed in the US who participate in this CME activity are eligible for a maximum of 15 *AMA PRA Category 1 Credits*™ for each issue, 60 credits per year.

Credit can be earned by reading the text material, taking the CME examination online at: http://www.theclinics.com/home/cme, and completing the evaluation. After taking the test, you will be required to review any and all incorrect answers. Following completion of the test and evaluation, your credit will be awarded and you may print your certificate.

FACULTY DISCLOSURE/CONFLICT OF INTEREST

The University of Virginia School of Medicine, as an ACCME accredited provider, endorses and strives to comply with the Accreditation Council for Continuing Medical Education (ACCME) Standards of Commercial Support, Commonwealth of Virginia statutes, University of Virginia policies and procedures, and associated federal and private regulations and guidelines on the need for disclosure and monitoring of proprietary and financial interests that may affect the scientific integrity and balance of content delivered in continuing medical education activities under our auspices.

The University of Virginia School of Medicine requires that all CME activities accredited through this institution be developed independently and be scientifically rigorous, balanced and objective in the presentation/discussion of its content, theories and practices.

All authors/editors participating in an accredited CME activity are expected to disclose to the readers relevant financial relationships with commercial entities occurring within the past 12 months (such as grants or research support, employee, consultant, stock holder, member of speakers bureau, etc.). The University of Virginia School of Medicine will employ appropriate mechanisms to resolve potential conflicts of interest to maintain the standards of fair and balanced education to the reader. Questions about specific strategies can be directed to the Office of Continuing Medical Education, University of Virginia School of Medicine, Charlottesville, Virginia.

The faculty and staff of the University of Virginia Office of Continuing Medical Education have no financial affiliations to disclose.

The authors/editors listed below have identified no professional or financial affiliations for themselves or their spouse/partner:

N. Scott Adzick, MD; Karel Allegaert, MD, PhD; Robert H. Ball, MD; Robert Boyle, MD (Test Author); Filip Claus, MD, PhD; Fergus V. Coakley, MD; Timothy M. Crombleholme, MD; Anne Debeer, MD; Jan A. Deprest, MD, PhD; Elise Done, MD; Diana L. Farmer, MD; Dario O. Fauza, MD; Vickie A. Feldstein, MD; Alan W. Flake, MD; Orit A. Glenn, MD; Eduardo Gratacós, MD, PhD; Léonardo Gucciardo, MD; Mounira Habli, MD; Richard Whit Hall, MD; Michael R. Harrison, MD; Shinjiro Hirose, MD; Carla Holloway (Acquisitions Editor); Linda M. Hopkins, MD; Lisa K. Hornberger, MD; Tim Jancelewicz, MD; Eric Jelin, MD; Russell W. Jennings, MD; Mark Paul Johnson, MD; Hanmin Lee, MD (Guest Editor); Foong Yen Lim, MD; Laurence B. McCullough, PhD; Tim Van Mieghem, MD; Kypros Nicolaides, MD, PhD; Larry Rand, MD; Irwin Reiss, MD, PhD; Jessica L. Roybal, MD; Matthew T. Santore, MD; Priya Sekar, MD, MPH; Rolla M. Shbarou, MD; Dick Tibboel, MD, PhD; Christopher G.B. Turner, MD; Wayne Tworetzky, MD; Danny Wu, MD; and Serena Wu, MD.

The authors/editors listed below identified the following professional or financial affiliations for themselves or their spouse/partner:

Frank A. Chervenak, MD serves on the Advisory Committee for Sequenom.
Louise E. Wilkins-Haug, MD, PhD serves on the Speakers Bureau for Up to Date.

Disclosure of Discussion of Non-FDA Approved Uses for Pharmaceutical Products and/or Medical Devices:

The University of Virginia School of Medicine, as an ACCME provider, requires that all faculty presenters identify and disclose any off-label uses for pharmaceutical and medical device products. The University of Virginia School of Medicine recommends that each physician fully review all the available data on new products or procedures prior to instituting them with patients.

TO ENROLL

To enroll in the *Clinics in Perinatology* Continuing Medical Education program, call customer service at 1-800-654-2452 or visit us online at: http://www.theclinics.com/home/cme. The CME program is available to subscribers for an additional fee of $195.00.

RELATED INTEREST

Surgical Clinics of North America, April 2006 (Vol. 86, Issue 2)
Current Practice in Pediatric Surgery
Mike K. Chen, MD, *Guest Editor*
www.surgical.theclinics.com

THE CLINICS ARE NOW AVAILABLE ONLINE!

Access your subscription at:
www.theclinics.com

Preface

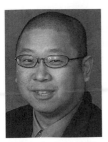

Hanmin Lee, MD
Guest Editor

Fetal surgery is a multidisciplinary field that relies on the participation and expertise of perinatologists, radiologists, neonatologists, pediatric/fetal surgeons, pediatric cardiologists, social workers, and a variety of other clinicians and support staff. Coordinating input from many different specialists is critical in overcoming the particular challenges of diagnosing and treating maternal–fetal patients. This issue of *Clinics in Perinatology* devoted to fetal surgery covers the history of the field, maternal considerations, diagnostic considerations, and ethical concerns, as well as specific diseases that may be amenable to fetal intervention. Finally, future possibilities in fetal intervention are discussed. Reflecting the multidisciplinary nature of our field, contributors to this edition include experts in perinatology, genetics, radiology, ethics, pediatric surgery, cardiology, and stem cell therapy.

Fetal surgery has evolved rapidly over the last three decades. Initially, animal models established the feasibility of fetal surgery, maternal safety, and efficacy of fetal intervention in ameliorating the profound physiologic consequences of simple anatomic defects. Establishing outcomes of fetal procedures in humans has evolved from the first case reports and small case series to large data registries and prospective randomized controlled trials, which will be discussed in several of the articles. These registries and prospective trials have, in large part, been facilitated by the emergence of fetal therapy organizations, such as Eurofoetus and the North American Fetal Therapy Network, whose registries and trials have led fetal surgical efforts in Europe and North America. The International Fetal Medicine and Surgery Society, the oldest of these organizations, is now approaching its 30th birthday. As the field progresses, these and other fetal therapy organizations will be central to the development of innovative practices and best practice guidelines.

Many of the world's experts in fetal surgery contributed to this issue of *Clinics in Perinatology*. In the first article, Dr. Harrison, widely regarded as the father of fetal surgery, and Dr. Jancelewicz recount the relatively short but rich and quickly evolving history of fetal surgery. Drs. Chervenak and McCullough give an excellent overview of the unique ethical considerations of fetal surgery. Drs. Wu and Ball review the critical issue of maternal management in fetal surgery, which is, in fact, *maternal–fetal* surgery.

Clin Perinatol 36 (2009) xv–xvi
doi:10.1016/j.clp.2009.03.017
0095-5108/09/$ – see front matter © 2009 Elsevier Inc. All rights reserved.

Fetal imaging and diagnosis is reviewed by Drs. Feldstein and Hopkins for ultrasound; Drs. Glenn and Coakley for MRI; and Drs. Hornberger and Sekar for echocardiography.

Opening the section on fetal diseases, Dr. Deprest, representing the Eurofoetus group, updates us on the European experience with tracheal occlusion for congenital diaphragmatic hernia, while Dr. Jelin and I review the U.S. experience. Dr. Adzick then reviews diagnosis and therapy for fetal lung lesions, including the use of steroids and open fetal lung resection; and Drs. Johnson and Wu discuss the challenges in diagnosis and appropriate treatment for lower urinary tract obstruction. Drs. Crombleholme, Habli, and Yen Lim describe diagnosis and stratification of disease severity for twin–twin transfusion syndrome along with the treatment options, including fetoscopic laser. Dr. Rand and I cover other complications of monochorionic twinning that may require fetal intervention. Next, Drs. Hirose and Farmer highlight the role of the NIH-funded prospective randomized controlled trial evaluating fetal surgery for myelomeningocele. Finally, Drs. Jennings, Tworetzky, and Turner give an update on the rapidly emerging area of fetal intervention for critical congenital cardiac defects.

Many impressive clinical and scientific accomplishments have been made in the short history of fetal surgery, largely due to the productive collaboration and cooperation among the specialists involved. For one, fetal surgery has mirrored surgery in general in its progression towards minimally invasive procedures. Initially, nearly all fetal surgical procedures required an open hysterotomy. Now, most procedures are performed percutaneously via sonographic or fetoscopic guidance with devices only 1 to 3 mm in diameter. The maternal benefits are obvious, with much quicker recovery and less morbidity. The benefits to the fetus are less obvious but potentially profound, as minimally invasive approaches appear to incite less preterm labor, a problem that has been the Achilles' heel of fetal surgery ever since its beginnings.

Looking forward, the future of fetal intervention seems boundless. In many ways, the fetal milieu will provide an ideal environment for the application of many areas of biomedical research that will become clinical reality in the next several decades. Drs. Flake, Santore, and Roybal discuss the current state of research on fetal stem cell transplantation and gene therapy: two areas poised to expand rapidly in terms of human clinical investigation in the next decade. In the final article, Drs. Fauza and Turner describe the exciting field of fetal tissue engineering and its potential applications for repairing prenatally diagnosed anomalies.

As fetal surgery evolves and advances, it will continue to be the responsibility of the clinicians involved to incorporate emerging technologies wisely and for the benefit of our patients. We must all keep in mind that the most important participants in this field are the pregnant women who selflessly undergo surgery for the potential benefit of their fetuses. This issue of *Clinics in Perinatology* is dedicated to these women and their families. I would like to acknowledge Elizabeth Gress, whose organizational and editorial abilities greatly enhanced this edition, and Jody Farrell, whose talent, work ethic, and professionalism drive the UCSF fetal treatment center.

Hanmin Lee, MD
Fetal Treatment Center
513 Parnassus Avenue, Suite HSW 1601
University of California, San Francisco
San Francisco, CA 94143

E-mail address:
Hanmin.Lee@ucsfmedctr.org (H. Lee)

Erratum

A drug dosage error appeared in the March 2009 issue of *Clinics in Perinatology*, Volume 36, No. 1, in the article "Drugs of Choice for Sedation and Analgesia in the Neonatal ICU" by R. Whit Hall and Rolla M. Shbarou. In Table 1, the dose for Remifentanil was listed as 1 mg/kg. **The correct dosage should be 1 mcg/kg.** As a matter of policy, this article has been removed from the March 2009 issue on record. A corrected version of the article is republished in its entirety in the June 2009 issue.

Clin Perinatol 36 (2009) xvii
doi:10.1016/j.clp.2009.05.001
0095-5108/09/$ – see front matter © 2009 Elsevier Inc. All rights reserved.

perinatology.theclinics.com

Drugs of Choice for Sedation and Analgesia in the Neonatal ICU

R. Whit Hall, MD[a],*, Rolla M. Shbarou, MD[b]

KEYWORDS

- Pain • Infant • Newborn • Premature • Analgesia • Sedation
- Opiate • Benzodiazepine • Barbituate

Before 1980, pain in the newborn period was infrequently recognized or treated.[1] The reference standard of pain assessment is self reporting which clearly is not possible in the newborn period; thus, clinicians can measure pain only indirectly. Animal and human studies have documented that neonatal pain is associated with both short- and long term consequences.[2,3] Further, the enhanced survival of extremely low birth weight babies makes them more susceptible to the effects of pain and stress because of increased exposure. Indeed, one study documented that neonates under 32 weeks' gestation were exposed to 10 to 15 painful procedures per day, and most of these procedures were untreated.[4] Unfortunately, this problem continues. A recent study by Carbajol and colleagues[5] has documented the increased occurrence and lack of treatment of neonatal pain in almost 80% of newborns in intensive care!

Analgesia and sedation in the neonatal ICU (NICU) has been fraught with controversy because of concern about the safety of these drugs in the neonatal population, the lack of adequate pharmacokinetic and pharmacodynamic data in this population, difficulty in assessing pain, and lack of long-term neurodevelopmental assessment of survivors for the pain experienced in the neonatal period.[6–9] Legitimate concern about safety has led to more governance for moderate sedation privileges for clinicians caring for neonates as well as more emphasis on obtaining consent for sedation,[10]

This article is being republished due to a drug dosage error that appeared in Clinics in Perinatology, Volume 36, No. 1 (2009), pp.15–26. In the originally published version of the article, Table 1 listed the dosage for Remifentanil as 1 mg/kg. The correct dosage is 1 mcg/kg. This article has been updated to reflect the correct dosage.

The author's (RWH) work was supported in part by funding from The Center for Translational Neuroscience by grant # RR 020,146 from the National Institutes of Health.

[a] Division of Neonatology, University of Arkansas for Medical Sciences, Slot 512B, 4301 W Markham, Little Rock, AR 72205, USA

[b] Division of Neurology, University of Arkansas for Medical Sciences, Arkansas Children's Hospital, Slot 512, 800 Marshall Street, Little Rock, AR 72202, USA

* Corresponding author.

E-mail address: hallrichardw@uams.edu (R.W. Hall).

creating roadblocks to giving sedation to neonates undergoing painful procedures. Further, individual differences and decreased morphine metabolism in neonates of younger gestational age may lead to the rapid development of tolerance as well as to the accumulation of the drug in extremely preterm neonates.[11] Thus, the use of sedation and analgesia in the neonatal population, although extremely important, must be done safely and effectively.

OPIOIDS

Opioids are used commonly in modern NICUs.[12] They provide relief from procedural pain (eg, medication before intubation)[13–15] and from chronic pain (eg, pain caused by necrotizing enterocolitis[16] or ventilation).[17–19] Several studies and reviews have concluded that opioids should be used selectively. A recent Cochrane review found insufficient evidence to recommend routine use of opioids in mechanically ventilated newborns.[19] The Cochrane review looked at pain scales and found an overall significant effect on pain in the treatment group. No significant effects were seen the treatment group with respect to neonatal mortality, duration of ventilation, short-term or long-term neurodevelopmental outcome, incidence of severe intraventricular hemorrhage (IVH), any IVH, or periventricular leukomalacia (PVL). Given the likely long-term adverse consequences associated with the chronic pain and stress of mechanical ventilation, it is reassuring that short-term adverse effects of analgesia are not more common in the opioid-treated groups.

Morphine

Morphine is the most frequently used opioid analgesic in patients of all ages and is the drug most commonly used for analgesia in ventilated neonates.[12] Morphine has a slow onset of analgesia. Its mean onset of action is 5 minutes, and the peak effect is at 15 minutes. It is metabolized in the liver into two active compounds, morphine-3-glucuronide and morphine-6-glucuronide. The former is an opioid antagonist, and the latter is a potent analgesic. Preterm infants mostly produce morphine-3-glucuronide, which explains why the infant develops tolerance after 3 to 4 days of morphine therapy.[20] Side effects of morphine include hypotension in neonates who have pre-existing hypotension and a gestational age less than 26 weeks,[21] prolonged need for assisted ventilation, and increased time to reach full feeds.[17,18] Others have suggested that morphine may have a specific effect on pulmonary mechanics, possibly resulting from some as yet undefined direct toxicity such as histamine release and/or bronchospasm.[22] There is even controversy as to whether morphine is effective in the treatment of acute pain.[23]

A randomized, controlled trial conducted in the Netherlands compared the analgesic effect of morphine versus placebo infusions for a duration of 7 days in 150 newborns who received mechanical ventilation. The findings of the study suggested that routine morphine infusion in preterm newborns who received ventilatory support neither improved pain relief nor protected against poor neurologic outcome (defined as severe IVH, PVL, or death within 28 days).[17]

The NEurologic Outcomes and Preemptive Analgesia in Neonates (NEOPAIN) trial included ventilated preterm neonates from 16 centers in the United States and Europe. It compared the effect of morphine versus placebo infusions, following a loading dose, on the neurologic outcomes of the ventilated neonates. The results suggested that continuous morphine infusion did not reduce early neurologic injury in ventilated preterm neonates. The poor neurologic outcome was defined as severe IVH, PVL, or death.[18,24] Hypotension occurred more frequently in the morphine group than the placebo group.

One study assessed the long-term outcome at age 5 to 6 years of prematurely born children (< 34 weeks' gestation) who by randomization received morphine in the neonatal period to facilitate mechanical ventilation. This study looked at children from two trials. The first included 95 infants who were assigned randomly to receive morphine alone, pancuronium alone, or both morphine and pancuronium. The second trial included 21 infants who received morphine and 20 infants who received placebo. Each child was assessed using three scales: the full-scale Weschler Preschool and Primary Scale of Intelligence, the Movement Assessment Battery for Children, and the Child Behavior Checklist. No adverse effects on intelligence, motor function, or behavior were found in the children treated with morphine.[25]

Fentanyl

Fentanyl is an opioid analgesic that is 50 to 100 times more potent than morphine.[26] It is used frequently because it provides rapid analgesia.[27] It may be used as a slow intravenous push every 2 to 4 hours or as a continuous infusion. Tolerance may develop, and withdrawal symptoms may occur after 5 or more days of continuous infusion.[26] In a blinded, randomized, controlled trial, a single dose of fentanyl given to ventilated preterm newborns significantly reduced pain behaviors and changes in heart rate. It also increased growth hormone levels.[28] In another study, fentanyl provided the same pain relief as morphine but with fewer side effects.[29] In other studies, fentanyl use resulted in lower heart rates and lower behavioral stress scores and pain scores than seen with placebo; however, the infants receiving fentanyl required higher ventilator rates and peak inspiratory pressures at 24 hours.[30] Fentanyl also may be used transdermally in patients who have limited intravenous access.

Side effects of fentanyl include bradycardia, chest wall rigidity, and opioid tolerance after prolonged therapy.[27]

Methadone

Methadone is a potent analgesic with a rapid onset of action and prolonged effect.[27] It has minimal side effects, high enteral bioavailability, and a low cost.

Other Opiates

Other opiates include the short-acting drugs sulfentanil, alfentanil, and remifentanil. All are useful for short procedures such as intubation. Sulfentanil and alfentanil are metabolized by the liver, which is immature in preterm neonates, resulting in increased drug levels with repeated infusions, especially in preterm neonates.[31] Remifentanil, on the other hand, is cleared rapidly by plasma esterases and is unaffected by the maturity of the liver enzyme system, making it attractive for short neonatal surgery or other procedures when rapid recovery is anticipated.[31]

BENZODIAZEPINES

The benzodiazepines are anxietolytic drugs that have limited analgesic effect but are commonly used in NICUs to produce sedation and muscle relaxation and to provide amnesia (in older patients). This class of drugs inhibits gamma aminobutyric acid A receptors.[32] The main complications include myoclonic jerking, excessive sedation, respiratory depression, and occasional hypotension.

Midazolam

The most commonly used benzodiazepine in the NICU is midazolam. When administered with morphine, it provides better sedation than morphine alone in ventilated patients, without adverse effects.[33] The minimal effective dose for most neonates is

200 µg/kg with a maintenance dose of 100 µg /kg/h.[34] It can be given orally, although in neonates the bioavailability of oral midazolam is only half that of intravenous midazolam.[35] Intranasal midazolam has been shown to be effective for fundoscopic examinations in older children, but this mode of delivery has not been tested in neonates.[36] One recent review found no apparent clinical benefit of midazolam compared with opiates in mechanically ventilated neonates.[37] Further, midazolam was associated with worse short-term adverse effects (death, severe IVH, or PVL) in the NOPAIN trial compared with morphine alone.[38] In summary, midazolam seems to provide sedative effects in mechanically ventilated neonates, but it should be used with caution because of reported adverse effects, particularly when used alone.

Lorazepam

Lorazepam is a longer-acting benzodiazepine that frequently is used in preterm neonates. Its duration of action is 8 to 12 hours. It also is an effective anticonvulsant for neonates refractory to phenobarbital. Unfortunately, one of its main side effects is myoclonic jerking, which mimics seizure activity.[12,39] It has been shown (along with morphine) to adhere to the tubing in patients treated with extracorporeal membrane oxygenation (ECMO), increasing dosing requirements by 50% in those patients.[40]

BARBITURATES

Barbiturates are used commonly in neonates for sedation and analgesic effects, despite a lack of evidence for pain relief.[12]

Phenobarbital

Phenobarbital usually is considered the drug of choice for seizure control. Despite minimal animal evidence for antinociception, it often is used for analgesia.[41] It also is used in conjunction with opioids for sedation,[18] although there is little recent evidence that it is effective. Classically, phenobarbital has been used for neonatal abstinence syndrome, but recent work by Ebner and colleagues[42] has demonstrated that opiates shorten the time required for treatment. Because of its anticonvulsant effects, however, phenobarbital is an attractive adjunct for patients who have seizures.

Thiopental

Thiopental is a short-acting barbiturate used for anesthetic induction. It is used sparingly in the NICU, but one randomized, controlled trial showed a decreased time needed for intubation and maintenance of heart rate and blood pressure with thiopental compared with placebo during nasotracheal intubation.[43]

Chloral Hydrate

Chloral hydrate is used for hypnosis when sedation but not analgesia is required for certain procedures such as MRI. Apnea and bradycardia may occur in ex-preterm infants undergoing procedural sedation with doses as little as 30 mg/kg. Side effects were inversely related to gestational age.[44] The usual dose is 50 to 100 mg/kg. A dose of 75 mg/kg administered orally is more efficacious than a 0.2-mg/kg dose of intravenous midazolam and has comparable side effects (apnea, bradycardia).[45]

KETAMINE

Ketamine is a dissociative anesthetic used for anesthesia, analgesia, and sedation. It causes bronchodilation and mild increases in blood pressure and heart rate.[46] Cerebral blood flow is relatively unaffected with ketamine, making it an attractive choice for some unstable hypotensive neonates requiring procedures such as cannulation for ECMO.[47] Animal studies have raised concern about the neurodegenerative effects of ketamine[48,49] although ketamine in clinically relevant doses is neuroprotective in the presence of inflammatory pain.[20] Nevertheless, extrapolating animal to human data is problematic at best, and there has been no credible evidence that ketamine is detrimental to the developing human brain in the presence of pain.[50] Clearly, more study is needed to determine the safety and efficacy of this anesthetic.

PROPOFOL

Propofol has become popular as an anesthetic agent for young children, but it has not been studied extensively in neonates.[51–53] One study compared propofol with morphine, atropine, and suxamethonium for intubation and found that propofol led to shorter intubation times, higher oxygen saturations, and less trauma than the combination regimen in neonates.[54] Propofol should be used with caution in young infants, however, because clearance is inversely related to neonatal and postmenstrual age. Thus with intermittent bolus or continuous administration this drug can accumulate in young immature neonates, leading to toxicity.[55]

ACETAMINOPHEN

Acetaminophen acts by inhibiting the cyclo-oxygenase (COX) enzymes in the brain and has been well studied in newborns.[16] It is useful for mild pain, in conjunction with other pain relief, or after circumcision.[56]

LOCAL ANESTHETICS
Lidocaine

Lidocaine inhibits axonal transmission by blocking Na^+ channels. Lidocaine is used commonly for penile blocks for circumcisions. In this circumstance, its use has demonstrated effectiveness in decreasing pain response to immunizations as long as 4 months after circumcision compared with neonates who received placebo.[57] The ring block has been shown to be a more effective than a dorsal penile root block or eutectic mixture of local anesthetics (EMLA) cream in relieving the pain of circumcision.[58]

Topical Anesthetics

Topical anesthetics have demonstrated effectiveness for certain types of procedural pain such as venipuncture,[59] lumbar puncture,[60] or immunizations.[61] Complications include methemoglobinemia and transient skin rashes.[62] In preterm neonates with thin skin, the concern for methemoglobinemia is accentuated.

Unfortunately, topical anesthetics are not effective in providing pain relief for the heel prick, one of the most common skin-breaking procedures, because of increased skin thickness.[63] Newer topical anesthetics include 4% tetracaine and 4% liposomal lidocaine. Although the newer agents have a shorter onset of action, they are no more effective in pain relief.

COMMON PROCEDURES

Common neonatal procedures and advantages and disadvantages of drug therapy are summarized in **Table 1**.

Table 1
Summary of procedures and treatment

Procedure	Drugs	Advantages of Treatment	Disadvantages of Treatment	Comments
Mechanical ventilation[17–19,29]	Fentanyl (1–3 µg/kg) Morphine (0.1 mg/kg) Midazolam (0.1–0.2 mg/kg)	Improved ventilator synchrony, lower pain scores	Prolonged time on assisted ventilation, prolonged time to full feeds, increased bladder catheterization, hypotension	Use sedation as needed, not preemptively; midazolam was associated with adverse short-term effects in NOPAIN trial.
Circumcision[58,62]	Lidocaine (1 mL) EMLA	Less pain response up to 4 months post-procedure	Allergic reaction, bruising at injection site	Ring block is more effective than dorsal penile nerve root block.
Heel lance[63]	Sucrose	Shorter crying, reduced changes in heart rate	None	EMLA cream is not effective.
Venipuncture, arterial puncture, lumbar puncture[60,61]	Topical anesthetic (EMLA) Sucrose	Lower Premature Infant Pain Profile scores, less crying	Local reaction, rare methemoglobinemia	Other nonpharmacologic treatments are effective.
Intubation[14,15,54,69,70]	Morphine (0.1 mg/kg) Fentanyl (1–3 µg g/kg) Remifentanil (1 mcg/kg) Midazolam (0.2 mg/kg) Propofol (2–6 mg/kg) Ketamine (1 mg/kg) Suxamethonium (2 mg/kg)	Shorter time to intubation, less trauma, less desaturation, better maintenance of vital signs	None	There is no accepted premedication. Opiates are the class most common used.

Indication	Drug (dose)	Benefit	Risk	Comment
More invasive procedures (eg, cannulation for ECMO)[71,72]	Propofol (2–6 mg/kg) Ketamine (1 mg/kg) Fentanyl (1–3 mcg/kg)	Maintenance of cardiovascular stability	Questionable neurotoxicity with ketamine	Ketamine may be neuroprotective.
Postsurgical pain[73]	Fentanyl (1–3 μg/kg) Morphine (0.1 mg/kg) Acetaminophen (15 mg/kg)	Lowered neuroendocrine response, faster recovery	Respiratory depression, hypotension with opiates	Use acetaminophen only for mild pain.
Endotracheal suctioning[34,74]	Midazolam (0.2 mg/kg) Morphine (0.1 mg/kg) Fentanyl (1–3 μg/kg)	Anxietolytic	Respiratory depression, hypotension, dependence	Pain usually is not treated.
Imaging (MRI)[45]	Chloral hydrate (50–100 mg/kg)	Sedation	Respiratory depression, hypotension	Chloral hydrate provides sedation only.

FUTURE DIRECTIONS
Nonsteroidal Anti-Inflammatory Drugs

Nonsteroidal anti-inflammatory drugs (NSAIDS) are used extensively for pain relief in children and adults, but they are used mainly for patent ductus arteriosus (PDA) closure in neonates. They act by inhibiting the COX-1 and COX-2 enzymes responsible for converting arachidonic acid into prostaglandins, thus producing their analgesic, antipyretic, and anti-inflammatory effects.[27] The analgesic effects of NSAIDS have not been studied in neonates, although both ibuprofen and indomethacin have been studied for use in PDA closure. Concern about side effects of renal dysfunction, platelet adhesiveness, and pulmonary hypertension have limited their study for this indication.[37,64,65] Ibuprofen, however, has demonstrated beneficial effects on cerebral circulation in human studies[66] as well as beneficial effects on the development of chronic lung disease in baboon experiments,[67] making it an attractive analgesic in preterm neonates. Nonpharmacologic approaches such as acupuncture, massage therapy, sucrose, and music are also safe and effective.[68]

ACKNOWLEDGMENTS

The authors thank Diana Hershberger for assistance in preparing this manuscript.

REFERENCES

1. Anand KJ, Hall RW. Controversies in neonatal pain: an introduction. Semin Perinatol 2007;31(5):273–4.
2. Anand KJ, Hickey PR. Pain and its effects in the human neonate and fetus. N Engl J Med 1987;317(21):1321–9.
3. Fumagalli F, Molteni R, Racagni G, et al. Stress during development: impact on neuroplasticity and relevance to psychopathology. Prog Neurobiol 2007;81(4):197–217.
4. Barker DP, Rutter N. Exposure to invasive procedures in neonatal intensive care unit admissions. Arch Dis Child Fetal Neonatal Ed 1995;72(1):F47–8.
5. Carbajal R, Rousset A, Danan C, et al. Epidemiology and treatment of painful procedures in neonates in intensive care units. JAMA 2008;300(1):60–70.
6. Jacqz-Aigrain E, Burtin P. Clinical pharmacology of sedatives in neonates. Clin Pharm 1996;31(6):423–43.
7. Anand KJ, Aranda JV, Verde CB, et al. Summary proceedings from the neonatal pain-control group. Pediatrics 2006;117(3 Pt 2):S9–22.
8. Ranger M, Johnston CC, Anand KJ. Current controversies regarding pain assessment in neonates. Semin Perinatol 2007;31(5):283–8.
9. Whitfield MF, Grunau RE. Behavior, pain perception, and the extremely low-birth weight survivor. Clin Perinatol 2000;27(2):363–79.
10. American Academy of Pediatrics, American Academy of Pediatric Dentistry, Charles J, et al. Guidelines for monitoring and management of pediatric patients during and after sedation for diagnostic and therapeutic procedures: an update. Pediatrics 2006;118(6):2587–602.
11. Saarenmaa E, Neuvonen PJ, Roseberg P, et al. Morphine clearance and effects in newborn infants in relation to gestational age. Clin Pharmacol Ther 2000;68(2):160–6.
12. Hall RW, Boyle E, Young T. Do ventilated neonates require pain management? Semin Perinatol 2007;31(5):289–97.

13. Whyte S, Birrell G, Wyllie J. Premedication before intubation in UK neonatal units. Arch Dis Child Fetal Neonatal Ed 2000;82(1):F38–41 [see comment].
14. Roberts KD, Leone TA, Edwards WH, et al. Premedication for nonemergent neonatal intubations: a randomized, controlled trial comparing atropine and fentanyl to atropine, fentanyl, and mivacurium. Pediatrics 2006;118(4):1583–91.
15. Sarkar S, Schumacher RE, Baumgart S, et al. Are newborns receiving premedication before elective intubation? J Perinatol 2006;26(5):286–9.
16. Menon G, Anand KJ, McIntosh N. Practical approach to analgesia and sedation in the neonatal intensive care unit. Semin Perinatol 1998;22(5):417–24.
17. Simons SH, van Dijk M, van Lingen RA, et al. Routine morphine infusion in preterm newborns who received ventilatory support: a randomized controlled trial. JAMA 2003;290(18):2419–27.
18. Anand KJ, Hall RW, Desai N, et al. Effects of morphine analgesia in ventilated preterm neonates: primary outcomes from the NEOPAIN randomised trial. Lancet 2004;363(9422):1673–82 [see comment].
19. Bellu R, de Waal KA, Zanini R. Opioids for neonates receiving mechanical ventilation. [update of Cochrane Database Syst Rev. 2005;(1):CD004212; PMID: 15674933]. Cochrane Database Syst Rev 2008;(1):CD004212.
20. Anand KJ. Pharmacological approaches to the management of pain in the neonatal intensive care unit. J Perinatol 2007;27(Suppl. 1):S4–11.
21. Hall RWKS, Barton BA, Kaiser JR, et al. Morphine, hypotension, and adverse outcomes in preterm neonates: who's to blame? Pediatrics 2005;115(5): 1351–9.
22. Levene M. Morphine sedation in ventilated newborns: who are we treating? Pediatrics 2005;116(2):492–3 [comment].
23. Carbajal R, Lenclen R, Jugie M, et al. Morphine does not provide adequate analgesia for acute procedural pain among preterm neonates. Pediatrics 2005; 115(6):1494–500.
24. Bhandari V, Bergqvist LL, Kronsberg SS, et al. Morphine administration and short-term pulmonary outcomes among ventilated preterm infants. Pediatrics 2005;116(2):352–9 [see comment].
25. MacGregor R, Evans D, sugden D, et al. Outcome at 5–6 years of prematurely born children who received morphine as neonates. Arch Dis Child Fetal Neonatal Ed 1998 Jul;79(1):F40–3.
26. Mitchell A, Brooks S, Roane D. The premature infant and painful procedures. Pain Manag Nurs 2000;1(2):58–65.
27. Anand KJ, Hall RW. Pharmacological therapy for analgesia and sedation in the newborn. [erratum appears in Arch Dis Child Fetal Neonatal Ed 2007 Mar;92(2):F156 Note: dosage error in text]. Arch Dis Child Fetal Neonatal Ed 2006;91(6):F448–53.
28. Guinsburg R, Kopelman BL, Anand KJ, et al. Physiological, hormonal, and behavioral responses to a single fentanyl dose in intubated and ventilated preterm neonates. J Pediatr 1998;132(6):954–9.
29. Saarenmaa E, Huttunen P, Leppaluoto J, et al. Advantages of fentanyl over morphine in analgesia for ventilated newborn infants after birth: a randomized trial. J Pediatr 1999;134(2):144–50 [see comment].
30. Orsini AJ, Leef KH, Costarino A, et al. Routine use of fentanyl infusions for pain and stress reduction in infants with respiratory distress syndrome. J Pediatr 1996;129(1):140–5 [see comment].
31. Berde CB, Jaksic T, Lynn AM, et al. Anesthesia and analgesia during and after surgery in neonates. Clin Ther 2005;27(6):900–21.

32. Blumer JL. Clinical pharmacology of midazolam in infants and children. Clin Pharm 1998;35(1):37–47.
33. Arya V, Ramji S. Midazolam sedation in mechanically ventilated newborns: a double blind randomized placebo controlled trial. Indian Pediatr 2001;38(9):967–72 [see comment].
34. Treluyer JM, Zohar S, Rey E, et al. Minimum effective dose of midazolam for sedation of mechanically ventilated neonates. J Clin Pharm Ther 2005;30(5): 479–85.
35. de Wildt SN, Kearns GL, Hop WC, et al. Pharmacokinetics and metabolism of oral midazolam in preterm infants. Br J Clin Pharmacol 2002;53(4):390–2.
36. Altintas O, Karabas VL, Demirci G, et al. Evaluation of intranasal midazolam in refraction and fundus examination of young children with strabismus. J Pediatr Ophthalmol Strabismus 2005;43(6):355–9.
37. Aranda JV, Carlo W, Hummel P, et al. Analgesia and sedation during mechanical ventilation in neonates. Clin Ther 2005;27(6):877–99.
38. Anand KJ, Baton BA, McIntosh N, et al. Analgesia and sedation in preterm neonates who require ventilatory support: results from the NOPAIN trial. Neonatal Outcome and Prolonged Analgesia in Neonates. [erratum appears in Arch Pediatr Adolesc Med 1999 Aug;153(8):895]. Arch Pediatr Adolesc Med 1999; 153(4):331–8.
39. Chess PR, D'Angio CT. Clonic movements following lorazepam administration in full-term infants. Arch Pediatr Adolesc Med 1998;152(1):98–9.
40. Bhatt-Meht V, Annich G. Sedative clearance during extracorporeal membrane oxygenation. Perfusion 2005;20(6):309–15.
41. Gonzalez-Darder JM, Ortega-Alvaro A, Ruz-Franzi I, et al. Antinociceptive effects of phenobarbital in "tail-flick" test and deafferentation pain. Anesth Analg 1992; 75(1):81–6.
42. Ebner N, Rohrmeister K, Winklbaur B, et al. Management of neonatal abstinence syndrome in neonates born to opioid maintained women. Drug Alcohol Depend 2007;87(2–3):131–8.
43. Bhutada A, Sahni R, Rastogi S, et al. Randomised controlled trial of thiopental for intubation in neonates. Arch Dis Child Fetal Neonatal Ed 2000;82(1):F34–7 [see comment].
44. Allegaert K, Daniels H, Naulaers G, et al. Pharmacodynamics of chloral hydrate in former preterm infants. Eur J Pediatr 2005;164(7):403–7.
45. McCarver-May DG, Kang J, Aouthmany M, et al. Comparison of chloral hydrate and midazolam for sedation of neonates for neuroimaging studies. J Pediatr 1996;128(4):573–6 [see comment].
46. Friesen RH, Henry DB. Cardiovascular changes in preterm neonates receiving isoflurane, halothane, fentanyl, and ketamine. Anesthesiology 1986;64(2): 238–42.
47. Betremieux P, Carre P, Pladys P, et al. Doppler ultrasound assessment of the effects of ketamine on neonatal cerebral circulation. Dev Pharmacol Ther 1993; 20(1–2):9–13.
48. Young C, Jevtovic-Todorovic V, Qin YQ, et al. Potential of ketamine and midazolam, individually or in combination, to induce apoptotic neurodegeneration in the infant mouse brain. Br J Pharmacol 2005;146(2):189–97.
49. Olney JW, Young C, wozniak DF, et al. Anesthesia-induced developmental neuroapoptosis. Does it happen in humans? Anesthesiology 2004;101(2):273–5 [see comment].

50. Bhutta AT, Venkatesan AK, Rovnaghi CR, et al. Anaesthetic neurotoxicity in rodents: is the ketamine controversy real? Acta Paediatr 2007;96(11):1554–6.
51. Disma N, Astuto M, Rizzo G, et al. Propofol sedation with fentanyl or midazolam during oesophagogastroduodenoscopy in children. Eur J Anaesthesiol 2005; 22(11):848–52.
52. Rigby-Jones AE, Nolan JA, Priston MJ, et al. Pharmacokinetics of propofol infusions in critically ill neonates, infants, and children in an intensive care unit. Anesthesiology 2002;97(6):1393–400.
53. Jenkins IA, Playfor SD, Bevan C, et al. Current United Kingdom sedation practice in pediatric intensive care. Paediatr Anaesth 2007;17(7):675–83.
54. Ghanta S, Abdel-Latif ME, Lui K, et al. Propofol compared with the morphine, atropine, and suxamethonium regimen as induction agents for neonatal endotracheal intubation: a randomized, controlled trial. Pediatrics 2007;119(6): e1248–55 [see comment].
55. Allegaert K, Peeters MY, Verbesselt T, et al. Inter-individual variability in propofol pharmacokinetics in preterm and term neonates. Br J Anaesth 2007;99(6):864–70.
56. Howard CR, Howard FM, Weitzman ML. Acetaminophen analgesia in neonatal circumcision: the effect on pain. Pediatrics 1994;93(4):641–6.
57. Taddio A, Katz J, Ilersich AL, et al. Effect of neonatal circumcision on pain response during subsequent routine vaccination. Lancet 1997;349(9052): 599–603 [see comment].
58. Lander J, Brady-Fryer B, Metcalfe JB, et al. Comparison of ring block, dorsal penile nerve block, and topical anesthesia for neonatal circumcision: a randomized controlled trial. JAMA 1997;278(24):2157–62 [see comment].
59. Garcia OC, Reichberg S, Brion LP, et al. Topical anesthesia for line insertion in very low birth weight infants. J Perinatol 1997;17(6):477–80.
60. Kaur G, Gupta P, Kumar A. A randomized trial of eutectic mixture of local anesthetics during lumbar puncture in newborns. Arch Pediatr Adolesc Med 2003; 157(11):1065–70.
61. Gradin M, Eriksson M, Holmqvist G, et al. Pain reduction at venipuncture in newborns: oral glucose compared with local anesthetic cream. Pediatrics 2002; 110(6):1053–7 [see comment].
62. Taddio A, Stevens B, Craig K, et al. Efficacy and safety of lidocaine-prilocaine cream for pain during circumcision. N Engl J Med 1997;336(17):1197–201 [see comment].
63. Larsson BA, Norman M, Bjerring P, et al. Regional variations in skin perfusion and skin thickness may contribute to varying efficacy of topical, local anaesthetics in neonates. Paediatr Anaesth 1996;6(2):107–10.
64. Allegaert K, Cossey V, DeBeer A, et al. The impact of ibuprofen on renal clearance in preterm infants is independent of the gestational age. Pediatr Nephrol 2005;20(6):740–3.
65. Ohlsson A, Walia R, Shah S. Ibuprofen for the treatment of patent ductus arteriosus in preterm and/or low birth weight infants. [update of Cochrane Database Syst Rev. 2005;(4):CD003481; PMID: 16235321]. Cochrane Database Syst Rev 2008;(1):CD003481.
66. Naulaers G, Delanghe G, Allegaert K, et al. Ibuprofen and cerebral oxygenation and circulation. Arch Dis Child Fetal Neonatal Ed 2005;90(1):F75–6.
67. McCurnin D, Seidner S, Chang LY, et al. Ibuprofen-induced patent ductus arteriosus closure: physiologic, histologic, and biochemical effects on the premature lung. Pediatrics 2008;121(5):945–56.

68. Golianu B, Krane E, Seybold J, et al. Non-pharmacological techniques for pain management in neonates. Semin Perinatol 2007;31(5):318–22.
69. Pereira e Silva Y, Gomez RS, Barbosa RF, et al. Remifentanil for sedation and analgesia in a preterm neonate with respiratory distress syndrome. Paediatr Anaesth 2005;15(11):993–6 [see comment].
70. Knolle E, Oehmke MJ, Gustorff B, et al. Target-controlled infusion of propofol for fibreoptic intubation. Eur J Anaesthesiol 2003;20(7):565–9.
71. Singh A, Girotra S, Mehta Y, et al. Total intravenous anesthesia with ketamine for pediatric interventional cardiac procedures. J Cardiothorac Vasc Anesth 2000; 14(1):36–9.
72. Oklu E, Bulutcu FS, Yalcin Y, et al. Which anesthetic agent alters the hemodynamic status during pediatric catheterization? Comparison of propofol versus ketamine. J Cardiothorac Vasc Anesth 2003;17(6):686–90 [see comment].
73. Bouwmeester JJ, Hop WC, van Dijk M, et al. Postoperative pain in the neonate: age-related differences in morphine requirements and metabolism. Intensive Care Med 2003;29(11):2009–15.
74. Simons SH, van Dijk M, Anand KS, et al. Do we still hurt newborn babies? A prospective study of procedural pain and analgesia in neonates. Arch Pediatr Adolesc Med 2003;157(11):1058–64.

A History of Fetal Surgery

Tim Jancelewicz, MD, Michael R. Harrison, MD*

KEYWORDS

- History fetal surgery • History prenatal intervention
- Fetal-maternal intervention • Fetal operation • Fetus

Quite pleasing is it, in the management of the fetus, to see how, when the fetus touches the surrounding air, it tries to breathe.
— *Vesalius, De Humani Corporis Fabrica (1543)*

Over the past 3 decades, fetal surgery for congenital disease has evolved from merely a fanciful concept to a medical field in its own right. Techniques for open hysterotomy, minimal-access hysteroscopy, and image-guided percutaneous fetal access have become well established, first in animal models and subsequently in humans. At the same time, major advances in fetal imaging and diagnosis, anesthesia, and tocolysis have allowed fetal intervention to become a vital tool for subsets of patients who would otherwise endure significant morbidity and mortality. This article offers a concise overview of the history of fetal surgery, from its tumultuous early days to its current status as an important means for the early treatment of potentially devastating congenital anomalies.

FETAL SURGERY: AN EXPERIMENTAL TIMELINE

Despite the early observations of the fetus by Vesalius in the sixteenth century, it was not until the nineteenth century that experimental animal preparations were used to make the first physiologic observations on the living mammalian fetus. Bichat in 1803 was the first to study fetal movements. Zuntz (1877) and later Preyer (1885) studied intact fetal guinea pigs suspended in warm saline. They noted that the fetus must be kept in warm physiologic salt solution and that a fetus, once allowed to breathe, could not be returned to its mother and survive. By 1920, the first successful nonhuman fetal operations had been performed: Mayer removed guinea pig fetuses from the uterus and placed them in the maternal abdominal cavity; a few guinea pigs survived for several days. Graham Brown studied fetal movements in the cat, and Lane in the rat. In the 1920s, Swenson demonstrated the first experimental in

Division of Pediatric Surgery, Department of Surgery, Fetal Treatment Center, University of California, San Francisco, 513 Parnassus Avenue, HSW-1601, San Francisco CA 94143-0570, USA
* Corresponding author.
E-mail address: fetus@surgery.ucsf.edu (M.R. Harrison).

Clin Perinatol 36 (2009) 227–236
doi:10.1016/j.clp.2009.03.007
0095-5108/09/$ – see front matter © 2009 Elsevier Inc. All rights reserved.

perinatology.theclinics.com

utero manipulation, and Nicholas established the possibility of normal delivery after in utero surgery.

In the 1930s and 1940s, experimental fetal observation gained momentum. Barcroft introduced the most productive fetal experimental model when he described operations on the lamb fetus using spinal anesthesia. Surgery was performed through a small uterine incision, without removing the fetus. Hall's work on development of the nervous system in the fetal rat and Barron's work on neurologic development in the fetal lamb extended the techniques for fetal surgery, including the use of purse-string sutures to avoid the loss of amniotic fluid.[1]

The first major dividend from experimental fetal manipulation came in 1946 when Jost demonstrated that removal of fetal rabbit testes had a profound influence on subsequent sexual development.[2] In the 1950s, Louw and Barnard produced intestinal atresia, similar to that seen in human neonates, by interrupting the mesenteric blood supply in fetal puppies.[3] This contribution was important because it not only established the ischemic pathogenesis of neonatal intestinal atresia but also demonstrated the feasibility of simulating human birth defects by appropriate fetal manipulation.

In the 1960s and 1970s, experimental fetal surgery was used to simulate various human congenital anomalies: coarctation of the aorta in the puppy,[4] congenital diaphragmatic hernia in the lamb,[5] congenital hydronephrosis in the rabbit[6] and lamb,[7] and congenital heart disease in the lamb.[8] The development of a chronically catheterized fetal lamb preparation led to intensive investigation of fetal cardiovascular, pulmonary, and renal physiology.[8,9] Experimental fetal surgery proved to be more difficult in the primate, where uterine contractility and preterm labor were more difficult to control. During the last 2 decades, however, advances in surgical and anesthetic techniques and in the pharmacologic control of labor have made experimental manipulation of even the primate fetus feasible.[10]

By the late 1970s, various experimental fetal models were being used widely in the study of normal developmental physiology and the pathophysiology of several congenital defects. These models proved to be both descriptive and predictive. For example, removal of a piece of diaphragm in the fetal lamb not only produced a lesion that mimicked the human disease analog of congenital diaphragmatic hernia (CDH), but also produced the associated developmental consequence (ie, pulmonary hypoplasia). In fact, use of the fetal lamb model of CDH is a microcosmic analogy for the evolution of the field of fetal surgery in general; the model has been used successfully to explore various types of fetal intervention aimed at reversing pulmonary hypoplasia: total repair in utero, maternal steroid treatment, and tracheal occlusion with clips and then removable balloons.[11,12] When fetal malformations, such as CDH, could be detected prenatally, fetal experiments designed to explore the pathophysiology of correctable congenital anomalies assumed some practical clinical significance. Our ability to detect malformations clinically and our ability to study them experimentally raise the question of what medical treatments can be applied to ameliorate these abnormalities.

By 1980, researchers were ready to attempt the correction of surgically created fetal anatomic defects. The focus of this experimentation occurred at the University of California, San Francisco (UCSF) where the right environment of multispecialty cooperation enabled productive study. Although many fetal anatomic malformations can be detected by sonography, only selected cases warranted consideration for intrauterine therapy because only a few have a compelling physiologic rationale for prenatal correction. Congenital hydronephrosis, diaphragmatic hernia, and obstructive hydrocephalus are examples of malformations in which a simple anatomic lesion interferes with organ development and, if the anatomic defect is corrected, fetal development may proceed normally. For each condition, the physiologic rationale for in utero correction of these lesions was first defined, and the feasibility of in utero correction was subsequently established in animal models.[13,14] Proof of concept in animal models was gradually followed by attempts at therapy for affected human pregnancies.

FETAL INTERVENTION IN THE HUMAN

Before the early ventures into human fetal surgery became a realistic possibility and the concept was able to move from the laboratory to the operating room, significant advances in imaging, assessment, and monitoring of the fetus were first necessary. There were some early endeavors, however. Hydrops fetalis, associated with maternal Rh sensitization, was the first fetal disorder to be treated successfully (**Table 1**). In the early 1960s, outcomes from available treatments of the neonate who had severe hydrops fetalis were so discouraging that Sir William Liley attempted to transfuse the fetus in utero. He demonstrated that intra-abdominal infusion of blood ameliorated severe hydrops; this procedure inaugurated human fetal intervention.[15] A little-known side to this story marked an inauspicious start for more invasive fetal treatment. A logical refinement in the treatment of the erythroblastotic fetus was complete exchange transfusion. This procedure required direct access to the fetal circulation, which prompted the first in utero fetal operations. Also in the early 1960s, obstetricians in New York and Puerto Rico exposed several fetuses through uterine incisions to cannulate femoral and jugular vessels for exchange transfusion. The overall experience was apparently discouraging. Reports are sketchy and this approach was quickly abandoned and lay dormant for the next decade. Surgical exposure of the living fetus would have to await development of better anesthetic agents and surgical techniques, but these initial experiences at least raised the notion of fetal surgical intervention.[16]

The next fetal disease to be approached therapeutically was the devastating respiratory distress syndrome of prematurity. Through a combination of clinical experience with severely premature infants and laboratory experiments using fetal lamb and rabbit preparations, surfactant deficiency was established as being the physiologic basis for respiratory distress syndrome. Effective treatment could then be devised. Glucocorticoid therapy to induce fetal lung maturation was first demonstrated by Liggins in 1972.[17] Prenatal therapy combined with improved methods of respiratory support for tiny premature infants has greatly reduced the mortality caused by this condition.

As summarized in **Table 1**, with time and experience, many different fetal diseases would be treated with prenatal intervention, and the field of fetal surgery would become the truly international movement it is today. But the fetus could not be truly considered a patient until prenatal ailments could be diagnosed, an ability that was slow to evolve. Fetal activity felt by the mother or palpated by her physician was the first crude measure of fetal well-being. Then the fetal heartbeat, detected at first by auscultation and later by sophisticated electronic monitors, was found to reflect fetal stress and distress. Later, minute amounts of gestational hormones were detected in maternal blood and urine. These levels correlated with the condition of the fetus. Still later came amniocentesis; analysis of the constituents of amniotic fluid made possible the prenatal diagnosis of many inherited metabolic and chromosomal disorders and permitted assessment of fetal pulmonary maturity and the severity of fetal hemolytic reactions.

Table 1
Milestones in fetal therapy

Rh disease—IUT	New Zealand	1961
Hysterotomy for fetal vascular access and IUT	Puerto Rico	1964
Respiratory distress syndrome of prematurity—prenatal steroids	London	1972
Fetoscopy—diagnostic	Yale	1974
Experimental pathophysiology (sheep model)	UCSF	1980
Hysterotomy & maternal safety (monkey model)	UCSF	1981
Uropathy—vesicoamniotic shunt	UCSF	1982
Hydrocephalus—vesicoamniotic shunt	Denver	1982
Uropathy—open fetal surgery	UCSF	1983
International Fetal Medicine and Surgery Society (IFMSS) founded	Santa Barbara	1982
CCAM—resection	UCSF	1984
Intravascular transfusion	London	1985
CDH—open repair	UCSF	1989
Anomalous twin—cord ligation	London	1990
CDH—NIH trial: open repair	UCSF	1990
Aortic valvuloplasty	London	1991
SCT—resection	UCSF	1992
Laser ablation of placental vessels	Milwaukee; London	1995
EXIT procedure for airway obstruction	UCSF	1995
Fetoscopic surgery (Fetendo)	UCSF	1996
XSCID—in utero stem cell transplant	Detroit	1996
Eurofoetus founded	Leuven	1997
CDH—Fetendo clip → balloon	UCSF	1997
Myelomeningocele—open repair	Vanderbilt	1997
CDH—NIH trial: Fetendo balloon	UCSF	1998
Twin reversed-arterial perfusion—radiofrequency ablation	UCSF	1998
Twin reversed-arterial perfusion—cord electrocautery	Leuven	1999
Resection of pericardial teratoma	UCSF	2000
CCAM—prenatal steroid therapy	UCSF	2001
Resection of cervical teratoma	UCSF	2001
CDH—fetoscopic tracheal occlusion (FETO) trial	Leuven; London; Barcelona	2002
Myelomeningocele—NIH trial: open repair	UCSF; CHOP; Vanderbilt	2002
Osteogenesis imperfecta—in utero stem cell transplant	Stockholm	2003
Twin–twin transfusion syndrome—amnioreduction v. laser	Poissy; Eurofetus	2004
Hypoplastic left heart syndrome—balloon septotomy; valve dilation	Boston	2004
Hypoplastic left heart syndrome—laser atrial septotomy	Tampa	2005
North American Fetal Therapy Network (NAFTNet) founded	United States and Canada	2005
Amniotic collagen plug	Leuven	2007
CCAM—sclerotherapy	Venezuela; Tampa	2007

Abbreviations: CCAM, congenital cystic adenomatoid malformation; CHOP, Children's Hospital of Philadelphia; EXIT, ex utero intrapartum treatment; IUT, intrauterine transfusion; NIH, National Institutes of Health; SCT, sacrococcygeal teratoma; X-SCID, X-linked severe combined immunodeficiency.

The development that had the most profound effect on our approach to the fetus was the introduction of a safe, noninvasive imaging technique that permitted direct visualization of the living fetus. Radiographs were recognized as being potentially harmful to the developing organism. Plain radiographs yielded little information, and introduction of radiopaque materials into the amniotic fluid (amniogram) increased the risk for premature rupture of the membranes or preterm labor without yielding much more diagnostic information. Sonography was then developed. This method enabled accurate delineation of normal and abnormal fetal anatomy with considerable detail and, later on, provided "live" moving pictures. Unlike previous techniques, ultrasonic imaging seems to have no harmful effect on the mother or on the fetus.

With prenatal ultrasound, the sonographer can make sophisticated observations of the developing heart and its valves. Fetal parts can be measured to assess fetal growth, and an increasing number of anatomic malformations can be accurately delineated. Sonography can be used to guide needle punctures of the amniotic cavity for amniocentesis, or needle aspiration of fetal urine, ascites, and cerebrospinal fluid. Real-time sonography can guide fetal endoscopic surgery and ensure the safe acquisition of fetal blood and other fetal tissues for biopsy (eg, skin, liver, muscle). Such samples enable the diagnosis of fetal hematologic disorders and enzymatic defects that cannot be detected by amniocentesis alone. In addition, the newest noninvasive imaging technique, nuclear magnetic resonance, promises not only definition of fetal anatomy but also actual chemical definition of fetal tissue without invasive sample.

While pediatric surgeons were exploring certain life-threatening neonatal problems that might lend themselves to correction before birth, obstetricians, geneticists, and sonographers were developing the techniques of prenatal diagnosis and were finding fetuses with similar defects. Although prenatal diagnosis by amniocentesis was aimed initially at potentially fatal fetal diseases, the refinement of ultrasonography allowed accurate delineation of other anomalies that were often found serendipitously during imaging performed for obstetric indications. Physicians primarily concerned with management of the mother and fetus through pregnancy (eg, perinatologists, geneticists, obstetric sonologists) could thus detect fetal lesions, such as hydronephrosis and hydrocephalus, and they could begin to wonder what they could do for the fetus and how they could best manage this pregnancy. Physicians interested in all phases of fetoneonatal development began sharing information and ideas about how the fetal condition might determine the place, timing, and mode of delivery. Detection of fetal defects also led to serial sonographic studies that defined the natural history and pathophysiology of an increasing number of human fetal diseases, including hydronephrosis, diaphragmatic hernia, hydrocephalus, and nonimmune hydrops. Fetal medicine was established.

The impetus provided by the neonate who had an uncorrectable disorder at birth combined with the fetus who had a birth defect detected before birth led to the realization that many fetal diseases may require medical management before birth. Although neither impetus was sufficient in itself to justify fetal intervention, together they spurred the necessary clinical and experimental studies that would lead to successful fetal treatment. When the baby's physician and the mother's physician together began to define the natural history of the disease by serial sonographic examination of untreated human fetuses and to study the pathophysiology and feasibility of fetal intervention in experimental animal models, the stage was set for a full consideration of the fetus as a patient. Fetal treatment is thus the flowering of a long history of clinical and experimental work in prenatal diagnosis and fetoneonatal physiology by physicians of diverse specialties and backgrounds.

THE EARLY DAYS: UNIVERSITY OF CALIFORNIA, SAN FRANCISCO AND BEYOND

Fetal therapy at UCSF was conceived and developed experimentally beginning in 1978 and came to fruition clinically in 1981. It was initially a rapidly growing enterprise with the exploration of many new therapies: decompression for obstructive uropathy and hydrocephalus, surgical treatment of severe sacrococcygeal teratoma and cystic adenomatoid malformation of the lung, pacing for congenital heart block, transamniotic fetal feeding for intrauterine growth retardation, and hematopoietic stem cell transplantation for various diseases. There was exciting work on the technical aspects of fetal access and control of preterm labor. Initially, a series of experiments was conducted at UCSF using the fetal lamb model for CDH, urinary tract obstruction, and hydrocephalus. In each case, the disease was first simulated by surgical intervention, then the consequences on target organ systems were studied, and finally the lesion was corrected and the developmental consequences of correction were ascertained. This pattern of investigation formed the basis of the fetal intervention enterprise for the next 2 decades and helped establish the fetal lamb model as the most widely used and widely accepted method of testing the physiologic rationale for fetal intervention in a host of diseases.

But the fetal lamb model had one grave deficiency: the sheep uterus is resistant to premature contraction and labor in response to an incision or trocar placement. This property made the sheep ideal for testing fetal pathophysiology, but completely inadequate for testing the safety of intervention for both mother and fetus and for developing techniques that would allow access to the fetus without precipitating preterm labor. It was decided early on that success in the fetal lamb model would not be enough to justify human intervention; instead, a proposed procedure first had to be established as safe for mother and fetus in the nonhuman primate model before it could be offered clinically. Fetal surgery experiments in rhesus monkeys occurred first at UCSF and then at the Primate Colony at the University of California, Davis, where the operated mothers could be followed for years and studied for the effects of intervention on fertility and reproductive potential. Availability of the facilities at UCSF and at Davis for sheep and primate work played a crucial role in the development of fetal surgery. In the 1980s, researchers operated on more than 2000 fetal lambs and 500 fetal monkeys at these institutions.

The first disease to attract serious attention as a possible target for fetal intervention was fetal hydronephrosis, specifically bladder outlet obstruction in a male with posterior urethral valves. This disease was one of the first and easiest to detect sonographically, and the disease was relatively well understood. First, it was demonstrated in the laboratory and in human fetuses that without intervention, a severe obstruction would produce oligohydramnios, pulmonary hypoplasia, and renal failure. Then it was proved in the laboratory that this clinical picture could be ameliorated by decompression before birth. The first successful fetal intervention for urinary tract obstruction was the placement of a double pigtail shunt in a procedure that involved the first orchestrated fetal surgery using the talents of a perinatologist (Golbus), sonographer (Filly), and surgeon (Harrison).[14] That boy and his family continue to communicate to the UCSF program 25 years later. The first open fetal surgery occurred almost simultaneously: a desperate case with complete oligohydramnios locking the fetus in a position where the only way to decompress the completely obstructed bladder at 18 weeks' gestation was through a hysterotomy and open vesicostomy. The procedure worked, but the fetus never made urine, undoubtedly because the intervention was too late and the kidneys were already dysplastic. Fortunately, both initial fetal operations were technical successes and, perhaps most importantly, they demonstrated the feasibility and initial safety for mothers. Of course, the techniques, the shunts, and the selection criteria have greatly improved through a vast amount of work that was initiated at UCSF and continues successfully around the world today.

With a growing number of catheter-shunts and the first open fetal surgery for obstructive uropathy at UCSF, and with the first news of catheter-shunt interventions for hydrocephalus in Denver[18] and then in several other centers in the United States, it became clear that fetal surgery was not only off to a fast start, but a precarious and vulnerable one. Recognizing that this fragile enterprise could easily be destroyed by too much exposure and that the enterprise would have to be nurtured carefully in dealing with ethical issues and public perception, we at UCSF and the other early practitioners around the world made a concerted and conscious effort to work together, share information, talk about new techniques, discuss treatment, hammer out ethical guidelines, and agree on some standards for intervention.

In early 1981, the Kroc Foundation (McDonald's Corporation) was persuaded to sponsor a symposium of fetal experts from around the world. This meeting in Santa Ynez, California, featured a frank, open, and honest discussion of every aspect of this embryonic enterprise from physiology to genetics to techniques of intervention. There was also debate about and acceptance of self-imposed "rules to live by": peer-reviewed publication before media exposure, attempting intervention only for lethal diseases in which the pathophysiology and natural history were understood, and strict adherence to ethical guidelines. Sir William Liley was the inspirational keynote participant, and it was a truly multidisciplinary collection of practitioners, which has set the tone of International Fetal Medicine and Surgery Society (IFMSS) meetings ever since: open and frank discussions, informality, lack of structural organizational rigidity, and a wonderfully unique ambiance. It also spawned the tradition of setting up future meetings; Bill Clewell agreed to host the subsequent session in Aspen, Colorado, where the organization was officially named, and the cycle of yearly meetings was initiated. Discussion of a new journal, spearheaded by Maria Michejda and Kevin Pringle, led to the founding of the journal *Fetal Diagnosis & Therapy* as the official voice of the IFMSS.

Perhaps the most important precedent set at the first meeting, and reinforced in subsequent meetings of the IFMSS, was that the participants willingly shoulder the heavy responsibility for stewardship of the enterprise. At that first meeting, a framework was created for fetal intervention (eg, requirements for undertaking fetal intervention and strictures about publishing all cases good or bad before they appear in the media), and this framework was published as a consensus in the *New England Journal of Medicine*, which set a high tone and a high standard for coming years.[19] A registry for fetal interventions was established and, later, the early results with shunts for hydrocephalus and hydronephrosis were published, again in the *New England Journal of Medicine*.[20] This widely referenced document laid out much of the collective thinking, but more importantly, it led to a voluntary moratorium on shunts for hydrocephalus that held for almost 2 decades, something for which the international fetal medicine community can be proud.

FETAL SURGERY: TRIALS, TRIBULATIONS, COMING OF AGE

Despite its many successes, the field of fetal surgery would not be what it is today without having endured significant failures. One good example of those tumultuous times was during the mid-1980s when the first National Institutes of Health (NIH)–sponsored CDH trial examining open fetal surgical repair was underway at UCSF. Although the trial was completed—confirming the important observation that prenatal open repair was no better than postnatal care—behind the scenes there were immense organizational difficulties and divisions among team members. This struggle, although painful, ultimately helped to mature the field of fetal surgery by strengthening the vital relationships between obstetricians, surgeons, and perinatologists, and forcing practitioners to hone their approaches to the unique aspects of fetal surgical research, including an overriding emphasis on maternal safety.

The three basic trends set in motion in San Francisco in the early turbulent times of fetal surgery continue to this day: (1) the move from anatomic repairs to physiologic manipulation (eg, from complete anatomic repair of diaphragmatic hernia to tracheal occlusion to promote fetal lung growth), (2) the move from open surgery by hysterotomy to less invasive fetoscopic techniques (Fetendo), and (3) the move from clinical descriptions and retrospective analysis to proper randomized controlled trials (see **Table 1**). While work at UCSF continued full-speed ahead in the 1990s, the worldwide fetal treatment enterprise was now in full swing and advances came from many centers.

By that time, it became clear that for fetal therapy to progress it would be necessary to determine the efficacy of intervention through properly controlled clinical trials. But they have proved incredibly difficult to execute. Two multicenter trials comparing vaginal to cesarean delivery for gastroschisis have not succeeded despite considerable effort. Single-center trials are much easier logistically. The first successful controlled trial compared open fetal surgical repair of CDH to optimal postnatal care, and as already noted it was successfully completed despite incredible logistical and bureaucratic challenges.[21] This trial provided a definitive answer to a difficult question and prevented further attempts at total repair of diaphragmatic hernias in fetuses without liver herniation. By stopping open fetal surgical repair, it directly spurred development of a new approach to reversing pulmonary hypoplasia by means of temporary tracheal occlusion. Subsequently, temporary tracheal occlusion was tested in a second successful randomized controlled clinical trial.[12] The results of this trial led to further refinements in the technique and a successful nonrandomized trial in Europe by the Eurofetus group.[22] This group also performed an informative trial comparing laser ablation to amnioreduction for twin–twin transfusion syndrome; this was followed by a prospective, randomized trial in North America.[23,24]

The success of the Eurofetus group inspired formation of the North American Fetal Therapy Network (NAFTNet) in 2005 to promote multi-institutional trials in the United States and Canada. The latest and most ambitious trial is the Management of Myelomeningocele Study (MOMS) comparing prenatal to postnatal repair of myelomeningocele (MMC). This trial is ongoing at this time. The UCSF struggle to complete a proper randomized trial for CDH ultimately paid off when NIH funding was secured for the MOMS trial. This achievement was pivotal in the development of the field because it spurred the development of a three-center trial (UCSF, Children's Hospital of Philadelphia, Vanderbilt) that, although agonizing to negotiate and implement, will have a profound effect not only on intervention for MMC but also (inadvertently) on determining how many fetal surgery centers are needed in the United States, how they should be organized and staffed, and who will pay for fetal intervention.

The short but eventful history of the field of fetal surgery reassures us that prenatal treatment offers new hope for the fetus with a correctable defect, but also reminds us that there is considerable potential for doing harm. We know that innovative fetal treatment must be fully tested in the laboratory, carefully considered in the light of current diagnostic and therapeutic uncertainties, honestly presented to the prospective parents, and finally undertaken only with trepidation. In the early harrowing days of fetal treatment, no one could be sure whether the enterprise would succeed or die.

We can now be confident that the enterprise itself has succeeded as reflected in the robustness of professional societies, such as IFMSS, the Fetus as a Patient Society, the Eurofetus group, and NAFTNet, and the proliferation of professional journals, such as *Fetal Diagnosis and Therapy* and *Ultrasound in Obstetrics and Gynecology*, and of textbooks, such as *The Unborn Patient: Prenatal Diagnosis and Therapy*, *Ultrasound in Obstetrics and Gynecology*, *Maternal and Fetal Medicine*, *Fetal Therapy*, and *Intensive Care of the Fetus and Newborn*. As the number of professionals devoted to fetal treatment increases, and the number and quality of fetal treatment teams and centers around the world continues to grow, the banner for fetal Surgery in the twenty-first century should read "Proceed with Caution...and Enthusiasm."

REFERENCES

1. Rosenkrantz JG, Simon RC, Carlisle JH. Fetal surgery in the pig with a review of other mammalian fetal technics. J Pediatr Surg 1968;3:392.
2. Jost A. Sur la différenciation sexuelle de l'embryon de lapin. I: Remarques au sujet de certaines operations chirurgicales sur l'embryon. II: Experiences de paraboise. C R Seances Soc Biol Fil 1946;140:461 [in French].
3. Louw JH, Barnard CN. Congenital intestinal atresia; observations on its origin. Lancet 1955;269:1065.
4. Jackson BT, Piasecki GJ, Egdahl RH. Experimental production of coarctation of the aorta in utero with prolonged postnatal survival. Surg Forum 1963;14:290.
5. Delorimier A, Tierney DF, Parker HR. Hypoplastic lungs in fetal lambs with surgically produced congenital diaphragmatic hernia. Surgery 1967;62:12.
6. Thomasson BH, Esterly JR, Ravitch MM. Morphologic changes in the fetal rabbit kidney after intrauterine ureteral ligation. Invest Urol 1970;8:261.
7. Beck AD. The effect of intra-uterine urinary obstruction upon the development of the fetal kidney. J Urol 1971;105:784.
8. Heymann MA, Rudolph AM. Effects of congenital heart disease on fetal and neonatal circulations. Prog Cardiovasc Dis 1972;15:115.
9. Assali NS. Biology of gestation. New York: Academic Press; 1968.
10. Suzuki K, Plentl AA. Chronic implantation of instruments in the neck of the primate fetus for physiologic studies and production of hydramnios. Am J Obstet Gynecol 1969;103:272.
11. Harrison MR, Jester JA, Ross NA. Correction of congenital diaphragmatic hernia in utero. I. The model: intrathoracic balloon produces fatal pulmonary hypoplasia. Surgery 1980;88:174.
12. Harrison MR, Keller RL, Hawgood SB, et al. A randomized trial of fetal endoscopic tracheal occlusion for severe fetal congenital diaphragmatic hernia. N Engl J Med 2003;349:1916.
13. Harrison MR, Filly RA, Parer JT, et al. Management of the fetus with a urinary tract malformation. JAMA 1981;246:635.
14. Harrison MR, Golbus MS, Filly RA. Management of the fetus with a correctable congenital defect. JAMA 1981;246:774.
15. Liley AW. Intrauterine transfusion of fetus in haemolytic disease. Br Med J 1963; 2:1107.
16. Adamsons K Jr. Fetal surgery. N Engl J Med 1966;275:204.
17. Liggins GC, Howie RN. A controlled trial of antepartum glucocorticoid treatment for prevention of the respiratory distress syndrome in premature infants. Pediatrics 1972;50:515.

18. Clewell WH, Johnson ML, Meier PR, et al. A surgical approach to the treatment of fetal hydrocephalus. N Engl J Med 1982;306:1320.
19. Harrison MR, Filly RA, Golbus MS, et al. Fetal treatment 1982. N Engl J Med 1982; 307:1651.
20. Manning FA, Harrison MR, Rodeck C. Catheter shunts for fetal hydronephrosis and hydrocephalus. Report of the international fetal surgery registry. N Engl J Med 1986;315:336.
21. Harrison MR, Adzick NS, Bullard KM, et al. Correction of congenital diaphragmatic hernia in utero VII: a prospective trial. J Pediatr Surg 1997;32:1637.
22. Deprest J, Gratacos E, Nicolaides KH. Fetoscopic tracheal occlusion (FETO) for severe congenital diaphragmatic hernia: evolution of a technique and preliminary results. Ultrasound Obstet Gynecol 2004;24:121.
23. Crombleholme TM, Shera D, Lee H, et al. A prospective, randomized, multicenter trial of amnioreduction vs selective fetoscopic laser photocoagulation for the treatment of severe twin-twin transfusion syndrome. Am J Obstet Gynecol 2007;197:396e1.
24. Senat MV, Deprest J, Boulvain M, et al. Endoscopic laser surgery versus serial amnioreduction for severe twin-to-twin transfusion syndrome. N Engl J Med 2004;351:136.

Ethics of Fetal Surgery

Frank A. Chervenak, MD[a],*, Laurence B. McCullough, PhD[b]

KEYWORDS

- Ethics • Human subjects research
- Fetal patient • Fetal research
- Fetal surgery • Informed consent

Progress in medical practice depends on innovation, which has brought many improvements to patient care in all specialties. Recently, attention has been called to the important distinction between managed and unmanaged innovation.[1] This is because medical innovation that is unmanaged has gone from innovation to standard of care without adequate scientific and ethical evaluation.[2] This is especially the case for surgery and surgically related specialties,[1] including fetal surgery.[3] Mammary artery ligation for the management of angina is a classic example of unmanaged innovation that can impair scientific progress and put the health and even lives of patients at unnecessary risk. Until recently, fetal surgery shared this history of unmanaged innovation, but with an impact on far fewer patients. Recent innovations in fetal surgery for spina bifida, a relatively common fetal anomaly that is usually diagnosed in the second trimester, raises the possibility of fetal surgery for a much greater number of patients.[4–6] These developments challenge the medical community to guide ongoing innovations in fetal surgery in an ethically responsible fashion,[7] for which there is widespread support in the professional community.[8] The purpose of this article is to provide a comprehensive ethical approach to the responsible management of fetal research from innovation to standard of care and to illustrate the clinical application of this approach to fetal surgery for spina bifida. This article is based on the authors' previous work on this topic.[9–12]

The proposed comprehensive ethical approach is based on a central concept of obstetric ethics: the concept of the fetus as a patient.[13] The authors identify ethical criteria for preliminary investigation for fetal surgery and ethical criteria for initiation of clinical trials and for assessment of the results of such trials (ie, whether they establish a standard of care). They then describe the informed consent process that should be followed for research in recruiting and enrolling subjects. They next consider whether selection criteria should include abortion preferences of the woman and address the question of whether practicing physicians have an obligation to offer

[a] Department of Obstetrics and Gynecology, New York Weill Cornell Medical Center, New York Presbyterian Hospital, 525 East 68th Street, J130, New York, NY 10065, USA
[b] Center for Medical Ethics and Health Policy, Baylor College of Medicine, One Baylor Plaza, Houston, TX 77030, USA
* Corresponding author.
E-mail address: fac2001@med.cornell.edu (F.A. Chervenak).

Clin Perinatol 36 (2009) 237–246
doi:10.1016/j.clp.2009.03.002
0095-5108/09/$ – see front matter © 2009 Elsevier Inc. All rights reserved.
perinatology.theclinics.com

referral to clinical trials of investigation of fetal surgery. They then apply this approach to investigational fetal surgery for spina bifida.

A COMPREHENSIVE APPROACH TO THE ETHICS OF FETAL RESEARCH
The Fetus as a Patient

The first component of the proposed comprehensive approach to the ethics of fetal surgery is the ethical concept of the fetus as a patient. The authors have argued elsewhere that this ethical concept should not be understood in terms of the independent moral status of the fetus. To say that an entity has moral status means that others have an obligation to protect and promote the interests of that entity. To say that the fetus has independent moral status means that there is some feature(s) of the fetus that, independent of other entities—including the pregnant woman, the physician, and the state—generates obligations of others to it. Unfortunately for its proponents, all attempts to establish such independent moral status have ended in failure and continue to do so. There are irreconcilable differences among philosophic and theologic methods that have been deployed over the centuries of debate about the independent moral status of the fetus.[12] This has the important implication that the divisive language of fetal rights has no place in the proposed comprehensive approach to the ethics of fetal surgery.

A philosophically more sound and clinically more useful line of ethical reasoning is that the moral status of the fetus depends on whether it is reliably expected later to achieve the relatively unambiguous moral status of becoming a child and, still later, the more unambiguous moral status of becoming a person. This is called the dependent moral status of the fetus.[13] The fetus is a patient when reliable links exist between it and its later achieving the moral status of a child, and then a person. There are two such links pertaining, respectively, to the viable fetus and to the previable fetus.

The first link between a fetus and its later achieving moral status as a child, and then a person, is viability, the ability of the fetus to exist ex utero with technologic support as necessary. Viability thus requires levels of technologic intervention necessary to support immature or impaired anatomy and physiology through delivery, when childhood exists, and into the second year of life, when, it has been argued, personhood exists.[13] Viability is therefore not an intrinsic characteristic of the fetus but a function of biology and technology. In developed countries, fetal viability occurs at about the 24th week of gestational age, as determined by competent and reliable ultrasound dating.[13–15] When the viable fetus and the pregnant woman are presented to the physician, the viable fetus is a patient.

The second link between a fetus and its later achieving moral status as a child, and then a person, is the decision of the pregnant woman to continue a previable pregnancy to viability, and thus to term. This is because the only link between a previable fetus and its later achieving moral status as a child, and then a person, is the pregnant woman's autonomy, exercised in the decision not to terminate her pregnancy, because technologic factors do not exist that can sustain the previable fetus ex utero. When the pregnant woman decides not to terminate her pregnancy and when the previable fetus and pregnant woman are presented to the physician, the previable fetus is a patient.[13]

The ethical concept of the fetus as a patient has the following implications for the moral status of the fetus. The viable fetus, when the pregnant woman presents for medical care, is a patient. The previable fetus is a patient as a function of the pregnant woman's decision to confer this status on the fetus and present herself for care. It cannot be overemphasized that the existence of a fetal research project does not establish that the fetus is a patient, because, by definition, research interventions have not been established as clinically beneficial to the fetus. A pregnant woman's decision to enroll in a clinical investigation of fetal surgery therefore does not mean that the previable fetus irrevocably has the status of being a patient, because before viability, the pregnant woman can withdraw the status of being a patient from her fetus even after having earlier conferred that status.

When the fetus is a patient, the physician has beneficence-based obligations to protect its life and health. This is not the whole of the story, however. These obligations must in all cases be considered along with beneficence-based and autonomy-based obligations to the pregnant woman[13]; that is, the fetus should not be considered a separate patient. Ethical criteria to guide innovation in fetal surgery must therefore take account of beneficence-based obligations to the fetal patient and beneficence-based and autonomy-based obligations to the pregnant woman. Failure to consider all these obligations results in an inadequate ethical approach to innovations in fetal surgery.

The Initiation and Assessment of Clinical Trials

The second component of the proposed comprehensive approach concerns the initiation and assessment of clinical trials. Innovation in fetal surgery should begin with the design of an intervention and its implementation in the form of a single case, and then a case series, preceded by work on appropriate animal models when they exist. This first stage is necessary to determine the feasibility, safety, and efficacy of innovations and to protect future research subjects from potentially harmful innovation. The authors identify three criteria, all of which must be satisfied to conduct such preliminary investigations in an ethically responsible fashion (ie, one that takes into account beneficence-based obligations to the fetal patient and beneficence-based obligations to the pregnant woman). The previable fetus is a patient in these cases because the woman has made a decision to continue her pregnancy, to have the opportunity to gain the potential benefits of the innovation. She remains free to withdraw that status before viability. The viable fetus is a patient in these cases by virtue of its viability.

1. The proposed fetal intervention is reliably expected on the basis of previous animal studies to be life saving or to prevent serious and irreversible disease, injury, or disability to the fetus.
2. Among possible alternative designs, the intervention is designed in such a way as to involve the least risk for mortality and morbidity to the fetal patient (which is required by beneficence and must satisfy the US research requirement of minimizing risk to the fetus).[16,17]
3. On the basis of animal studies and analysis of theoretic risks for the current and future pregnancies, the mortality risk to the pregnant woman is reliably expected to be low and the risk for disease, injury, or disability to the pregnant woman is reliably expected to be low or manageable.[9]

The first two criteria implement beneficence-based obligations to the fetal patient. Research on animal models should suggest that there would be therapeutic benefit without disproportionate iatrogenic fetal morbidity or mortality. If animal studies result in high rates of mortality or morbidity for the fetal subject, innovation should not be introduced to human subjects until these rates improve in subsequent animal studies.

The third criterion is important because surgery for potential fetal benefit is also maternal surgery. This criterion reminds investigators that the willingness of a subject, in this case, the pregnant woman, to consent to risk does not establish whether the risk/benefit ratio is favorable. Investigators have an independent benef-icence-based obligation to protect human subjects from unreasonably risky research and should use beneficence-based risk-benefit analyses. The phrase "maternal-fetal surgery" is useful if it reminds investigators of the need for such comprehensive analysis. If it is used systematically to subordinate fetal interests to maternal interest and rights, thus undermining the concept of the fetus as a patient in favor of the concept that the fetus is merely a part of the pregnant woman, the authors reject this phrase.

Preliminary innovation should cease and randomized clinical trials should begin when there is clinical equipoise. One approach to clinical equipoise holds that it exists when there is "a remaining disagreement in the expert clinical community, despite the available evidence, about the merits of the intervention to be tested".[14] Brody[17] notes that one challenge here is identifying how much disagreement can remain for there still to be equipoise. Lilford[18] has suggested that when two thirds of the expert community, measured reliably, no longer disagrees, equipoise is not satisfied. A newly emerging scientifically and ethically more appropriate concept of equipoise is known as norma-tive equipoise. More accurately, this is evidence-based equipoise: investigators should judge equipoise to exist when a rigorous evidence-based evaluation of outcomes supports the judgment that neither intervention is better than the other.[19] When the experimental intervention should be judged to be clinically more harmful than nonintervention, equipoise cannot be achieved.

The authors propose that the satisfaction of the previous three criteria, with slight modifications, should count as normative equipoise in the expert community:

1. The initial case series indicates that the proposed fetal intervention is reliably expected to be life saving or to prevent serious and irreversible disease, injury, or disability.
2. Among possible alternative designs, the intervention continues to involve the least risk for morbidity and mortality to the fetus.
3. The case series indicates that the mortality risk to the pregnant woman is reliably expected to be low and the risk for disease, injury, or disability to the pregnant woman, including for future pregnancies, is reliably expected to be low or manageable.[9]

One good test for the satisfaction of the first and third criteria is significant trends in the data from the case series. When normative evidence-based equipoise has been achieved on the basis of these three criteria, randomized clinical trials should commence, as the means to innovate responsibly, and thus improve patient care. Trials should have relevant and clearly defined primary and secondary end points and a design adequate to measure these end points.

These three criteria can be used in a straightforward manner to define stopping rules for clinical trials. When the data support a rigorous clinical judgment that the first or third criterion is not satisfied, the trial should be stopped, because normative evidence-based equipoise can no longer exist. When the clinical trial is completed, its outcome can be assessed to determine whether the innovative fetal surgery should be regarded as standard of care. The trial results should meet the following three criteria to establish the innovation as standard of care:

1. The fetal surgery has a significant probability of being life saving or preventing serious or irreversible disease, injury, or disability to the fetus.
2. The surgery involves low mortality and low or manageable risk for serious and irre-versible disease, injury, or disability to the fetus.

3. The mortality risk to the pregnant woman is low and the risk for disease, injury, or disability is low or manageable, including for future pregnancies.[9]

Brody[17] has underscored the value of data safety and monitoring boards to prevent investigator bias and to protect subjects. Such boards should be used in fetal surgical research, especially to ensure adherence of the previously mentioned ethical criteria as a basis for monitoring such research.

The Informed Consent Process

The third component of the proposed comprehensive approach is the informed consent process. The informed consent process should always be led by a physician competent to explain the interventions, its alternatives, and their benefits and risks. This requirement means that, as a rule, the physician-investigator should lead the consent process or be readily available to answer questions. Having a physician lead the consent process who is not involved in the research project is an acceptable alternative only if that physician possesses the requisite competence and experience with the procedure under investigation.

Like all consent processes for human subject research,[17,20] counseling the pregnant woman about initial innovation or clinical trials should be rigorously nondirective; participation should only be offered and not recommended. Investigators should be sure to emphasize the distinction between research and treatment to prevent therapeutic misconception. Technically, "therapeutic misconception" occurs when the potential subject thinks that all aspects of research design are based on judgments of clinical benefit. This is not the case for research design components, such as randomization and blinding, however. More recently, therapeutic misconception has come also to refer to the belief of potential subjects that research, like treatment, is going to be beneficial and does not exclude advantages of the therapeutic setting (eg, beliefs that the purpose of a randomized trial is to treat her condition and that her physician is going to select the best treatment for her condition).[21] To prevent therapeutic misconception in both of its meanings, the terms *treatment* and *therapy* should never be used by investigators to describe the intervention. The investigators should be explicit about the fact that the surgical technique is research or experimentation. Potential subjects in a case series should be told about the results of animal studies, and potential subjects in clinical trials should be told about the results of the case series. The nature of the surgical procedure should be described to the pregnant woman in detail, including the risks to future pregnancies. The alternatives of termination of pregnancy and postpartum management should be presented, along with their benefits and risks.

In the consent process, word choice is extremely important. Terms like *mother*, *father*, and *baby* should not be used by investigators because these suggest moral relationships and moral status that do not apply.[22] Terms like *pregnant woman*, *potential father*, *fetus*, and *fetal patient* should be used instead. The pregnant woman should be clearly informed that she is under no obligation to the fetal patient to enroll it in a clinical research project.

Clinical experience teaches that there can be considerable internal and external pressure on women to enroll in fetal research. The consent process should be altered to mitigate these effects. The woman should have time for reflecting on her decision, asking questions, and having her questions answered to her satisfaction. To protect the woman from being coerced, her husband or partner and other family members should be reminded that although they may have strong views for or against her participation, their role should be to support and respect the woman's decision-making process and its outcome. Their relationship to her is primarily one of obligation to respect and support her decision. Family members do not have the right to make decisions for her. When necessary, this aspect of the informed consent process should be made clear to family members.

Clinical investigators should ensure that everyone involved in the consent process takes a strictly nondirective approach. Although not currently required in federal consent regulations, prospective monitoring of the consent process (eg, in random sampling) could be used to enforce the nondirective approach.

Publicity about a case series investigation or a clinical trial should be nondirective because it is the first step in the informed consent process. Press releases, media interviews, patient education materials, Web sites, and other forms of publicity should be strictly nondirective; this is an especially important consideration because Web sites are now often the first point of contact for potential subjects to learn about clinical trials. These restrictions on word choice should be followed strictly. "Science by press conference" should be avoided. The data and safety monitoring board should assume oversight responsibilities in these areas.

Investigators face an ethical challenge when a pregnant woman refuses to enter a randomized trial and insists on fetal surgery. The investigator should explain that the assumption that surgery would benefit the fetal patient has no scientific basis and that, on balance, fetal surgery could turn out to be harmful, depending on the results of the trial. Acquiescing to such requests only encourages and potentially exploits false hopes. The ethically justified response is to refuse all such requests, no matter how insistent. Institutional review boards should refuse requests for compassionate exceptions unless a compelling case can be made for them, a steep burden of proof.

US federal regulations are distinctive in the international context in continuing to require the consent of the father for fetal research, including fetal surgery.[16] It should be clear from the preceding discussion that this requirement lacks ethical foundations. Indeed, it is unethical in that it allows for undue influence or even control over the pregnant woman's autonomy by someone who, although he surely has an interest in the woman's decisions, bears none of the medical risks.[9–12]

Selection Criteria and Abortion Preference

The fourth component of the proposed comprehensive approach concerns potential subjects' views on abortion. It is an accepted feature of study design in general that clinical trials should be conducted in such a way as to control for the idiosyncratic effects of patients' preferences on results. This, for example, justifies such strategies as randomization and blinding.

For fetal surgery, this general rule of study design raises significant ethical issues. From the perspective of investigators, to obtain the cleanest results about outcomes for fetuses and future children, one would not want any pregnancies in which fetal surgery occurred to result in elective abortions. From the perspective of pregnant women who would accept elective termination, it might be desirable to prevent, through abortion before viability, adverse outcomes of fetal surgery.

To address the first problem, the study design could exclude women who indicated any willingness to consider elective abortion. To address the second problem, the study design could exclude women who were opposed to abortion. These solutions share a disabling ethical problem: such study designs, in effect, decide for the pregnant woman whether the previable fetus is or is not a patient, an unjustifiable violation of her autonomy in favor of research considerations.

To avoid such ethically unacceptable study designs, there should be no exclusion criteria in research on fetal surgery based on the willingness of potential subjects to countenance elective abortion. Study designs should therefore include elective abortion and birth of adversely affected infants as end points. In addition, investigators should understand that the decision of a pregnant woman to enroll herself and her previable fetus in research does not mean that she has irrevocably conferred the status of being a patient on the previable fetal subject. The informed consent process should make this clear to all pregnant women recruited to fetal surgery research.

Physician Obligation to Refer to Clinical Trials

The fifth component of the proposed comprehensive approach concerns referral of potential subjects to clinical trials of fetal surgery. It is widely accepted that practicing physicians are justified in informing their patients about relevant clinical investigation, and, with the patient's consent, in referring them to the investigators.[17] In the authors' view, there is also an ethical obligation to do so in the case of fetal surgery. The justification for this ethical obligation cannot appeal to benefit to the pregnant woman or fetal patient, because, by definition, the existence of clinical investigation means there is no established clinical benefit. Nevertheless, there is an obligation to future patients, pregnant and fetal alike, to establish whether investigative fetal intervention improves the current standard of care or not. All physicians should take seriously their obligation to pregnant and fetal patients of the future to ensure that innovation has the opportunity to be validated scientifically and ethically rather than introduced in an unmanaged fashion or simply ignored.

APPLICATION OF THE COMPREHENSIVE APPROACH TO EXPERIMENTAL SURGERY FOR SPINA BIFIDA

Animal investigation of fetal surgery for spina bifida suggested that there would be therapeutic benefit without disproportionate morbidity or mortality.[23] The three criteria for investigation with human subjects of feasibility, safety, and efficacy were therefore satisfied.

The results of the case series reported in the literature and clinical experience meet the three criteria for equipoise. There has been reduction in the Arnold-Chiari malformation and subsequent reduction in the necessity for shunt placement. Improvements in spinal cord function, overall functional status, and quality of life have not been clearly demonstrated. The intervention continues to have low rates of fetal mortality and maternal morbidity.[4,5]

With normative evidence-based equipoise having been established, it is ethically justified and warranted to undertake a well-designed randomized clinical trial in the few centers qualified to perform the procedure. Such a trial should have well-defined end points. There are two main clinical concerns about spina bifida. First, it results in loss of motor and sensory function of the lower extremities, in addition to bowel and bladder impairment. Second, the associated Arnold-Chiari malformation results in hydrocephalus, with its resultant shunt dependency and complications. The primary end points of the clinical trial should therefore address both outcomes, in addition to short-term and (to the extent possible) long-term rates of fetal and maternal surgical complications, and iatrogenic prematurity.

Normative evidence-based equipoise means that there is no established benefit for the procedure and that it should be investigated according to scientific standards. This means that the procedure should not be offered outside the context of a clinical trial, even in response to the most urgent requests of pregnant women or referral by colleagues for the procedure. This restriction is a powerful antidote to the problem of the technologic imperative and to unmanaged innovation in fetal surgery.

Stopping rules should be established at the beginning of the trial, and their application should be based on statistical evidence of clear net benefit or net harm. The data and safety monitoring board should approve the study design and end points, define the stopping rules, and set up a procedure to monitor the trial closely, including recruitment and the informed consent process.

The informed consent process should be rigorously nondirective, which is likely to be challenging for physicians who have participated in the innovation phase and have championed the procedure. Expressions of clinical judgment about the benefits of the procedure or other forms of enthusiasm have no place in the informed consent process for a randomized clinical trial. Consent forms, in addition to Web sites and other marketing materials, should take great care with word choice, as described previously. In particular, there should be no use of such terms as *treatment* and *therapy*. Instead, the terms *research*, *experimental intervention*, and the like should be used. The use of such language in oral and written communication is a powerful antidote to the problem of therapeutic misconception.[21] It should also be made abundantly clear to the pregnant woman and her partner that she is under no obligation to place herself or her fetus in the clinical trial, because no benefit from the procedure has been established and it might prove, on balance, to be harmful.

Selection criteria should make no reference to the woman's willingness to terminate or continue her pregnancy before or during the trial. The consent process should make clear to her that her preferences for the disposition of her pregnancy are going to be respected, just as they would in the nonexperimental clinical setting.

Participating centers should report the results of the research at professional meetings and in the scientific literature. Only after reports have appeared in the scientific literature should inquiries by the lay press be accommodated and addressed. Science by press conference should be assiduously avoided.

Referring physicians should be clear that the procedure remains experimental and is available in a clinical trial. They should emphasize that this means the benefits and risks of the procedure have not been established and there is therefore no obligation on the part of the pregnant woman to her fetus or future child to enroll in the trial. Her judgment about the importance of her obligation to future pregnant and fetal patients should be explored nondirectively.

SUMMARY

It has long been recognized that fetal surgery is fraught with ethical issues.[24,25] This article has provided a comprehensive responsible approach to managing the transition from innovation in fetal surgery, to clinical trials, to offering fetal surgery to pregnant women as a standard of care for the management of fetal anomalies. This article has argued that the informed consent process for innovation and research should be strictly nondirective and has emphasized that the pregnant woman has no ethical obligation to the fetal patient to enroll it and herself in such investigations. This article has shown that selection criteria based on abortion preference, pro or con, have no place in the ethical design of research on fetal surgery. This article has also argued that the practice community has an obligation to offer referral to clinical investigation of fetal surgery. The ethical integrity of all forms of fetal research is just as important as their scientific integrity. The current controversy concerning clinical investigation of fetal surgery for spina bifida can be reliably addressed using this ethical framework.

REFERENCES

1. Reitsma A, Moreno JD, editors. Guidelines for innovative surgery. Hagerstown (MD): University Publishing Group; 2006.
2. Frader JE, Caniano DA. Research and innovation in surgery. In: McCullough LB, Jones JW, Brody BA, editors. Surgical ethics. New York: Oxford University Press; 1998. p. 216–41.
3. Harrison MR, Evans MI, Adzick NS, et al. The unborn patient: the art and science of fetal therapy. Philadelphia: WB Saunders Company; 2001
4. Bruner JP, Iulipan N, Paschall RL, et al. Maternal-fetal surgery for myelomeningocele and the incidence of shunt-dependent hydrocephalus. JAMA 1999;282: 1819–25.
5. Sutton LN, Adzick NS, Bilanivic LT, et al. Improvement in hindbrain herniation demonstrated by serial fetal magnetic resonance imaging following maternal-fetal surgery for myelomeningocele. JAMA 1999;282:1826–31.
6. Simpson JL. Maternal-fetal surgery for myelomeningocele: promise, progress and problems. JAMA 1999;282:1873–4.
7. Lyerly AD, Gates EA, Cefalo RC, et al. Toward the ethical evaluation and use of maternal-maternal-fetal surgery. Obstet Gynecol 2001;98:689–97.
8. Lyerly AD, Cefalo RC, Socol M, et al. Attitudes of maternal-fetal specialists concerning maternal-maternal-fetal surgery. Am J Obstet Gynecol 2001;185:1052–8.
9. Chervenak FA, McCullough LB. A comprehensive ethical framework for fetal research and its application to fetal surgery for spina bifida. Am J Obstet Gynecol 2002;187:10–4.
10. McCullough LB, Coverdale JH, Chervenak FA. A comprehensive ethical framework for responsibly designing and conducting pharmacologic research that involves pregnant women. Am J Obstet Gynecol 2005;193:901–7.
11. McCullough LB, Coverdale JH, Chervenak FA. Preventive ethics for including women of childbearing potential in clinical trials. Am J Obstet Gynecol 2006; 194:1221–7.
12. Chervenak FA, McCullough LB. Ethics of maternal-fetal surgery. Semin Fetal Neonatal Med 2007;12:426–31.
13. McCullough LB, Chervenak FA. Ethics in obstetrics and gynecology. New York: Oxford University Press; 1994.
14. Chervenak FA, McCullough LB. The limits of viability. J Perinat Med 1997;25: 418–20.
15. Chervenak FA, McCullough LB, Levene MI. An ethically justified, clinically comprehensive approach to peri-viability: gynaecological, obstetric, perinatal, and neonatal dimensions. J Obstet Gynaecol 2007;27:3–7.
16. Department of Health and Human Services. Regulations for the protection of human subjects. 45 CFR 46.
17. Brody BA. The ethics of biomedical research: an international perspective. New York: Oxford University Press; 1998.
18. Lilford RJ. The substantive ethics of clinical trials. Clin Obstet Gynecol 1992;35: 837–45.
19. Brody BA, McCullough LB, Sharp RR. Consensus and controversy in research ethics. JAMA 2005;294:1411–4.
20. Faden RR, Beauchamp TL. A history of theory of informed consent. New York: Oxford University Press; 1986.
21. Appelbaum PS, Roth LH, Lidz CW, et al. False hopes and best data: consent to research and the therapeutic misconception. Hastings Cent Rep 1987;17:20–4.

22. DeCrespigny L, Chervenak F, McCullough L. Mothers and babies, pregnant women and fetuses. Br J Obstet Gynaecol 1999;106:1235–7.
23. Meuli M, Meuli-Simmen C, Hutchins GM, et al. In utero surgery rescues neurological function at birth in sheep with spina bifida. Nat Med 1995;1:342–7.
24. Barclay WR, McCormick RA, Sidbury JB, et al. The ethics of in utero surgery. JAMA 1981;246:1551–2, 1554–5.
25. Fletcher JC, Jonsen AR. Ethical considerations of fetal therapy. In: Harrison MR, Golbus MS, Filly RA, editors. Unborn patient. 2nd edition. Orlando: Grune & Stratton; 1990. p. 159–70.

The Maternal Side of Maternal–Fetal Surgery

Danny Wu, MD[a],*, Robert H. Ball, MD[b]

KEYWORDS

- Maternal–fetal surgery • Maternal morbidity
- Fetal surgical techniques • Fetoscopic surgery
- Percutaneous ultrasound-guided procedures

The term fetal surgery is used widely for fetal intervention during pregnancy; maternal–fetal surgery may be more appropriate, because all these invasive procedures also affect the mother. Although there is no direct benefit to the mother from these procedures, the risk to her is for a purely altruistic purpose. It is therefore important to understand the potential complications of maternal–fetal surgery, so physician can provide accurate counseling to the patient.

When fetal surgeries were first performed, they all involved maternal laparotomy and hysterotomy. There has been an evolution of approach from open procedures, such as laparotomy, to less invasive approaches, such as uterine endoscopy and most recently percutaneous procedures using devices with diameters of 3 mm or less. This progression to microinvasive, fetoscopic approaches has been associated with a reduction of morbidity (**Table 1**).[1] Maternal complications associated with these various approaches are discussed in detail.

HYSTEROTOMY

After the patient has been given general anesthesia and intubation has been initiated, the surgical field is prepared and draped in sterile fashion. Ultrasound is then used to determine fetal lie and presentation. External manipulation under ultrasound guidance allows positioning of the fetal surgical site near the fundus. Once fetal positioning is optimized, laparotomy is then performed. Covered in a sterile sleeve, an ultrasound transducer is placed directly on the uterine serosal surface. The position of the placental edge is mapped. This step is crucial because uterine incision should be centered as far from the placental edge as possible. The uterine cavity often contracts

[a] Department of Obstetrics, Gynecology, and Reproductive Sciences, University of California, San Francisco, 505 Parnassus Avenue, Box 013, San Francisco, CA 94143-0132, USA
[b] HCA Fetal Therapy Initiative, Maternal-Fetal Services of Utah, St Mark's Hospital, 1140 E. 3900 South, Suite 390, Salt Lake City, UT 84124, USA
* Corresponding author.
E-mail address: wudw@obgyn.ucsf.edu (D. Wu).

Clin Perinatol 36 (2009) 247–253
doi:10.1016/j.clp.2009.03.012
0095-5108/09/$ – see front matter
© 2009 Elsevier Inc. All rights reserved.

Table 1
Maternal morbidity and mortality for 178 interventions at University of California, San Francisco with postoperative continuing pregnancy, divided into operative subgroups

	Open Hysterotomy	Endoscopy FETENDO/ Lap-FETENDO	Percutaneous FIGS/Lap-FIGS	All Interventions
Patients with postop continuing pregnancy	79	68	31	178
Gestational age at surgery (wk)	25.1	24.5	21.1	24.2
Range (wk)	17.6–30.4	17.9–32.1	17.0–26.6	17.0–32.1
Gestational age at delivery (wk)	30.1	30.4	32.7	30.7
Range (wk)	21.6–36.7	19.6–39.3	21.7–40.4	19.6–40.4
Interval surgery to delivery (wk)	4.9	6.0	11.6	6.5
Range (wk)	0–16	0–19	0.3–21.4	0–21.4
Pulmonary edema	22/79 (27.8%)	17/68 (25.0%)	0/31 (0.0%)	39/178 (21.9%)
Bleeding requiring blood transfusion	11/87 (12.6%)	2/69 (2.9%)	0/31 (0.0%)	13/187 (7.0%)
PTL leading to delivery	26/79 (32.9%)	18/68 (26.5%)	4/31 (12.9%)	48/178 (27.0%)
PPROM	41/79 (51.9%)	30/68 (44.1%)	8/31 (25.8%)	79/178 (44.4%)
Chorioamnionitis	7/79 (8.9%)	1/68 (1.5%)	0/31 (0.0%)	8/178 (4.5%)

Abbreviations: FETENDO, fetal endoscopic procedure; FIGS, fetal image–guided surgery; Lap-FETENDO, laparotomy and fetal endoscopic procedure; Lap-FIGS, laparotomy and fetal image guided surgery; PPROM, preterm premature rupture of membranes; PTL, preterm labor.

after hysterotomy is made and the placental edge can get very close to the incision. Every effort should be made to avoid interfering with the placenta because this may cause abruption and subsequent bleeding. If significant bleeding occurs and cannot be controlled, immediate delivery is sometimes required for the safety of the mother. Another factor in deciding the site of the incision is access to the targeted fetal surgical site. Fetal heart rate is monitored by ultrasound during the procedure. Once the fetal procedure is completed, the membranes and myometrium are closed with several layers of suture. A catheter is left in the uterine cavity to allow lactated Ringer solution to be infused together with antibiotics. The volume of amniotic fluid is usually maintained at a low-normal level to minimize stress on the suture line.

Postoperatively the mother is usually given a 24-hour course of tocolysis with magnesium sulfate. In addition, oral indomethacin is given for a total of 48 hours. Maintenance tocolysis until delivery is given with nifedipine. Prophylactic antibiotics are continued for 24 hours. The patient also undergoes daily ultrasound by which fetal well-being, fluid volume, and ductal patency are assessed. Most patients recover in the hospital for 4 to 5 days after surgery. The patient is then seen on a weekly basis with ultrasound evaluation.

Our experience at the University of California, San Francisco (UCSF) with maternal hysterotomy is summarized in a recent publication (see **Table 1**).[1] Between 1989 and 2003, 87 hysterotomies were performed in total. We found significant maternal morbidities. In the early experience when multiple tocolytics were used, particularly nitroglycerin together with aggressive fluid management, there was significant risk for pulmonary edema.[2] Twenty-eight percent of patients suffered this complication.

Thirteen percent of the patients required blood transfusion. Pregnancy outcomes were also significantly affected with premature rupture. Preterm labor was also a significant problem: we found a preterm premature rupture of membranes (PPROM) rate of 52%. Thirty-three percent of patients delivered preterm despite tocolytic therapy. The mean time from hysterotomy to delivery was 4.9 weeks (range 0–16 weeks). The mean gestational age at the time of delivery was 30.1 weeks (range 21.6–36.7 weeks). Increased risk for preterm delivery after hysterotomy was also observed in other fetal surgery centers.[3,4]

Compared with early experiences with hysterotomy, some of the associated morbidities have now decreased. Significant pulmonary edema or blood loss is now relatively rare. In the report by Bruner and colleagues[4], in 178 cases of open repair of myelomeningocele, the rate of pulmonary edema was 5.1% and transfusion was only 2.2%. The mean gestational age at the time of delivery for repair of myelomeningocele is now around 34 weeks.

With these facts in mind, the patient should be carefully counseled before the procedure regarding the risks, benefits, and alternatives to the procedure. She should also understand the experimental nature of the surgery. Preoperative counseling of risks can be divided toward mother, the fetus, and the pregnancy.

The risks to the mother are similar to any major abdominal surgery: bleeding, infection, and damage to adjacent organs. The mother should understand that the procedure carries no direct physical benefit to her. In addition there are the risks associated with aggressive tocolytic therapy and bed rest in a hypercoagulable state. The risks to the fetus can result from intraoperative vascular instability and hypoperfusion leading to injury or death. The result is also at risk for preterm delivery. The risks to the pregnancy are primarily PPROM and preterm delivery. If prolonged PPROM occurs, the pregnancy is also at risk for infection. To avoid the risk of uterine scar rupture, all subsequent deliveries, including the index pregnancy, must be by cesarean section. Experience from Children's Hospital of Philadelphia suggests the risk for uterine rupture/dehiscence in subsequent pregnancies is up to 6% to 12%,[5] which would be considerably higher than the risk after one prior low transverse cesarean section (1% or less)[6] or classic cesarean section (5%–10%).[7] In theory, there is an increased risk for placenta accreta if in subsequent pregnancy the placenta implantation is in an area of uterine scarring. To date, however, we have not identified any case of placenta accreta in a fetal surgical patient of ours in a subsequent pregnancy. We also could not identify any report of such case in the literature. Data regarding future fertility is reassuring, with no increased incidence of infertility in the UCSF experience in those patients attempting pregnancy.[8]

FETOSCOPY

Endoscopic fetal surgery developed as a result of the advances in videoendoscopic surgery and experience with fetoscopy. Access to the fetus is achieved with a tiny puncture of the amniotic cavity. The idea is that with this less-invasive approach, some of the major limiting steps in fetal surgery can be overcome: (1) preterm labor, which was believed to be triggered by the large uterine incision of open fetal surgery; and (2) significant maternal morbidity associated with a large laparotomy. With advances in technology, the hope is that fetoscopic intervention would be done through a percutaneous approach.

Preoperatively, patients are premedicated with a tocolytic, often indomethacin, and given prophylactic intravenous antibiotics. The procedures are performed under local or regional anesthesia. Depending on the gestational age and the tradition of the center, the surgery may be performed in the surgical operating rooms, labor and delivery rooms, or the ultrasound suite. Ultrasound is performed at the same time so that the surgical team can see the ultrasound and fetoscopic images simultaneously. There has been tremendous evolution of the cannulas, instruments, and fetoscopes over the last 10 years. Purpose-designed embryo- or fetoscopes typically have remote eyepieces, to reduce weight and facilitate precise movements. Nearly all are bendable fiber endoscopes rather than conventional rod lens scopes, and as the number of pixels increases over time, image quality improves. Typical diameters are between 1.0 and 2.0 mm. Thin-walled semiflexible plastic cannulas are used to create amniotic access, so that instrument changes are possible. Sharp trocars have been developed to accommodate the wide range of diameters used for different operations. Alternatively one introduces the endoscope sheath loaded with a sharp obturator.

Entry point is determined with the help of ultrasound. Under ultrasound guidance the trocar is inserted into the amniotic cavity, avoiding the placenta, the fetus, and other maternal organs. Transplacental approach is generally avoided despite one group reporting its safety.[9] The trocar is then replaced by the fetoscope. Ultrasound guidance is continued to help direct the scope around the uterus, because the field and depth of the fetoscopic field can be limited. These procedures are therefore considered "sono-endoscopic." For twin-to-twin transfusion syndrome (TTTS) cases the endoscope is in the sac of the recipient twin where there is more fluid. The entry point is determined by the factors noted earlier. In addition the entry site should allow good visualization of the vascular equator of the twins. Any unpaired vessels along the equator consistent with abnormal communications are ablated using the laser fiber that is advanced through the operating channel of the endoscope sleeve. When successful ablation of these vessels is achieved, the endoscope is withdrawn and amnioreduction is performed by draining amniotic fluid through the cannula under ultrasound guidance. The aim of amnioreduction is to reach a normal level (deepest vertical pocket of around 5–6 cm).This amnioreduction reduces the rate of complication of port site leaking, which can lead to amniotic fluid irritation of the peritoneal cavity, causing postoperative pain. It may also improve placental perfusion. In contrast to hysterotomy, many of these fetoscopic cases require little or no tocolytic medication and patients are generally discharged within 24 hours.

The risks of fetoscopy are associated with the uterine puncture and underlying pathology that is being treated. For example, some of the adverse outcomes are inherent to conditions such as TTTS rather than attributable to the procedure itself. According to our experience at UCSF, the morbidities were in some cases similar to the more invasive procedure of hysterotomy and in some cases much more akin to the pattern seen in fetal image–guided surgery (FIGS).[1] A potential explanation is that the UCSF approach has evolved from the initial phase of macro-invasive endoscopy, including laparotomy, uterine exteriorization, and general anesthesia. With the current approach being much more minimally invasive, with a percutaneous approach and smaller instruments, there is much less morbidity.[10] This change has translated into a much lower rate of preterm labor and even PPROM.

Preoperative cervical length assessment has been shown to predict premature delivery.[11] With a cervix less than 30 mm the risk for delivery before 34 weeks is about 74%. If it is shorter than 20 mm the vast majority of patients miscarry. The risk for PPROM is estimated to be around 10% or less; the risk for abruption is 1% to 2% but is probably related to the amnioreduction part of the procedure. Other less common complications are chorioamnionitis and hemorrhage.

Similar outcomes were observed in the randomized trial of laser treatment versus amnioreduction in TTTS conducted in Europe.[12] They reported in the laser group a 1% rate of placental abruption, which led to delivery. They also observed a 3% rate of abdominal pain related to amniotic fluid leakage, which all resolved with expectant management. PPROM rate was 6% with 7 days and 9% within 28 days after the procedure. Overall delivery before 34 weeks' gestation was 53%.

SHUNTS AND RADIOFREQUENCY ABLATION

In cases such as obstructed bladders, pleural effusion, and large macrocystic Congenital Cystic Adenomatoid Malformation, shunts can be useful for chronic drainage. The first shunt was developed by Harrison[13] at UCSF in the early 1980s. It is basically a double pigtail shunt, which is introduced through a 14-gauge introducer. A double-pigtail shunt was developed during a similar time period in the United Kingdom; it is longer and has a greater diameter.[14]

Radiofrequency ablation (RFA) is most commonly used for destruction of tumor tissue in solid organs, such as the liver. The group at the UCSF Fetal Treatment Center was first in using it for ablating the feeding vessels to the anomalous fetus in twin reversed arterial perfusion.[15,16] Currently other indications include selective reduction in monochorionic twin gestations discordant for severe anomalies and in severe TTTS in which one of the twins is near demise.

Many of these cases are performed as outpatient procedures. A single dose of indomethacin is given to suppress uterine activities. Routine preoperative antibiotic prophylaxis is also given. These procedures are performed completely under ultrasound guidance (FIGS). These procedures can be performed under either spinal or local anesthesia. For shunts, a tiny incision is made in the maternal skin, and then the introducer with the trocar in place is advanced into the amniotic cavity. Under ultrasound guidance we generally avoid entry through the placenta. In addition, with color flow Doppler with low flow settings, we can identify an entry point through the myometrium to avoid large veins. The trocar and introducer are then advanced into the area to be drained. Once in position the trocar is removed and care taken to not allow the fluid to be drained or to escape, by placing one's finger over the end. The shunt is then loaded into the introducer and advanced using a pusher. These pushers either are of a certain length or have marks on them, to advance just the internal coils out of the introducer. It is critical to image this with ultrasound also. Once the inner coils are appropriately positioned, the introducer is carefully withdrawn, while at the same time advancing the shunt farther so that the outer coil is positioned on the skin of the fetus, within the amniotic cavity. The operator has to make sure that there is enough of a fluid gap between the fetus and the wall of the uterus; otherwise the outer end of the shunt can be stuck in the myometrium or maternal abdominal wall, resulting in an amnio-peritoneal shunt. Despite in utero shunt placement being one of the more commonly performed fetal interventions, its experience and associated outcomes are not well reported.

Postoperative management involves maternal and fetal monitoring. Use of tocolytic management depends on contraction activity. Often, no further medication is needed. Maternal vital signs should be followed carefully; confirmation of hemostasis of the uterine puncture by visualization is not possible because of the percutaneous approach.

At UCSF, we use an RFA 17-gauge needle device. Most of these procedures can be done under local anesthesia. The instrument is guided into the tissue of the targeted twin at the level of the cord insertion. The prongs are deployed and energy transmission to the device initiated. Out-gassing from the tissue caused by the heat is readily visible with ultrasound. Color and pulse Doppler ultrasound are used to confirm cessation of flow in the targeted twin or the cord. The prongs are then retracted and the device withdrawn. Postoperative monitoring is similar to shunt placement and rarely tocolysis is necessary. The patients can generally be discharged within hours of the procedure.

Not surprisingly, with a less invasive approach, the risk for complication of shunt placement and RFA are lower than for fetal surgical interventions, such as hysterotomy. In our experience, bleeding and infection occurred at a much lower frequency with these percutaneous procedures (see **Table 1**).[1] The rate of preterm delivery is also lower with these procedures, although the risk for PPROM remains. Regarding fetal risk to the surviving twin in cases of monochorionic twins, exsanguination into the placental vascular bed and the other fetus can occur, leading to hypovolemia and hypotension resulting in damage. Long-term neurologic outcome in the surviving twin after RFA reduction is currently lacking.

SUMMARY

Many fetal and particularly placental procedures can now be performed using micro-endoscopes. Hysterotomies are reserved only for a few rare indications. The wider use of minimally invasive approaches has improved the rate and severity of maternal complications. Nevertheless these procedures are not completely risk-free and there have been intraoperative maternal deaths reported. Maternal complications from fetal surgery must therefore be discussed with a patient and her family in balancing the risks and benefits of a prospective intervention.

REFERENCES

1. Golombeck K, Ball RH, Lee H, et al. Maternal morbidity after maternal-fetal surgery. Am J Obstet Gynecol 2006;194(3):834–9.
2. DiFederico EM, Burlingame JM, Kilpatrick SJ, et al. Pulmonary edema in obstetric patients is rapidly resolved except in the presence of infection or of nitroglycerin tocolysis after open fetal surgery. Am J Obstet Gynecol 1998;179(4):925–33.
3. Wilson RD, Johnson MP, Crombleholme TM, et al. Chorioamniotic membrane separation following open fetal surgery: pregnancy outcome. Fetal Diagn Ther 2003;18(5):314–20.
4. Bruner JP, Tulipan N, Richard WO, et al. In utero repair of myelomeningocele: a comparison of endoscopy and hysterotomy. Fetal Diagn Ther 2000;15(2):83–8.
5. Wilson RD, Johnson MP, Flake AW, et al. Reproductive outcomes after pregnancy complicated by maternal-fetal surgery. Am J Obstet Gynecol 2004;191(4): 1430–6.
6. Macones GA, Peipert J, Nelson DB, et al. Maternal complications with vaginal birth after cesarean delivery: a multicenter study. Am J Obstet Gynecol 2005; 193(5):1656–62.
7. McMahon MJ. Vaginal birth after cesarean. Clin Obstet Gynecol 1998;41(2): 369–81.
8. Farrell JA, Albanese CT, Jennings RW, et al. Maternal fertility is not affected by fetal surgery. Fetal Diagn Ther 1999;14(3):190–2.
9. Yamamoto M, Albanese CT, Jennings RW, et al. Incidence and impact of perioperative complications in 175 fetoscopy-guided laser coagulations of chorionic plate anastomoses in fetofetal transfusion syndrome before 26 weeks of gestation. Am J Obstet Gynecol 2005;193(3 Pt 2):1110–6.

10. Gratacos E, Deprest J. Current experience with fetoscopy and the Eurofoetus registry for fetoscopic procedures. Eur J Obstet Gynecol Reprod Biol 2000; 92(1):151–9.
11. Robyr R, Boulvain M, Lewi L, et al. Cervical length as a prognostic factor for preterm delivery in twin-to-twin transfusion syndrome treated by fetoscopic laser coagulation of chorionic plate anastomoses. Ultrasound Obstet Gynecol 2005; 25(1):37–41.
12. Senat MV, Deprest J, Boulvain M, et al. Endoscopic laser surgery versus serial amnioreduction for severe twin-to-twin transfusion syndrome. N Engl J Med 2004;351(2):136–44.
13. Harrison MR, Golbus MS, Filly RA, et al. Management of the fetus with congenital hydronephrosis. J Pediatr Surg 1982;17(6):728–42.
14. Nicolini U, Rodeck CH, Fisk NM. Shunt treatment for fetal obstructive uropathy. Lancet 1987;2(8571):1338–9.
15. Tsao K, Feldstein VA, Albanese CT, et al. Selective reduction of acardiac twin by radiofrequency ablation. Am J Obstet Gynecol 2002;187(3):635–40.
16. Lee H, Wagner AJ, Sy E, et al. Efficacy of radiofrequency ablation for twin-reversed arterial perfusion sequence. Am J Obstet Gynecol 2007;196(5): 459e1–e4.

The Use of Ultrasound in Fetal Surgery

Linda M. Hopkins, MD[a], Vickie A. Feldstein, MD[b], *

KEYWORDS

- Fetal surgery • Ultrasound • Fetal anomalies • Fetal MRI
- Fetoscopy

Ultrasound (US) has been instrumental in the development of fetal diagnosis, intervention, and treatment and remains the cornerstone in identifying the need for and guiding appropriate fetal surgery. Before surgery, precise determination of the correct diagnosis is pivotal in directing possible interventions, and in utero US remains the sole method of evaluation in many conditions. Once a diagnosis is established, sonography can reveal additional findings and can provide important prognostic information. This information can be used to characterize the condition better, predict outcome, and help to guide families weighing options regarding pregnancy management and physicians determining the potential benefits of fetal intervention. When fetal surgery is pursued, real-time intraoperative US guidance assists in the technical aspects of the procedure and in fetal monitoring. After surgery, US is performed to assess the fetal response to the intervention, identify any procedural complications, and continue to monitor fetal growth and well-being.

Because the indications for and types of fetal intervention have increased over the past few years, this article includes sections covering the types and indications for fetal surgery. Further details about the role of US are presented for each specific fetal condition considered.

HYSTEROTOMY

With the development of successful minimally invasive techniques for fetal surgery, the role and frequency of open hysterotomy, with inherent higher maternal and fetal risk, have decreased. Currently, at the authors' institution, the few fetal indications for hysterotomy include prenatal repair of myelomeningocele (**Fig. 1**) and surgical resection of a large congenital cystic adenomatoid malformation (CCAM) (**Fig. 2**) or of a large sacrococcygeal teratoma (SCT) associated with fetal hydrops. Before

[a] Division of Perinatal Medicine and Genetics, University of California, San Francisco, 350 Parnassus Avenue, Suite 810, Campus Box 0705, San Francisco, CA 94143, USA
[b] Department of Radiology, University of California, San Francisco, Box 0628, San Francisco, CA 94143–0628, USA
* Corresponding author.
E-mail address: hopkinsl@obgyn.ucsf.edu (L.M. Hopkins).

Clin Perinatol 36 (2009) 255–272
doi:10.1016/j.clp.2009.03.009   perinatology.theclinics.com
0095-5108/09/$ – see front matter © 2009 Elsevier Inc. All rights reserved.

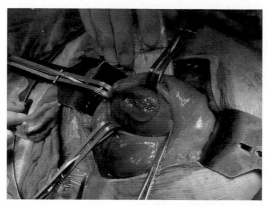

Fig. 1. Intraoperative view during hysterotomy with fetal exposure for myelomeningocele repair.

hysterotomy, targeted US evaluation includes confirmation of the suspected fetal diagnosis and detection of possible associated hydrops; determination of size, extent, or severity of the lesion; measurement of baseline cervical length; and documentation of placental location.

Open hysterotomy is usually performed under general anesthesia. Intraoperative US is used to establish the fetal position and lie. Laparotomy is performed, and surgical exposure of the uterus is accomplished. With a sterile cover applied, a linear-array transducer is placed directly on the uterine surface. The placental edge is identified and carefully "mapped." A uterine incision can then be made, avoiding the placenta

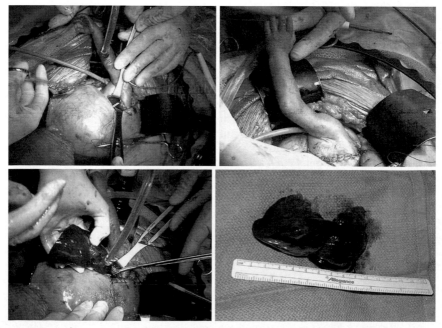

Fig. 2. Images from open fetal surgery with thoracotomy and resection of CCAM.

by an appropriate and safe margin. Once the uterus is opened and the fetus is appropriately positioned for optimal exposure, sometimes necessitating external or internal manipulation, surgical intervention (myelomeningocele repair or tumor resection) can proceed. During the repair, US is used to monitor the fetal heart rate and contractility and to assess for potential complications, including placental abruption.

While the uterine incision remains open, a sterile catheter is used to instill lactated Ringer's solution into the amniotic cavity. Before closure, fluid, combined with an appropriate dose of antibiotics, is instilled, aiming for a "low-normal" level of intra-amniotic fluid, as determined by US. The uterus, amnion, and chorion are then closed in one layer with a second imbricating suture that is placed for myometrial strength and hemostasis.

Possible risks of the open procedure are significant.[1] For some conditions, the degree of benefit to the fetus is under investigation and must be weighed against potential harm. Preterm delivery may result from preterm labor (PTL), premature rupture of membranes, or nonreassuring fetal status prompting urgent delivery. Chorion-amnion separation with or without overt vaginal leakage of amniotic fluid can occur, requiring prolonged hospitalization or delivery. Potential maternal complications include pulmonary edema, significant bleeding, abruption, and infection (chorioamnionitis). Given the significant risk in the current or future pregnancies of uterine rupture at the hysterotomy site, patients must be delivered at 36 to 37 weeks of gestation by cesarean section. In future pregnancies, there is a risk for placenta accreta should the placental implantation overlie the myometrial scar.

After surgery, US is an adjunct to the clinical assessment of PTL or preterm rupture of membranes (PPROM), and it can be used to assess for chorion-amnion separation. Transient mild oligohydramnios without overt rupture of membranes is not uncommon in this group of postsurgical patients, possibly caused by leakage of amniotic fluid through the hysterotomy site or transient fetal renal injury with oliguria (**Fig. 3**).

PRENATAL REPAIR OF MYELOMENINGOCELE

Prenatal surgical repair of fetal myelomeningocele is currently under investigation as part of a National Institutes of Health (NIH)-sponsored randomized controlled trial. Thus, the use of US in this setting is protocolized as per study guidelines. Prenatal US is used in the evaluation of myelomeningocele to confirm the diagnosis (given the potential for meningocele only), with a targeted attempt to identify any other

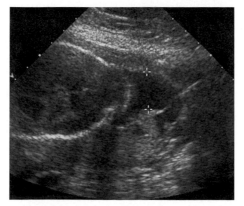

Fig. 3. US demonstration of low normal amniotic fluid level in a postoperative patient.

anomalies, related or unrelated, that may indicate an increased risk for aneuploidy or genetic syndrome. Assessment includes attention to intracranial anatomy, including the ventricles (with measurement of the atrial diameter of the lateral ventricle) and posterior fossa, and to the lower extremities. US is also helpful in obtaining prognostic information by assessing the level of the spinal defect (**Fig. 4**). This information is used to inform and counsel the family about the spectrum of disabilities anticipated. MRI of the fetal brain and spine may be performed as an adjunct to US, particularly in the evaluation of structural brain abnormalities (eg, heterotopias).

Intraoperative US considerations include those outlined previously. Selecting and directing a uterine incision remote from the placental edge is particularly important for this condition, which may require prolonged fetal surgical repair with ongoing fetal heart rate monitoring. Postoperative US assessment of the fetus includes views of the surgical site, lateral cerebral ventricles, posterior fossa, and lower extremities.

CONGENITAL CYSTIC ADENOMATOID MALFORMATION RESECTION

Sonographic considerations in the evaluation of CCAM include confirmation of the diagnosis and assessment of possible fetal compromise, specifically hydrops, which might prompt fetal surgery despite the otherwise favorable outcomes associated with this lesion.[2] The differential diagnosis for fetal chest lesions includes CCAM, pulmonary sequestration (which may be recognized if a feeding vessel arising from the descending thoracic aorta is detected), and congenital diaphragmatic hernia (CDH). CCAM size is measured because it is a useful prognostic indicator. Two methods of assessing chest mass size have been proposed, including CCAM volume ratio (CVR) and mass-thorax ratio. CVR is calculated by measuring the product (in centimeters) of the width $\times$ length $\times$ height of the CCAM. This value is then multiplied by 0.52 to generate a volume (in cubic centimeters), and the result is divided by the head circumference (in centimeters). A CVR value greater than 1.6 is associated with an increased risk for fetal hydrops (**Fig. 5**).[3] The presence and size of cysts help to categorize a CCAM as predominantly microcystic (echogenic, solid-appearing) or macrocystic (with visible discrete cysts on US), which also influences prognosis and possible response to in utero steroids. Microcystic lesions tend to peak in size at 25 to 26 weeks of gestation and then plateau or seem to involute; macrocystic lesions may demonstrate a rapid change in size at any point in pregnancy. Based on preliminary evidence and pilot studies, a multicenter trial is currently underway to investigate the efficacy of steroids in managing large microcystic fetal CCAMs.[4]

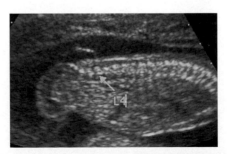

Fig. 4. Sagittal sonogram of the distal fetal spine with assessment of level of myelomeningocele defect (*arrow*).

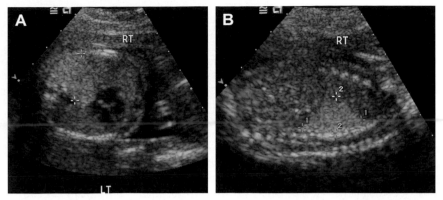

Fig. 5. US determination of CVR measurement. An echogenic right-sided (RT) chest mass is measured, using electronic calipers, in the transaxial (A) and sagittal (B) planes.

Intraoperative US considerations during hysterotomy include those described previously. After fetal thoracotomy and CCAM resection, US is used to assess for fetal response, including residual evidence of hydrops.

RESECTION OF SACROCOCCYGEAL TERATOMA

Similar to CCAMs, SCTs only rarely warrant prenatal intervention with surgical resection. Initial sonographic evaluation involves confirmation of the diagnosis and determination of lesion size, morphology, and presence of intrapelvic involvement and extent. Helpful morphologic features include lesion characterization (cystic versus solid) and assessment with Doppler flow of degree of vascularity (**Fig. 6**). As expected, large, predominantly solid, highly vascular lesions are more frequently associated with fetal decompensation and hydrops before 30 weeks of gestation. Fetal MRI can be performed, particularly if hydrops develops, for enhanced assessment and delineation of the lesion and its extent before prenatal surgery. If hydrops develops after 30 weeks of gestation, premature delivery and postnatal resection are typically recommended.

After surgery and SCT resection, if there is concern for possible fetal anemia, fetal middle cerebral artery peak systolic velocity can be measured and compared with expected values, based on gestational age.

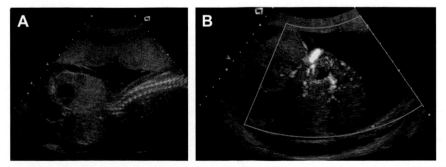

Fig. 6. (A) Obstetric sonogram demonstrates a large exophytic predominantly solid SCT. (B) Power Doppler US interrogation reveals increased vascularity within the mass.

FETOSCOPY

Clinical indications for fetoscopy and fetal intervention include laser ablation of inter-twin vascular connections to treat twin-twin transfusion syndrome (TTTS), tracheal balloon occlusion for CDH, ablation of posterior urethral valves (PUVs) causing bladder outlet obstruction, and umbilical cord occlusion for selective monochorionic fetal reduction (although this is accomplished using US-guided percutaneous radio-frequency ablation [RFA] in some instances and at some institutions).

Before fetoscopic intervention, US is used to diagnose and assess the degree of severity of the fetal condition. The cervical length is routinely measured, as a baseline and to identify women who may be at increased risk for PTL or in need of cerclage placement. Placental location is documented, and a "window" for fetoscopic access is sought. Lack of an appropriate window can mean weighing the potential risks and benefits of delaying a procedure until later in gestation, when safe access may become possible, versus selecting a transplacental approach.

At the authors' institution, fetoscopy is typically performed under regional anes-thesia in the operating room or labor and delivery unit. The US transducer is prepared, covered, and draped in the usual sterile fashion and is used to document placental location, fetal position, umbilical cord insertion site, and maternal anatomy so as to select a safe optimal entry point for introduction of the scope. A small 3-mm incision is made in the skin, and uterine entry is performed under direct real-time US guidance, using the Seldinger technique or a sharp obturator with an endoscopic sheath. The trocar or obturator is then removed, and the fetoscope is inserted.

Intraoperative US is used for fetal heart rate monitoring and screening for abruption or bleeding. After surgery, examinations document the response to intervention; assess fetal well-being; and detect possible complications, including PTL, PPROMs, and chorion-amnion separation.

LASER ABLATION FOR TWIN-TWIN TRANSFUSION SYNDROME

Twin gestations with apparent discrepancy in amniotic fluid volume should undergo careful US examination to evaluate for and possibly confirm the diagnosis of TTTS.[5] This assessment requires determination of chorionicity and amnionicity (if not previ-ously established), estimation of fetal weights, measurement of the deepest vertical pocket of amniotic fluid for each twin, and evaluation of fetal anatomy. In some cases, discordance in estimated fetal weights of monochorionic twin pairs may be explained by unequal placental sharing, particularly if the cord insertion sites are noted to be central and velamentous or marginal.

TTTS, a significant potential complication of monochorionic (MC) twinning, is mani-fest on prenatal US as concomitant oligohydramnios of the donor twin and polyhy-dramnios of the recipient twin (**Fig. 7**), and it is covered in detail in another article in this issue. Sonographic assessment of MC twins can include a search, using careful Doppler technique, for an artery-to-artery (A-A) anastomosis. This is recognized as a vessel coursing between the cord insertion sites along the fetal surface of the placenta with characteristic bidirectional pulsatile flow on spectral Doppler interroga-tion (**Fig. 8**). The presence of an A-A anastomosis has been shown to be useful in prog-nosis and risk stratification.[6] Its presence identifies pregnancies at lower risk for developing overt TTTS. Should TTTS develop, MC pregnancies with an A-A anasto-mosis seem to respond better to amnioreduction. If in utero demise of an MC twin should occur, the presence of an A-A anastomosis is associated with greater risk for neurologic injury to the surviving cotwin. Sonographic assessment of an MC preg-nancy complicated by TTTS should include targeted evaluation of fetal anatomy,

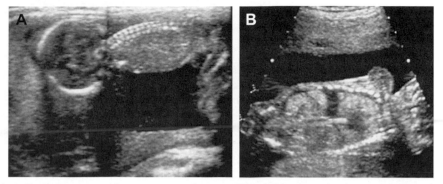

Fig. 7. Typical sonographic appearance of severe TTTS. (*A*) Donor twin appears "stuck" within an oligohydramniotic sac and is closely apposed to the anterior uterine wall. (*B*) Recipient twin is dependent within a polyhydramniotic sac with pleural effusions and ascites, indicating hydrops.

because both twins are at risk for end-organ injury, with particular attention to the recipient heart and Doppler assessment of umbilical cord flow.

In TTTS, preprocedural US determination of placental location and documentation of donor and recipient cord insertion sites are valuable. Once an optimal entry site is identified and the device is safely inserted, the fetal vessels and intertwin vascular connections along the placental surface can be directly visualized through the fetoscope. Laser ablation is performed using a thin fiber that is advanced through the operating channel of the scope. After ablation of vascular connections, the fetoscope is removed and US is used during large-volume amnioreduction (performed through the port site) of the recipient's sac.

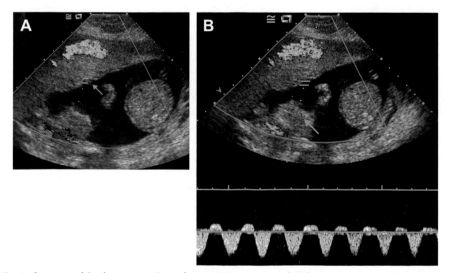

Fig. 8. Sonographic demonstration of an artery-to-artery (AA) anastomosis in a monochorionic placenta. (*A*) Color Doppler US reveals a prominent vessel on the fetal surface of the shared placenta (*arrow*). (*B*) Spectral Doppler evaluation of this vessel (*arrow*) reveals a characteristic bidirectional pulsatile flow pattern.

Risks and potential complications of fetoscopy for laser ablation to treat TTTS include limited visualization of the vessels because of bleeding or previous amnioreduction (for which amnioinfusion may be helpful), recurrence or role reversal of TTTS after intervention, fetal neurologic injury or demise of one or both twins, miscarriage or premature delivery related to PTL, PPROMs or infection, maternal bleeding, or placental abruption.[7–12]

US evaluation of the fetal response to laser ablation includes measurement of the deepest vertical pocket of amniotic fluid for each twin, attempted bladder visualization in the donor, and cardiac assessment in the recipient. As for other interventions, post-procedural US should include detection of possible chorioamniotic separation and, unique to twins, determination of possible disruption of the intertwin membrane (septostomy).

Appropriate evaluation of a surviving twin after cotwin demise is an area under current investigation. Evaluation for possible fetal anemia by measuring peak systolic flow velocity in the middle cerebral artery may be considered, and in utero transfusion may be prompted in some cases.[13]

TRACHEAL BALLOON OCCLUSION FOR CONGENITAL DIAPHRAGMATIC HERNIA

The diagnosis of CDH warrants multidisciplinary evaluation and counseling. Once this major defect is identified, careful US is performed to evaluate for other anomalies, the presence of which portends a dismal prognosis and, most would argue, excludes a patient from consideration for fetal surgery. A fetal echocardiogram is performed to assess for a possible concomitant cardiac defect(s) and to evaluate the size of the pulmonary arteries, which can be helpful in determining the degree of associated pulmonary hypoplasia. Karyotype analysis and genetic consultation are useful, because the risk for aneuploidy and genetic syndromes is significant with this anomaly. In the setting of a large apparently isolated left-sided CDH, fetal intervention is considered.[14] At the authors' institution, US is used to determine whether a portion of the liver is herniated into the chest and to calculate the lung-to-head ratio (LHR). A transaxial view of the fetal chest at the level of the four-chamber view of the heart at 22 to 26 weeks of gestation is obtained. The visualized right lung is measured in two perpendicular axes: anterior-posterior and transverse dimensions. These lengths (in millimeters) are multiplied, and the product is divided by the head circumference (in millimeters) (**Fig. 9**). The presence of a herniated liver in the chest and LHR measurements of 1.0 or less are features associated with high mortality and are used to identify those fetuses most likely to benefit from in utero intervention.[15–17]

Tracheal balloon occlusion for large fetal CDH is typically performed at 26 to 28 weeks of gestation. A 1.2-mm endoscope within a 3.0-mm sheath is introduced into the fetal trachea to position a detachable fluid-filled balloon between the carina and vocal cords. Using fetoscopy in a similar fashion, the balloon is later deflated and retrieved, generally at 32 to 34 weeks of gestation.

The procedure requires US guidance and direct visualization by fetoscopy and fetal bronchoscopy. US is used to guide the endoscope toward the fetal mouth and, at the conclusion of the intervention, to confirm adequate positioning of the balloon within the fetal trachea (**Fig. 10**). After surgery, US is used to assess balloon size and location and to evaluate lung size and echogenicity. US cannot reliably determine fetal lung growth, maturity, or postnatal function, however.

Potential risks of fetoscopic tracheal balloon occlusion for CDH are similar to those for fetoscopic treatment for TTTS; however, because of the difference in gestational stage, premature delivery is a more likely possibility than miscarriage. Difficulties in

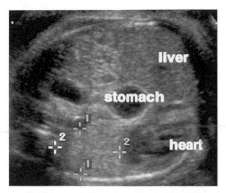

Fig. 9. Transaxial sonographic image of the chest in a fetus that has a left diaphragmatic hernia (liver, stomach, and heart labeled). Measurements of the right lung are made using electronic calipers to calculate the LHR.

balloon placement and deployment can occur, resulting in suboptimal positioning and incomplete response.

ABLATION OF POSTERIOR URETHRAL VALVES

Cases of fetal lower urinary tract obstruction (LUTO) pose vexing clinical dilemmas. Determining prognosis is difficult; thus, selecting appropriate patients for fetal intervention can be challenging. In utero ablation of PUVs is reserved for patients in whom significant LUTO results solely from PUVs and renal function remains reasonable but who are suspected of progressing to irreversible renal damage if the lesion is not corrected before birth.

US is used to identify the level and cause of LUTO. Bladder outlet obstruction attributable to PUVs is manifest by a distended urinary bladder with a classic "keyhole" configuration and dilatation of the posterior urethra in a male fetus (**Fig. 11**). Evaluation of fetal kidneys may be difficult, particularly in the setting of oligohydramnios. Typically, there is significant associated bilateral hydroureteronephrosis. Thorough assessment for possible small renal cortical cysts is crucial, because the presence of cysts indicates irreversible renal parenchymal injury (**Fig. 12**). The lack of visualization of renal cysts does not, however, reliably indicate normal kidney function. These patients are typically managed with serial US-guided bladder taps with laboratory

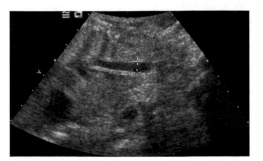

Fig. 10. Sonographic findings after tracheal occlusion in a fetus that has a CDH. Electronic calipers delineate the margins of the fluid-filled balloon on this coronal US image.

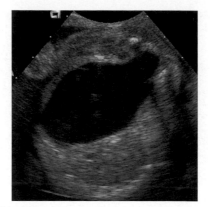

Fig. 11. Markedly dilated bladder with a "keyhole" configuration in a fetus with PUVs.

analysis and measurement of urine electrolytes and β_2-microglobulin.[18] US can be used to assess amniotic fluid volume, degree of hydroureteronephrosis, echogenicity of the renal parenchyma, presence of renal cysts, response to bladder drainage, and measurement of thoracic circumference as an indirect indicator of pulmonary hypoplasia.

Intraoperative US can be used for guiding instillation of fluid into the amniotic cavity and introduction of the device through the maternal anterior abdominal wall, myometrium, and fetal abdominal wall and into the bladder (**Fig. 13**). Postprocedural sonographic assessment includes measurement of amniotic fluid volume, detection of fetal urinary ascites, and visualization of the fetal kidneys and bladder.

RADIOFREQUENCY ABLATION

RFA has been used at the authors' institution for performing selective termination of an anomalous twin in a complicated monochorionic twin gestation (in which intracardiac injection cannot safely be performed because of vascular connections in the shared placenta) and for obliterating blood flow to an acardiac twin in cases of a twin-reversed arterial perfusion (TRAP) sequence. RFA uses high-frequency alternating currents to induce temperature changes by means of electrodes placed directly into fetal tissue. This results in local coagulation and tissue desiccation. Favorable outcomes using this technique have been reported.[19–21]

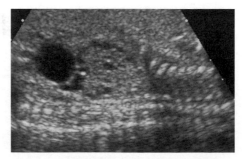

Fig. 12. Sagittal sonogram of the fetal kidney revealing variably sized cortical cysts, indicating dysplasia resulting, in this case, from bladder outlet obstruction.

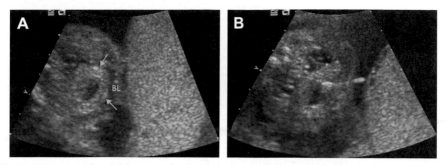

Fig. 13. Intraoperative US images obtained during fetal intervention and ablation of PUVs. (*A*) Arrows indicate thick-walled fetal urinary bladder (BL). (*B*) Linear echogenic structure represents a portion of the T-bar extending from the partially decompressed bladder into the amniotic cavity.

RFA procedures are performed in the operating room under regional anesthesia (although local anesthesia alone is used in some institutions). Under real-time sonographic guidance, a 17-gauge RFA needle device is introduced percutaneously into the uterus and directed into the fetal abdomen at the level of the umbilical cord insertion (**Fig. 14**). Needle tines are deployed, and energy is applied until a temperature of approximately 105°C is achieved and cessation of blood flow within the umbilical cord of the anomalous fetus is observed by US (**Fig. 15**).

The associated procedural risks are small and include pregnancy loss, PPROMs, chorioamnionitis, bleeding, maternal injury (eg, thermal burn from the grounding pad), membrane separation or disruption, and injury to or demise of the cotwin.

Preprocedural US assessment includes confirmation of the diagnosis and determination of severity. Targeted intraoperative US is done to determine the optimal location for device entry and device deployment. Care is taken to avoid traversing the placenta and intertwin membrane if at all possible and to guide entry of the device

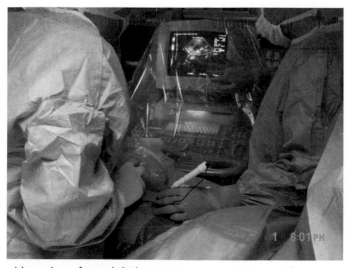

Fig. 14. US guidance is performed during a percutaneous RFA procedure.

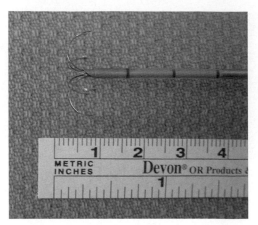

Fig. 15. Photograph of a RFA device with tines deployed.

directly into the amniotic sac of the anomalous twin (**Fig. 16**). After appropriate energy is applied, Doppler US is used to detect any residual flow within the umbilical cord of the anomalous twin (which would prompt additional energy application) or to document complete cessation of flow, the end point for the intervention. This is confirmed by means of repeat targeted Doppler US performed on postoperative day 1.

TWIN-REVERSED ARTERIAL PERFUSION SEQUENCE AND RADIOFREQUENCY ABLATION

Preoperative US evaluation is done to confirm the diagnosis of TRAP and to provide prognostic information so as to select cases best suited for RFA over expectant management. TRAP is manifest as a monochorionic twin gestation with a morphologically normal "pump" twin and an anomalous and typically anencephalic fetus that lacks a beating heart. Blood flow within the acardiac fetus is provided by the pump twin by means of A-A and vein-to-vein connections in the shared placenta. Color and spectral Doppler US shows reversed flow direction with pulsatile flow in the umbilical artery of the acardiac twin directed away from the placenta and toward the anomalous fetus (**Figs. 17** and **18**). US is used to determine amnionicity (because monoamniotic twins are reported to have poorer outcomes than diamniotic MC twins

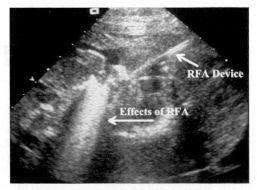

Fig. 16. Intraoperative US image shows adequate position of the RFA device, with evidence of effects on the fetal tissues (regional increased echogenicity) as energy is applied.

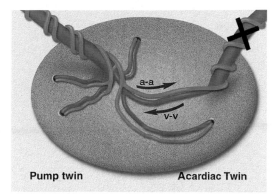

Fig. 17. Simplified schematic representation of placental vascular anatomy in the setting of twin reversed arterial perfusion (TRAP) with a pump and an acardiac twin. v-v, vein-to-vein. (*Courtesy of* V.A. Feldstein, MD, San Francisco, CA.)

after RFA), evaluate for polyhydramnios or hydrops in the pump twin, and calculate the size and volume of the acardiac twin.[22] As expected, increased size or mass of the acardiac twin has been reported in association with increased risk for decompensation of the pump twin, thereby identifying those cases warranting intervention.

EX UTERO INTRAPARTUM TREATMENT PROCEDURE

The ex utero intrapartum treatment (EXIT) procedure is used to deliver a fetus at risk for significant airway compromise at birth (**Fig. 19**). This delivery approach has been performed for fetuses with large neck masses (eg, teratomas) or high airway obstruction (attributable to tracheal or laryngeal atresia). The procedure requires a multidisciplinary team, including radiologist, anesthesiologist, obstetrician, pediatric/fetal surgeon, and neonatologist, and specific equipment, including a fetal pulse oximetry device, tracheal intubation materials, a US machine, and cesarean section equipment. US

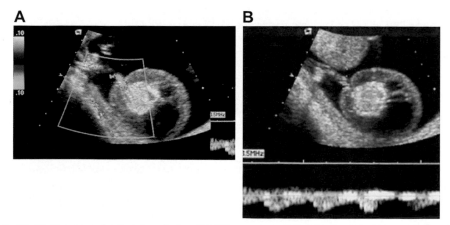

Fig. 18. Twin reversed arterial perfusion (TRAP) sequence. (*A*) Color Doppler US reveals blood flow (*coded blue*) directed away from the transducer toward the fetus. (*B*) Reversed pulsatile arterial flow, directed toward the fetal abdomen, is shown by spectral Doppler interrogation.

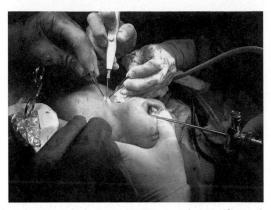

Fig.19. Intraoperative photograph during an EXIT procedure performed to access the airway safely.

is used to document fetal presentation and position and to assist with external cephalic version, if required. US is also used before uterine entry to map the placenta and guide selection of a safe incision site. After hysterotomy, the fetal head and neck are exposed to the level of the chest and intubation is performed or airway access is established in some way. The umbilical cord can then be cut, and the fetus can be delivered and cared for by the neonatology team.

Risks of the EXIT procedure include those inherent in cesarean section delivery. If uterine entry can be accomplished by a low transverse incision, there are minimal risks to future pregnancies. However, if a vertical or classic incision is required, this necessitates repeat cesarean delivery at 36 to 37 weeks of gestation in future pregnancies because of the increased risk for uterine rupture at or near term. Other potential complications include placental abruption, maternal bleeding, and fetal bradycardia, which could prompt urgent delivery of the fetus before securing airway access.[23]

Preoperative US evaluation includes careful assessment of the fetal neck and airway to establish the need for this intervention. In some instances, fetal MRI is also performed to delineate anatomy and demonstrate the trachea. Documentation of placental location is used to determine the approach for the uterine incision, which is helpful in counseling patients regarding implications for future pregnancies.

SHUNT PLACEMENT

Shunt placement to drain fluid from fetal compartments is used for a variety of conditions, with several reports in the literature regarding its applications.[24–26] A comprehensive list of possible indications for this intervention is beyond the scope of this article; therefore, only a general discussion of the role of US is included here.

The two most common indications for fetal shunt placement at the authors' institution are large pleural effusion and bladder outlet obstruction. US helps to assess the etiology of fluid accumulation and the presence and severity of associated sequelae, such as hydrops or oligohydramnios.

As in other applications, US documents fetal position and placental location and is used to guide catheter placement. The Harrison shunt, a double-pigtail catheter advanced and deployed by means of a 14-gauge introducer, is used at the authors' institution. Potential complications unique to these procedures include suboptimal catheter positioning or dislodgement and failure of the shunt to drain the accumulated fluid fully.

FETAL PLEURAL EFFUSION

US assesses the presence and size of fetal pleural effusion, addressing whether it is uni- or bilateral and whether it is associated with a cardiac lesion, chest mass, or any other fetal morphologic abnormality. Large pleural effusion may lead to fetal decompensation with development of hydrops. Full evaluation into the possible etiology of pleural effusion is necessary because it can be related to aneuploidy or genetic syndromes. Real-time US guidance is provided during introduction and deployment of the thoracoamniotic shunt, with a portion of the catheter coiled in the pleural space and the other portion curled within the amniotic fluid (**Fig. 20**).

Postprocedural US assessment of the fetal chest after fluid removal and re-expansion of the lung may reveal an underlying lesion not previously appreciated. A fetal echocardiogram can also be performed. Follow-up US surveillance is useful to detect possible catheter migration or fluid reaccumulation and to assess the need for repeat shunt placement.

FETAL BLADDER OUTLET OBSTRUCTION

Considerations in US assessment of bladder outlet obstruction before catheter placement are similar to those described before fetoscopic cystoscopy. US may be used to guide instillation of fluid into the amniotic cavity before device entry. After the procedure, US is used to assess the response to shunt drainage; to evaluate the kidneys, bladder, and amniotic fluid volume; and to detect the need for repeat intervention should the shunt become occluded or dislodged.

FETAL CARDIAC INTERVENTIONS

Fetal intervention for severe congenital cardiac defects is a more recent pursuit undergoing active investigation. The conditions for which fetal treatment has been pursued include significant aortic stenosis and hypoplastic left heart syndrome with intact atrial septum.[27,28] Preoperative assessment includes careful scrutiny of fetal anatomy, searching for other structural defects, and detailed evaluation of the cardiac abnormality. A targeted fetal echocardiogram is necessary for precise diagnosis and determination of the need for and potential benefit from in utero intervention.

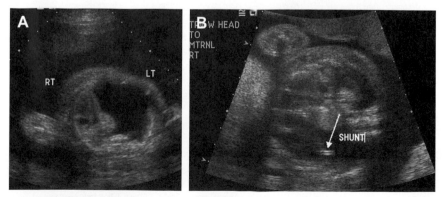

Fig. 20. Fetal pleural effusions. (*A*) Transaxial sonogram of the fetal chest shows a large left-sided (LT) pleural effusion with associated marked rightward (RT) cardiac shift. (*B*) Transaxial US view of the chest in a different fetus with a portion of a thoracoamniotic shunt shown in the pleural space (*arrow*).

Typically, the procedure requires a minilaparotomy for adequate uterine exposure and for facilitating placement and movement of an intracardiac wire or catheter. US is used to identify the appropriate laparotomy and uterine entry site, based on placental location and fetal position, and to guide insertion and placement of the wire. After surgery, fetal echocardiography is performed to assess the response to the cardiac intervention.

MRI OF THE FETAL BRAIN

MRI of the fetal brain is offered at the authors' institution to assess developing intracranial anatomy, particularly if there is concern about a possible intra- or postoperative complication related to fetal intervention. US is less sensitive than targeted MRI in the detection of possible hypoxic or ischemic injury to the developing fetal brain. It has been shown that MRI, typically done approximately 2 weeks after an event like profound bradycardia or cotwin demise, may reveal brain injury not appreciated on US.[29] Patients are counseled about this adjunctive imaging technique for evaluating the fetal brain, and it is offered, particularly if neurologic injury is suspected.

SUMMARY

Obstetric US is an integral part of fetal surgery for open and minimally invasive techniques. With advances in US imaging, the ability to refine diagnosis, predict prognosis, and contribute to fetal treatment continues to grow. Current research in fetal diagnosis and treatment includes identifying the most reliable sonographic features for determining prognosis before and after surgery, understanding the role of three-dimensional and four-dimensional US, and correlating US and fetal MRI findings with long-term neurologic outcome. Even as newer less invasive techniques and technologies, such as gene therapy, for fetal intervention are developed, there should continue to be high demand for and reliance on high-quality US in these applications.

REFERENCES

1. Golombeck K, Ball RH, Lee H, et al. Maternal morbidity after maternal-fetal surgery. Am J Obstet Gynecol 2006;194:834–9.
2. Grethel EJ, Wagner AJ, Clifton MS, et al. Fetal intervention for mass lesions and hydrops improves outcome: 15-year experience. J Pediatr Surg 2007;42(1): 117–23.
3. Crombleholme TM, Coleman BG, Hedrick HL, et al. Cystic adenomatoid malformation volume ratio predicts outcome in prenatally diagnosed cystic adenomatoid malformation of the lung. J Pediatr Surg 2002;37:331–8.
4. Tsao K, Hawgood S, Hirose S, et al. Resolution of hydrops fetalis in congenital cystic adenomatoid malformation after prenatal steroid therapy. J Pediatr Surg 2003;38(3):508–10.
5. Feldstein VA, Filly RA. Complications of monochorionic twins. Radiol Clin North Am 2003;41(4):709–27. Review.
6. Feldstein VA. Understanding twin-twin transfusion syndrome: role of Doppler sonogram. Ultrasound Q 2002;18(4):247–54.
7. Chmait RH, Quintero RA. Operative fetoscopy in complicated monochorionic twins: current status and future directions. Curr Opin Obstet Gynecol 2008; 20(2):169–74.
8. Roberts D, Neilson JP, Kilby M, et al. Interventions for the treatment of twin-twin transfusion syndrome. Cochrane Database Syst Rev 2008;(1):CD002073. Review.

9. Crombleholme TM, Shera D, Lee H, et al. A prospective, randomized, multicenter trial of amnioreduction vs selective fetoscopic laser photocoagulation for the treatment of severe twin-twin transfusion syndrome. Am J Obstet Gynecol 2007;197(4):396.e1–9.

10. Hecher K, Plath H, Bregenzer T, et al. Endoscopic laser surgery versus serial amniocenteses in the treatment of severe twin-twin transfusion syndrome. Am J Obstet Gynecol 1999;180(3 Pt 1):717–24.

11. Rossi AC, D'Addario V. Laser therapy and serial amnioreduction as treatment for twin-twin transfusion syndrome: a metaanalysis and review of literature. Am J Obstet Gynecol 2008;198(2):147–52. Review.

12. Senat MV, Deprest J, Boulvain M, et al. Endoscopic laser surgery versus serial amnioreduction for severe twin-twin transfusion syndrome. N Engl J Med 2004; 351(2):136–44 [Epub 2004 Jul 6].

13. Quarello E, Stirnemann J, Nassar M, et al. Outcome of anaemic monochorionic single survivors following early intrauterine rescue transfusion in cases of feto-fetal transfusion syndrome. BJOG 2008;115(5):595–601.

14. Grethel EJ, Nobuhara KK. Fetal surgery for congenital diaphragmatic hernia. J Paediatr Child Health 2006;42(3):79–85. Review.

15. Jani J, Nicolaides KH, Keller RL, et al. Observed to expected lung area to head circumference ratio in the prediction of survival in fetuses with isolated diaphragmatic hernia. Ultrasound Obstet Gynecol 2007;30(1):67–71.

16. Lipshutz GS, Albanese CT, Feldstein VA, et al. Prospective analysis of lung-to-head ratio predicts survival for patients with prenatally diagnosed congenital diaphragmatic hernia. J Pediatr Surg 1997;32:1634–6.

17. Keller RL, Glidden DV, Paek BW, et al. The lung-to-head ratio and fetoscopic temporary tracheal occlusion: prediction of survival in severe left congenital diaphragmatic hernia. Ultrasound Obstet Gynecol 2003;21:244–9.

18. Johnson MP, Corsi P, Bradfield W, et al. Sequential fetal urine analysis provides greater precision in the evaluation of fetal obstructive uropathy. Am J Obstet Gynecol 1995;173:59–65.

19. Tan TY, Sepulveda W. Acardiac twin: a systematic review of minimally invasive treatment modalities. Ultrsound Obstet Gynecol 2003;22:409–19.

20. Lee H, Wagner AJ, Sy E, et al. Efficacy of radiofrequency ablation for twin-reversed arterial perfusion sequence. Am J Obstet Gynecol 2007;196(5): 459.e1–4.

21. Livingston JC, Lim FY, Polzin W, et al. Intrafetal radiofrequency ablation for twin reversed arterial perfusion (TRAP): a single-center experience. Am J Obstet Gynecol 2007;197(4):399.e1–3.

22. Moore TR, Gale S, Benirschke K. Perinatal outcome of forty-nine pregnancies complicated by acardiac twinning. Am J Obstet Gynecol 1990;163:907–12.

23. Noah MM, Norton ME, Sandberg P, et al. Short-term maternal outcomes that are associated with the EXIT procedure, as compared with cesarean delivery. Am J Obstet Gynecol 2002;186:773–7.

24. Wilson RD, Baxter JK, Johnson MP, et al. Thoracoamniotic shunts: fetal treatment of pleural effusions and congenital cystic adenomatoid malformations. Fetal Diagn Ther 2004;19(5):413–20.

25. Wilson RD, Johnson MP. Prenatal ultrasound guided percutaneous shunts for obstructive uropathy and thoracic disease. Semin Pediatr Surg 2003;12(3):182–9.

26. Biard JM, Johnson MP, Carr MC, et al. Long-term outcomes in children treated by prenatal vesicoamniotic shunting for lower urinary tract obstruction. Obstet Gynecol 2005;106:503–8.

27. Kohl T, Sharland G, Allan LD, et al. World experience of percutaneous ultrasound-guided balloon valvuloplasty in human fetuses with severe aortic valve obstruction. Am J Cardiol 2000;85:1230–3.

28. Marshall AC, Van der Velde ME, Tworetzky W, et al. Creation of an atrial septal defect in utero for fetuses with hypoplastic left heart syndrome and intact or highly restrictive atrial septum. Circulation 2004;110:253–8.

29. Jelin AC, Norton ME, Bartha AI, et al. Intracranial magnetic resonance imaging findings in the surviving fetus after spontaneous monochorionic cotwin demise. Am J Obstet Gynecol 2008;199(4):398.e1–5.

MRI of the Fetal Central Nervous System and Body

Orit A. Glenn, MD*, Fergus V. Coakley, MD

KEYWORDS

• MRI • Prenatal diagnosis • Fetal abnormalities
• Central nervous system

Fetal MRI is increasingly used in clinical practice, partly because of the increasing interest in fetal surgery and fetal medicine. It is a powerful modality to evaluate the fetal brain, fetal spine, and fetal body, and is a valuable complement to prenatal ultrasound. The development of ultrafast- imaging techniques has contributed to the increasing clinical use of fetal MRI. Fetal MRI allows direct visualization of certain structures, such as the developing brain parenchyma, is not susceptible to the same limitations as ultrasound, and has higher contrast resolution than prenatal ultrasound, thereby allowing better differentiation of normal from abnormal tissue. Structural brain abnormalities, such as developmental malformations and destructive lesions, can be sonographically occult on prenatal ultrasound, yet detectable by fetal MRI. Fetal body abnormalities can also be well characterized using fetal MRI. As fetal-surgical techniques are increasingly developed, fetal MRI is also useful in evaluation of patients before and following surgery. Moreover, fetal MRI offers the promise of contributing to our understanding of normal and abnormal fetal development with continued advances in MRI techniques.

INDICATIONS

Fetal MRI is primarily used to evaluate abnormalities of the fetal central nervous system (CNS) or fetal body that are detected by routine prenatal sonography. Most commonly, fetal MRI is performed to evaluate suspected brain abnormalities. In these cases, it is performed to confirm the sonographically detected abnormality, further characterize it, and identify any additional sonographically occult CNS abnormalities.[1,2] Although no formal data exist, it is well accepted that prenatal ultrasound is limited in its ability to detect many of the destructive and developmental lesions that occur prenatally.[3,4] MRI of the fetal brain is most commonly performed for prenatally

Department of Radiology, University of California, San Francisco, 505 Parnassus Avenue, Room L358, San Francisco, CA 94143, USA
* Corresponding author.
E-mail address: orit.glenn@radiology.ucsf.edu (O.A. Glenn).

Clin Perinatol 36 (2009) 273–300
doi:10.1016/j.clp.2009.03.016
0095-5108/09/$ – see front matter © 2009 Elsevier Inc. All rights reserved.

detected ventriculomegaly, followed by abnormalities of the corpus callosum and posterior fossa, including Chiari II malformations.

Fetal MRI is also used to detect brain abnormalities in cases where the fetus is at increased risk for brain abnormalities, even if the prenatal ultrasound of the brain is normal. This includes complicated twin pregnancies and patients with a history of a prior child or fetus with developmental brain abnormalities. In these cases, fetal MRI is performed even when the prenatal sonogram is normal, since many brain abnormalities can be difficult to detect with sonography.

With recent advances in fetal surgical techniques, fetal MRI is being increasingly used to evaluate the fetal brain and spine before or following surgical intervention. In particular, fetal MRI is used to evaluate the fetal brain in complicated monochorionic twin pregnancies, including twin-twin transfusion syndrome or co-twin demise. Because complicated monochorionic twin pregnancies are associated with higher risk of neurodevelopmental childhood disabilities, fetal MRI is used to evaluate these fetuses, even when the prenatal ultrasound of the brain is normal. Fetal MRI is also performed to evaluate the brain and spine in cases of myelomeningocele. In centers that perform in utero repair of myelomeningoceles, it is typically performed before surgery.

Fetal MRI is also performed for evaluation of fetal masses, including neck masses, thoracic masses, and abdominal masses. In cases of congenital diaphragmatic hernia, congenital cystic adenomatoid malformation, neck masses, and urinary tract obstruction, fetal MRI can provide important diagnostic information which can be used to evaluate for fetal surgery.[1]

Fetal MRI can also be useful in situations where the fetus is difficult to image by ultrasound. These include cases of decreased amniotic fluid, such as in urinary tract obstruction, large maternal body habitus; and when fetal position makes it difficult to evaluate the structure of interest. In cases of suspected brain abnormalities, fetal MRI is also useful at advanced gestational ages when shadowing from the calvarium can interfere with ultrasound images.

SAFETY OF FETAL MRI

There are no known deleterious effects of fetal MRI on the fetus when performed on MRI scanners that are 1.5 Tesla strength or lower.[5–12] Recent guidelines by the American College of Radiology on safe MRI practice states that "Pregnant patients can be accepted to undergo MRI scans at any stage of pregnancy if, in the determination of a Level Two MRI Personnel designated attending radiologist, the risk/benefit ratio to the patient warrants that the study be performed."[9] When performing fetal MRI, sedating agents are not administered during the examination. Intravenous contrast is also not recommended in fetal MRI because of the potential risk to the fetus. Prior to the examination, all patients are screened for possible contraindications to MRI. It is also recommended that all patients sign a consent form at the time of the fetal MRI. Because of the current technical limitations of fetal MRI, it is preferable to wait until at least 20 to 22 weeks gestation to minimize the difficulties created by the small size of the fetus and the excessive motion of younger fetuses.

IMAGING TECHNIQUES

Fetal MRI is routinely performed on 1.5 Tesla scanners. There are several limitations to fetal MRI, including fetal motion, the small size of the structure being imaged (particularly at younger gestational ages), and the distance between the receiver coil and the structure being imaged. Because of this, fetal MRI is usually not performed until 20 gestational weeks for evaluation of the fetal body and until 22 gestational weeks for evaluation of the fetal brain and spine. An 8-channel torso phased array coil is used to allow increased coverage and increased signal-to-noise ratio over more standard pelvic phased array coils. The mother lies supine during the course of the examination, which typically lasts 45 minutes. If the mother cannot tolerate lying on her back (eg, because of back pain or compression of the inferior vena cava), then the examination can be performed with the mother lying on her left side. To reduce fetal motion, the mother is kept n.p.o. for 4 hours before the MRI examination.

Image acquisition is susceptible to fetal motion because fetal MRI is performed without maternal or fetal sedation. For that reason, fetal MRI is performed primarily with ultrafast MRI techniques, known as single-shot rapid acquisition with refocused echoes, (ie, single-shot fast spin-echo [ssFSE] or half-Fourier acquired single-shot turbo spin-echo [HASTE]). Using these techniques, a single T2-weighted image can be acquired in less than one second, decreasing sensitivity to fetal motion. Because each image is acquired separately, fetal motion will affect only the particular image that was acquired while the fetus moved.

Typically, an initial localizer is obtained in three orthogonal planes with respect to the mother, using 6 to 8 mm thick ssFSE T2-weighted slices with 1 to 2 mm gap and a large field of view (**Fig. 1**). The localizer is useful for visualizing the position of the fetus and determining fetal sidedness. We also use this localizer to ensure that maximal signal is obtained from the area of interest. In certain cases, such as twins and Chiari II

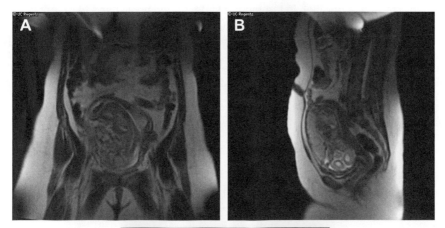
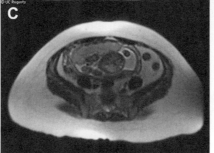

Fig. 1. Initial 3-plane localizer obtained using 8mm thick ssFSE T2-weighted slices in coronal (A) sagittal (B) and axial (C) planes with respect to the mother. (*From* Glen OA. Fetal central nervous system MR imaging. Neuroimaging Clinics of North America 2006;16(1):1–17; with permission.)

malformations, the coil may need to be repositioned in the middle of the examination (eg, when switching from one twin to the other, or from the fetal brain to the spine). From this localizer, the ssFSE T2-weighted images of the fetal area of interest are prescribed. Images are then obtained in the axial, sagittal, and coronal planes.

For imaging of the fetal brain and neck, ssFSE T2-weighted images are obtained using a slice thickness of 3 mm with no gap (**Fig. 2**). For the fetal spine, 2 mm slice thickness is used. For imaging the fetal body, 4 to 7 mm slice thickness is used. Images are acquired during free maternal breathing. For the fetal brain and spine, imaging parameters include TE_{eff} = 90 milliseconds, TR = 4500 milliseconds, bandwidth = 25 kHz, matrix = 192×160, field of view = 24 cm and number of excitations = 0.5. For the fetal body, imaging parameters include TE_{eff} =100 milliseconds, TR = ∞, bandwidth = 62.5 kHz, matrix = 192×128, field of view = 20 cm, and number of excitations = 0.5. Field of view may need to be increased for increased fetal or maternal size or when aliasing artifact is problematic. To reduce potential signal loss caused by cross talk between slices, images are acquired in an interleaved manner. Steady state-free procession gradient echo sequences can also result in high-quality T2-weighted images (the FIESTA sequences using General Electric equipment or the TRUE FISP sequence using Siemens equipment)[13] of fetal body structures, and some sites may prefer this type of T2 sequence for fetal body indications.

The application of T1-weighed imaging to fetal MRI is more limited. Fast multiplanar gradient recalled echo techniques, such as fast multi-planar spoiled gradient-recalled acquisition in the steady state, are primarily used to detect hemorrhage or calcification in the fetal brain (**Fig. 3**). They are also used to evaluate fetal body structures. Images are of lower signal-to-noise ratio and require longer acquisition times (18 seconds), and are therefore susceptible to maternal and fetal motion. Scanning parameters include TR = 120 milliseconds, TE = minute, flip angle = 70, field of view = 24 cm, matrix = 256 × 160, number of excitations = 1, slice

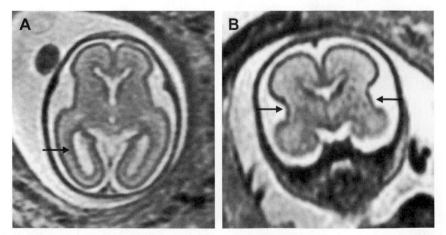

Fig. 2. (*A*) Axial ssFSE T2-weighted image demonstrates normal appearance of the fetal brain at 23 gestational weeks. The germinal matrix appears as a band of low signal surrounding the lateral ventricles (*arrow*). The Sylvian fissures appear box-like on both axial and coronal (*B*) images at 23 week's gestation (*arrows*). (*From* Glen OA. Fetal central nervous system MR imaging. Neuroimaging Clinics of North America 2006;16(1):1–17; with permission.)

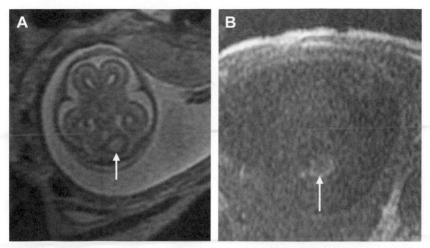

Fig. 3. (*A*) Cerebellar hemorrhage is identified on axial ssFSE T2-weighted image as primarily high signal intensity with low signal intensity rim (*arrow*). (*B*) Axial FMPSPGR T1-weighted image at corresponding level confirms the hemorrhage, which demonstrates high signal intensity (*arrow*). (*From* Glen OA. Fetal central nervous system MR imaging. Neuroimaging Clinics of North America 2006;16(1):1–17; with permission.)

thickness = 5 mm, skip = 0 to 1 mm, bandwidth = 31.25 kHz. This sequence yields eight slices in the axial plane. Images are acquired during a single maternal breath hold.

Gradient echo echo-planar T2-weighted images are used to detect intracranial hemorrhage, and are typically acquired in the axial and coronal planes. Scanning parameters include TR = 5290 milliseconds, TE = 94, flip angle = 90, field of view = 30 cm, matrix = 256 × 256, number of excitations = 1, slice thickness = 3 mm, skip = 0 mm. Images are acquired in 7 seconds, during a single maternal breath hold. It is important to note that hemorrhage and normal intracranial vessels appear hypointense on this sequence. T2-weighted gradient-echo sequence (long repetition and echo times and a small flip angle, eg, 130/20 ms, 20° flip angle) can also be used to demonstrate low signal in the liver in cases of suspected congenital hemochromatosis.[14,15]

Advanced MRI techniques, such as diffusion-weighted imaging and parallel imaging, have also recently been successfully applied to fetal MRI.[16–20] Diffusion-weighted imaging provides quantitative information about water motion and tissue microstructure. Fetal diffusion-weighted imaging has applications for both developmental and destructive brain processes. At our institution, single-shot echo planar diffusion-weighted images are acquired in 18 seconds during a single maternal breath hold (**Fig. 4**). Scanning parameters include TR = 4500 milliseconds, TE = minimum, Field of View = 32, matrix = 128 × 128, slice thickness = 5 mm, skip = 2 mm, bandwidth = 167 kHz. Gradients are applied in three orthogonal directions using a b-value of 0 and 600 sec/mm². Because of the longer scan time, images are susceptible to fetal and maternal motion. With increasing gestational age and engagement of fetal head in the pelvis, the amount of motion is decreased. Diffusion-weighted imaging can be used to identify focal areas of injury and to assess brain development. Parallel imaging can also be applied to fetal MRI to decrease the scan time, increase image resolution, or decrease specific absorption rate.

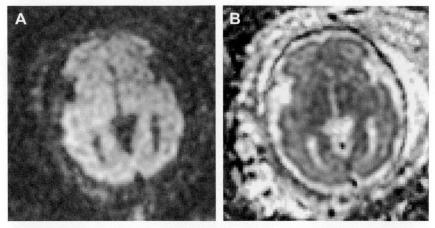

Fig. 4. (*A*) Diffusion-weighted image obtained at 29 gestational weeks. (*B*) Corresponding Apparent Diffusion Coefficient Map. (*From* Glen OA. Fetal central nervous system MR imaging. Neuroimaging Clinics of North America 2006;16(1):1–17; with permission.)

Some manufacturers have, or are developing, interactive scanning programs that can be applied to fetal MRI. Such programs allow adjustment of scanning parameters in real time.[21] Thus, the technologist can rapidly adjust the angle of a prescribed image when the fetus moves without having to exit and reprogram a new ssFSE T2 sequence. This is critical for obtaining true midline sagittal images of the fetal brain and spine, and true, nonoblique axial and coronal images, which results in more accurate identification of abnormalities. As a result, overall image quality is improved, and scan time is reduced.

Advanced postprocessing techniques, such as the formation of high-resolution three-dimensional structural images of the fetal brain, can be used to study fetal morphometry and have recently been developed.[22,23] Because fetal MR images are typically acquired as contiguous slices with no gap, fetal volumetry can also be performed of the entire fetus and of individual fetal body organs.[24–29] This is applied to fetuses with congenital diaphragmatic hernia, where lung volumetry can be of prognostic significance.[28] In addition, assessment of fetal liver volume by prenatal MRI may facilitate recognition of intrauterine growth retardation, which is difficult to diagnose accurately using clinical or sonographic criteria. In a study of 32 high-risk pregnancies, 11 resulted in the birth of a fetus with intrauterine growth retardation.[25] Ten of these eleven fetuses had an abnormally small-liver volume at prenatal MRI, while the remaining 21 fetuses had normal liver volumes.

CLINICAL APPLICATIONS OF FETAL MRI

It is important to be familiar with the normal appearance of fetal structures before interpreting images for the presence of any fetal abnormalities. This is especially important when evaluating the fetal brain, which is a very dynamic structure whose appearance on fetal MRI changes on a weekly basis. The reader is referred to several excellent reviews of the normal appearance of the fetal brain on MRI.[30–35] Although the neurologic and body indications for clinical fetal MRI will be discussed below, this list is by no means a complete list of the indications for fetal MRI.

Ventriculomegaly

Ventriculomegaly is the most common CNS abnormality identified on prenatal sonography,[36] and is one of the most common indications for fetal MRI. It is defined as atrial width equal to or greater than 10 mm on sonogram. Measurements of the atrial width on axial images have been more recently reported using fetal MRI,[37–39] however ventricular size can differ on MRI compared with US by up to 1 to 2 mm when measured in the axial plane.[37] When the ventricular atrium is measured in the coronal plane, US and MRI measurements are highly concordant.[40]

Ventriculomegaly can be the result of developmental, destructive and obstructive processes. Indeed, additional abnormalities are seen in up to 84% of fetuses with ventriculomegaly and include CNS, extra-CNS and chromosomal anomalies.[41–47] In cases of sonographically diagnosed ventriculomegaly, fetal MRI is used to identify additional brain abnormalities. Studies have shown that fetal MRI can detect additional brain abnormalities in up to 50% of cases of sonographically-diagnosed ventriculomegaly.[46–49] Sonographically occult findings include developmental abnormalities, such as agenesis of the corpus callosum, cortical malformations, periventricular heterotopia, and cerebellar dysplasia. Sonographically occult findings also include destructive abnormalities, such as periventricular leukomalacia, porencephaly, multicystic encephalomalacia, intraventricular hemorrhage, and subependymal hemorrhage.[14,46–52]

The neurodevelopmental outcome of fetal ventriculomegaly is better when the ventriculomegaly is an isolated finding.[36,53–55] In a large study of sonographically isolated ventriculomegaly, Gupta and colleagues reported that the incidence of developmental delay was 37% in children with isolated ventriculomegaly, as compared with 84% in children in whom additional abnormalities were identified at birth.[53] Additionally, the outcome of fetal ventriculomegaly is better when the ventricles are only mildly dilated, defined as measuring less than 15 mm in diameter.[44,54,56] In fetuses with both isolated and mild ventriculomegaly on prenatal ultrasound, the risk of neurodevelopmental abnormalities is reported to range from 0% to 36%.[53,57–64] One likely explanation for the variable outcome of fetuses with sonographically-diagnosed isolated mild ventriculomegaly is that those who will experience neurodevelopmental disabilities actually have additional brain abnormalities that are not detected on prenatal ultrasound. Thus, fetal MRI is routinely performed in fetuses diagnosed with isolated mild ventriculomegaly on prenatal ultrasound. In a recent prospective study of 101 fetuses with isolated mild ventriculomegaly on prenatal US, and confirmed by fetal MRI, normal neurodevelopmental outcome was observed in 85% to 94%.[64] Neurodevelopmental outcome was worse for those fetuses with ventricular size of 12 mm to 15 mm compared with those fetuses with ventricular size of 10 mm to 11.9 mm, but did not differ for unilateral versus bilateral ventriculomegaly, or for stable versus regressive ventriculomegaly.[64]

Because the prognosis of ventriculomegaly is related to the presence of additional abnormalities, fetal MRI is performed to evaluate for any additional brain abnormalities. Fetal MRI can directly visualize the developing structures of the fetal brain, such as the ventricles, ventricular walls, germinal matrix, developing white matter, and cortex, and offers better tissue contrast compared with ultrasound, thereby allowing improved identification of fetal brain abnormalities. Fetal MRI can directly visualize the corpus callosum and detect callosal agenesis, which is often seen in association with ventricular dilatation. Fetal MRI can also detect periventricular nodular heterotopia in cases of ventriculomegaly. Periventricular nodular heterotopia appear as nodules along the margins of the lateral ventricles which are isointense to the germinal matrix (**Fig. 5**). Cortical malformations can also be detected with fetal MRI, and include lissencephaly and polymicrogyria. Lissencephaly appears as a smooth brain, with absence of the expected sulci for the fetus' gestational age (**Fig. 6**). Polymicrogyria appears as multiple abnormal infoldings of the developing cortex (**Fig. 7**). The identification of polymicrogyria in the setting of ventriculomegaly should raise the possibility of a genetic component, including metabolic disturbances, or an infectious component of the ventriculomegaly.

Fetal MRI can also be used to detect destructive brain lesions, which can appear as small, focal areas of increased T2 signal in the developing white matter or as larger areas involving the overlying cortex (**Fig. 8**). More subtle irregularity of the ventricular margin may also be an indication of injury to the overlying developing white matter. Hemorrhage is usually detected as areas of decreased signal on ssFSE T2-weighted images, marked decreased signal on gradient EPI T2-weighted images, and increased signal on T1-weighted images, although the signal intensity can vary depending on the stage of hemorrhage. Hemorrhage can occur within the germinal matrix or adjacent brain parenchyma, or within the ventricle, appearing as debris layering within the ventricle or as a focal hematoma (see **Fig. 7**).

Abnormalities of the Corpus Callosum

The corpus callosum can be directly visualized on fetal MRI as a curvilinear T2 hypointense structure located at the superior margin of the lateral ventricles, superior to the fornix (**Fig. 9**). The corpus callosum is best assessed by fetal MRI using thin (3 mm) midline sagittal images. Callosal abnormalities include agenesis, hypogenesis (or partial agenesis), dysgenesis, and hypoplasia, and these can be diagnosed by fetal MRI.

Fetal MR is useful in the evaluation of sonographically suspected callosal anomalies because (1) the corpus callosum can be directly visualized in the sagittal and coronal planes after 20 weeks, and (2) associated anomalies are more easily detected as compared with ultrasound. Fetal MRI has been reported to identify an intact corpus

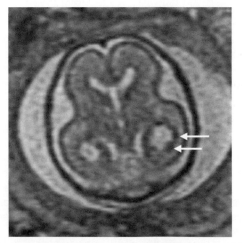

Fig. 5. Axial ssFSE T2-weighted image of a 22-gestational-week-old fetus shows several nodular areas of low signal intensity (isointense to the germinal matrix) along the margin of the left lateral ventricle (*arrows*). This is consistent with periventricular nodular heterotopia; and was confirmed at autopsy. (*From* Glen OA. Fetal central nervous system MR imaging. Neuroimaging Clinics of North America 2006;16(1):1–17; with permission.)

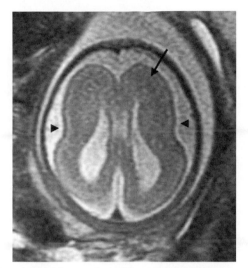

Fig. 6. Axial ssFSE T2-weighted image in a 34-gestational-week fetus demonstrates near complete absence of sulcation, with extremely shallow Sylvian fissures bilaterally (*arrowheads*). A thick band of low-signal intensity is seen in the developing fetal white matter consistent with arrested migration of neurons in classical lissencephaly (*arrow*). (*From* Glen OA. Fetal central nervous system MR imaging. Neuroimaging Clinics of North America 2006;16(1):1–17; with permission.)

callosum in approximately 20% of cases referred for sonographically suspected callosal abnormalities, which has significant implications for patient counseling.[65] Fetal MRI has also been reported to have a greater detection of callosal agenesis as compared with prenatal ultrasound.[66]

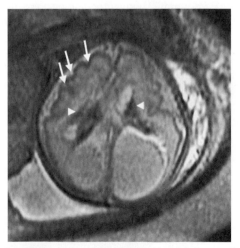

Fig. 7. Axial ssFSE T2-weighted image in a 27-gestational-week fetus referred for ventriculomegaly and choroid plexus cysts demonstrates multiple abnormal infoldings of the developing cortex bilaterally for expected gestational age, representing polymicrogyria (*arrows*). Areas of low signal consistent with hemorrhage are also seen along the lateral ventricles and in the adjacent parenchyma (*arrowheads*). (*From* Glen OA. Fetal central nervous system MR imaging. Neuroimaging Clinics of North America 2006;16(1):1–17; with permission.)

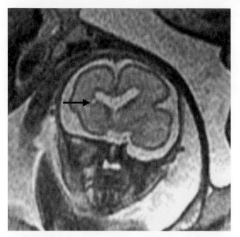

Fig. 8. Coronal ssFSE T2-weighted image in a 25-gestational-week fetus referred for isolated mild ventriculomegaly on prenatal sonogram. A single focus of T2 hyperintensity is identified adjacent to the frontal horn of the lateral ventricle (*arrow*), consistent with an area of parenchymal injury. This was also confirmed on axial image (not shown). (*From* Glen OA. Fetal central nervous system MR imaging. Neuroimaging Clinics of North America 2006;16(1):1–17; with permission.)

Detection of associated brain anomalies in callosal agenesis is also greater with fetal MRI as compared with prenatal ultrasound.[65–69] Additional brain anomalies have been detected by fetal MRI in up to 93% of cases of callosal agenesis.[65,69–71] These include abnormal sulcation in nearly all fetuses, characterized by either too numerous cortical infoldings or delayed sulcation, abnormalities of the cerebellum and vermis in about 50% of fetuses, and abnormalities of the brainstem in about 33% of fetuses.[71] Less frequently, periventricular nodular heterotopia, dysplastic ventricular system, abnormal deep gray nuclei, and intraparenchymal hemorrhage

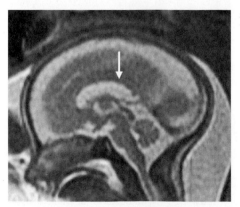

Fig. 9. Normal appearance of the corpus callosum on midline sagittal ssFSE T2-weighed image of a 26-gestational-week fetus (*arrow*). Obtaining a thin-section (3mm), nonoblique-midline image is critical to evaluating the corpus callosum. (*From* Glen OA. Fetal central nervous system MR imaging. Neuroimaging Clinics of North America 2006;16(1):1–17; with permission.)

or injury have been detected by fetal MRI (**Fig. 10**).[71] In 17% of cases, the identification of additional findings by fetal MRI may suggest a specific disorder; this has implications both for the current pregnancy and for future pregnancies.[71]

Complications of Monochorionic Twin Pregnancies

Fetal MRI is used to identify parenchymal injury in monochorionic twin pregnancies that are at increased risk for brain injury, such as co-twin demise and twin-twin transfusion syndrome. Monochorionic twins share a common placenta which often contains abnormal intertwin vascular connections. Because of the placental vascular anatomy, the overall morbidity and mortality of monochorionic twins is much higher than that of diamniotic twins.[72–74] Thus fetal MRI is used to evaluate these fetuses, even when the brain appears normal on prenatal ultrasound.

In utero death of a co-twin is associated with increased risk of neurologic impairment in the surviving co-twin, most likely caused by acute cerebral hypoperfusion at the time of demise, or possibly thromboemboli.[75] Fetal MRI can identify destructive parenchymal lesions that may not be detected by prenatal sonography, such as those that may result following co-twin demise.[51,66,67,76–78] On fetal MRI, ischemic injuries can appear as focal or diffuse areas of increased T2 signal in the germinal matrix, developing white matter, or cortex. Ischemic injury can also result in cortical malformations that are detectable by fetal MRI, such as polymicrogyria (**Fig. 11**),[76] which are associated with developmental delay, epilepsy, and focal neurologic deficits. In a recent study of survivors of spontaneous monochorionic co-twin demise, fetal MRI detected sonographically occult abnormalities in one third of patients, including polymicrogyria, encephalomalacia, germinolytic cysts, hemorrhage, ventriculomegaly, and delayed sulcation.[77] More acute areas of injury can be identified immediately following co-twin demise using fetal diffusion-weighted imaging.[79] Thus, fetal MRI is

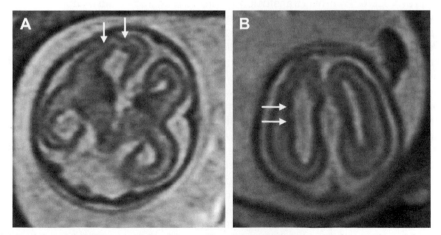

Fig. 10. (A) Axial ssFSE T2-weighted image in a 20-gestational-week fetus referred for suspected callosal agenesis demonstrates absence of the corpus callosum and enlargement of the right lateral ventricle. Abnormal infoldings of the right-frontal developing cortex are consistent with polymicrogyria (*arrows*). (B) Axial ssFSE T2-weighted image demonstrates multiple nodules along the wall of the right-lateral ventricle consistent with periventricular nodular heterotopia (*arrows*). Unilateral microphthalmia and cerebellar hypoplasia (not shown) was also identified by fetal MRI, and led to the diagnosis of Aicardi syndrome. (*From* Glen OA. Fetal central nervous system MR imaging. Neuroimaging Clinics of North America 2006;16(1):1–17; with permission.)

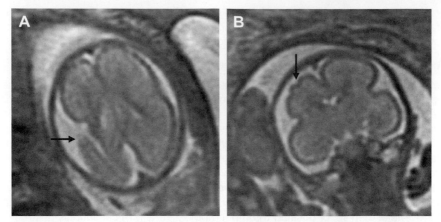

Fig. 11. Monochorionic twin pregnancy complicated by co-twin demise. (*A*) Axial ssFSE T2-weighted image of the surviving 23-gestational-week fetus demonstrates a large area of encephalomalacia involving the left frontal and parietal lobes (*arrow*). (*B*) Coronal image demonstrates several abnormal infoldings of the developing cortex (*arrow*) consistent with polymicrogyria (confirmed on postnatal MRI). (*From* Glen OA. Fetal central nervous system MR imaging. Neuroimaging Clinics of North America 2006;16(1):1–17; with permission.)

best performed immediately after co-twin demise to identify acute abnormalities in the surviving co-twin, and then repeated at 2 to 3 weeks after the demise to detect subacute/chronic sequelae of intracranial injury.

Another serious complication of monochorionic twin pregnancies is twin-twin transfusion syndrome. Twin-twin transfusion syndrome is characterized by abnormal blood flow from the smaller donor twin to the larger recipient twin by way of placental vascular connections. The recipient twin develops polyhydramnios caused by volume overload, and the donor twin develops oligohydramnios resulting in a stuck twin. The exact pathophysiology underlying twin-twin transfusion syndrome is complex, however it appears to be related to the types of intertwin vascular connections.[80] The morbidity rate is very high in twin-twin transfusion syndrome; the recipient and donor twin are at risk for cerebral ischemia or hemorrhage.[77,81–88] Fetal MRI can be used to identify brain injury in twins affected by twin-twin transfusion syndrome; although imaging the polyhydramniotic twin can be challenging because of excessive fetal motion (**Fig. 12**). Brain abnormalities detected by fetal MRI are similar to those seen in survivors of co-twin demise and include encephalomalacia, periventricular white matter injury, germinal matrix hemorrhages, intraventricular hemorrhage, intraparenchymal hemorrhage, and cortical malformation.[77,79,83,86,89,90] In cases where placental laser ablation is being performed, fetal MRI is often used to evaluate the fetal brain before and following surgical intervention.

Myelomeningoceles/Chiari II Malformations

Myelomeningoceles are almost always seen in association with a small posterior fossa and herniation of cerebellar tissue into the cervical subarachnoid space, and are referred to as Chiari II malformations. Fetal MRI is performed to evaluate the brain and spine in sonographically detected myelomeningoceles (**Fig. 13**). Fetal MRI is used to characterize the severity of the hindbrain herniation. It is also used to characterize the ventricular size and morphology, with ventricles often appearing angular in

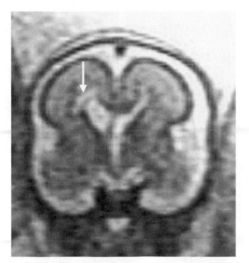

Fig. 12. Monochorionic-twin pregnancy complicated by twin-twin transfusion syndrome. Coronal ssFSE T2-weighted image at 24 week's gestation shows a focal area of T2 hyperintensity adjacent to the frontal horn (*arrow*), with ex-vacuo enlargement of the frontal horn. Findings are consistent with parenchymal injury; and were confirmed at autopsy. (*From* Glen OA. Fetal central nervous system MR imaging. Neuroimaging Clinics of North America 2006;16(1):1–17; with permission.)

their morphology.[37] Additional developmental brain abnormalities are frequently seen in children with Chiari II malformations and they can be detected using fetal MRI. In particular, 57% of children with Chiari II malformations have abnormalities of the corpus callosum, most commonly hypoplasia or dysplasia,[91] and fetal MRI allows direct visualization of corpus callosal abnormalities (see **Fig. 13**). Periventricular nodular heterotopia is present in about 20% of patients with Chiari II malformation[91] and they can be detected with fetal MRI, appearing as nodules along the ventricular walls that are similar in signal intensity to the germinal matrix (see **Fig. 13**). In addition to callosal abnormalities and periventricular nodular heterotopia, microgyria, polymicrogyria, cerebellar dysplasia, syringohydromyelia, and diastematomyelia are seen in association with Chiari II malformations.[92,93] Rarely, destructive lesions can be detected in the fetuses with Chiari II malformations, such as germinal matrix hemorrhage. Following in utero repair of the myelomeningocele, improvement of hindbrain herniation can be observed on fetal MRI.[94]

The fetal spine is also imaged in cases of myelomeningoceles, to identify any additional spinal malformations, such as diastematomyelia, which may be occult on ultrasound.[95] MRI does not seem to offer any additional information about the level of the spinal defect when compared with prenatal US.[96] However, fetal MRI can be especially helpful when the fetal spine is positioned posteriorly with respect to the mother.

Neck Masses

Fetal MRI is used to evaluate sonographically detected masses of the fetal neck, most commonly venolymphatic malformations and teratomas.[97] It is used to provide additional imaging characteristics of the mass, which may help to narrow the diagnosis, and thereby influence counseling on prognosis. Both congenital teratomas and venolymphatic malformations can appear very heterogeneous on MRI, although increased

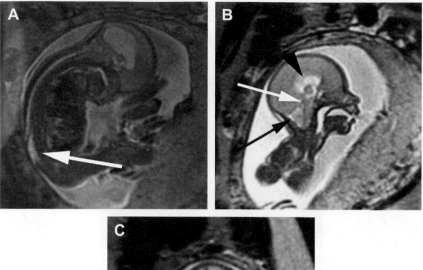

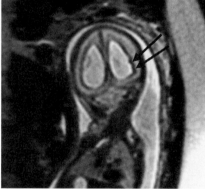

Fig. 13. (*A*) Sagittal ssFSE T2-weighted image in a 22-gestational-week fetus demonstrates a bony spina bifida involving the lumbar and sacral spine with neural placode extending dorsally, consistent with a myelomeningocele (*arrow*); a small posterior fossa is also seen. (*B*) Sagittal ssFSE T2-weighted image of the brain demonstrates stigmata of Chiari II malformation including a small posterior fossa (*black arrow*), beaking of the midbrain tectum (*white arrow*), and hypogenesis of the posterior corpus callosum (*arrowhead*). (*C*) Coronal ssFSE T2-weighted image demonstrates two nodular areas of decreased signal along the lateral ventricular margin (*arrows*), consistent with periventricular nodular heterotopia. Findings were confirmed on postnatal MRI.

heterogeneity favors the diagnosis of a congenital teratoma, and primarily cystic composition with fluid-fluid levels favors the diagnosis of venolymphatic malformations. Moreover, although both can appear large and infiltrative, venolymphatic malformations tend to preserve the overall morphology of the involved structures (**Fig. 14**).

Because of its larger field of view and high tissue contrast, fetal MRI is also particularly helpful in delineating the extent of the mass and identifying structures that may be involved or displaced by the mass, such as the oral cavity (including the tongue), orbit, neck vessels, and mediastinum. Moreover, the fetal airway structures, including the pharynx and trachea, appear hyperintense on ssFSE T2-weighted images because of their fluid content, and can be separated from adjacent soft tissues. Evaluation of the fetal airway for any evidence of obstruction or compression by the mass is particularly important for planning surgical delivery options, including identifying

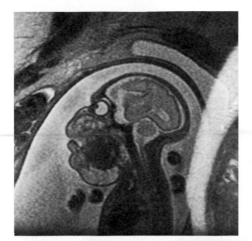

Fig.14. Sagittal ssFSE T2-weighted image demonstrates a large hyperintense infiltrative mass involving the mid and lower face of a 27-gestational-week fetus. The tongue is hypointense within the oral cavity, and is surrounded, but not displaced, by the mass. The infiltrative nature of the mass with preservation of anatomic structures favors a venolymphatic malformation.

cases where an ex-utero intrapartum treatment (EXIT) procedure may be needed because of anticipated difficult endotracheal intubation or need for immediate surgical resection of the mass.[98–103]

Congenital High Airway Obstruction Syndrome

Congenital high airway obstruction syndrome (CHAOS) is a rare intrinsic form of obstruction of the larynx or upper trachea[104] that results in retention of bronchial secretions and pulmonary distension by the retained fluid. Over inflation of the lungs, with flattening or inversion of the diaphragm, is thought to impair venous return to the heart, resulting in fetal hydrops and ascites. The result is a combination of characteristic features at ultrasound, consisting of large bilateral-echogenic fetal lungs, flattening or inversion of the diaphragm, dilated fluid-filled airways below the level of obstruction, and fetal hydrops or ascites. MRI can also demonstrate these features **(Fig. 15)**.[14] The EXIT procedure is a form of surgical delivery that can be used for fetuses with a prenatal diagnosis of upper airway obstruction, whether extrinsic or caused by CHAOS.[98] During the EXIT procedure, the mother is deeply anesthetized to promote uterine relaxation, and the fetal head and neck are delivered through a hysterotomy. The fetus is supported by the placental circulation while the airway is secured in a controlled fashion. Bronchoscopy, endotracheal intubation, and tracheostomy can be performed as appropriate. The EXIT procedure was developed to deliver fetuses with congenital diaphragmatic hernia after therapeutic tracheal occlusion, but the technique has also been successfully applied to fetuses with large neck masses.[105,106] CHAOS has been successfully managed by a combination of fetal tracheostomy and delivery using the EXIT procedure.[107]

Pulmonary Sequestration

Pulmonary sequestration consists of a developmental mass of nonfunctioning-bronchopulmonary tissue that is not connected to the tracheobronchial tree and is fed by systemic arterial blood (usually from the aorta). Postnatal pulmonary

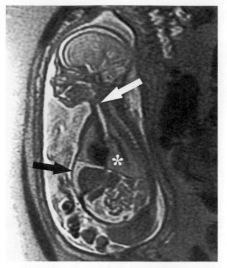

Fig. 15. Sagittal ssFSE T2-weighted image of a fetus with CHAOS at 26 week's gestation. Note the lungs (*asterisk*) are overexpanded with inversion of the diaphragm, large volume ascites (*black arrow*), and a blind-ending airway (*white arrow*) in the neck.

sequestrations are classified as extralobar (15%–25%) or intralobar (75%–85%), depending on whether the sequestration has a separate pleural investment or is within the pleura of the lung, respectively. Most, if not all, prenatal sequestrations are extralobar and are characterized pathologically by diffuse dilation of bronchioles, alveoli, and subpleural lymphatic vessels. Cysts are occasionally present. Pulmonary sequestration accounts for 6% of congenital thoracic lesions and over 75% of prenatally detected lung lesions.[108] MRI can be used as an adjunct to ultrasound in the evaluation of congenital thoracic anomalies.[105] At MRI, sequestration appears as a well-defined chest mass that is of higher T2-signal intensity than normal lung **(Fig. 16)**,[105] but lower than amniotic fluid. The frequency with which MRI identifies a feeding vessel is not known,[105,109] and the incremental benefit of MRI over ultrasound remains under investigation. We have found MRI helpful in the prenatal distinction of subdiaphragmatic sequestration from neuroblastoma (see abdominal masses, below).[109]

Congenital Cystic Adenomatoid Malformation

Congenital cystic adenomatoid malformation is a developmental lung mass composed pathologically of a proliferation of terminal bronchioles. The blood supply is usually from the pulmonary arteries. Communication with the bronchial tree or gastrointestinal tract may be present. Congenital cystic adenomatoid malformations may consist of a few large or medium sized cystic spaces (macrocystic type) or of multiple tiny cysts (microcystic type). The microcystic type may appear solid at prenatal sonography. Small to moderate sized congenital cystic adenomatoid malformations usually have a benign course and are treated by postnatal resection. Large congenital cystic adenomatoid malformations are increasingly recognized as a cause of prenatal demise, because progressive enlargement can lead to compression of the esophagus, vena cava, and lungs, resulting in impaired swallowing, reduced venous return, pulmonary hypoplasia, polyhydramnios, and hydrops fetalis. Prenatally detected congenital cystic adenomatoid malformations, especially if large, should be

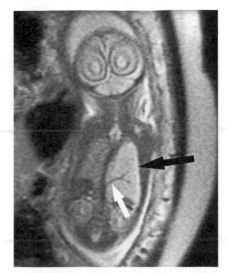

Fig. 16. Coronal ssFSE T2-weighted image of a fetus at 23 week's gestation with a large left-sided pulmonary sequestration (*black arrow*), which is of higher T2 signal intensity than the normal contralateral right lung. A feeding vessel (*white arrow*) can be seen arising from the descending thoracic aorta. (*From* Dhingsa R, Coakley FV, Albanese CT, et al. Prenatal sonography and MR imaging of pulmonary sequestration. AJR Am J Roentgenol 2003;180(2): 433–7; with permission.)

closely monitored for the development of polyhydramnios or hydrops, indication for early delivery in a mature fetus and for prenatal resection in an immature fetus.[106,110] On prenatal MRI, congenital cystic adenomatoid malformations are seen as intrapulmonary masses of increased T2 signal intensity.[105] Discrete cysts may be identified (**Fig. 17**). In the absence of a visible feeding artery from the aorta suggesting the diagnosis of sequestration, congenital cystic adenomatoid malformation and sequestration may be indistinguishable.

Congenital Diaphragmatic Hernia

Congenital diaphragmatic hernia is a developmental defect in the posterolateral diaphragm with herniation of abdominal viscera into the thorax. Congenital diaphragmatic hernia has an incidence of 1 in 3000 to 4000 live births, and 90% of cases are left-sided.[111] The etiology is unknown, but one third of cases are associated with chromosomal or additional anatomic abnormalities and have a mortality of 76%.[112] The position of the liver and the degree of pulmonary hypoplasia are important prognostic factors in isolated congenital diaphragmatic hernia, because mortality is predominantly caused by compression of the lungs by the herniated abdominal viscera. Sixty to eighty-six percent of left-sided congenital diaphragmatic hernias[111,113] are liver-up and have a mortality of 57% compared with 7% for liver-down cases.[112,113] The sonographic diagnosis of congenital diaphragmatic hernia and the evaluation of liver position can be difficult, because lung and liver are of similar echogenicity. At prenatal MRI, lung, liver, stomach, and bowel are easily identified. Because of this excellent soft-tissue contrast, MRI can be used to confirm the diagnosis, evaluate liver position (**Fig. 18**), and perform lung volumetry.[27] Lung volume measured by planimetry on MRI can be expressed as a percentage of the expected lung volume based on fetal size, a measurement known as the relative lung volume.[29] This measurement appears

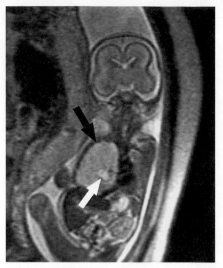

Fig. 17. Coronal ssFSE T2-weighted image of a fetus at 21 week's gestation with a large right-sided congenital cystic adenomatoid malformation (*black arrow*). Note the mass is of increased T2 signal intensity and contains a discrete macrocyst (*white arrow*). The presence of identifiable cysts within the lesion helps in the distinction from pulmonary sequestration.

to be of prognostic importance; in a preliminary study of isolated left congenital diaphragmatic hernia, three of four fetuses with a relative lung volume less than 40% died postnatally despite intensive treatment, while all seven fetuses with a relative lung volume greater than 40% survived.[28]

Abdominal Masses

Fetal abdominal disease encompasses a wide array of conditions that can arise from nearly every structure in the abdominal cavity. The prognosis and treatment of these diseases is equally variable. Management options include corrective fetal surgery (eg, bladder outlet obstruction), postnatal resection, chemotherapy (eg, neuroblastoma), and surveillance (eg, small ovarian cysts).[114–116] Accordingly, accurate diagnosis is crucial for optimal treatment planning and parental counseling, and prenatal ultrasound is the primary modality for the detection and characterization of these anomalies.[117] Fetal abdominal disease is a rare indication for MRI; our research suggests the primary supplemental value of MRI relative to ultrasound lies in the improved tissue characterization, rather than improved anatomic characterization.[118] In eight of 422 fetuses (1.9%) that underwent MRI referred for evaluation of abdominal disease, we found MRI was of supplemental value relative to ultrasound because of improved tissue characterization in three of the six cases with established diagnoses, specifically, in the fetuses with congenital hemochromatosis, subdiaphragmatic sequestration, and cecal atresia with proximal bowel dilatation.[118]

Upper quadrant masses

Upper quadrant masses seen in the fetus are usually caused by subdiaphragmatic extra lobar pulmonary sequestration or neuroblastoma. Subdiaphragmatic extralobar pulmonary sequestration on ultrasound examination is typically echogenic, left sided, and identified in the first trimester, and with neuroblastoma it is cystic, right sided, and recognized in the third trimester.[119] However, the distinction can be very difficult at

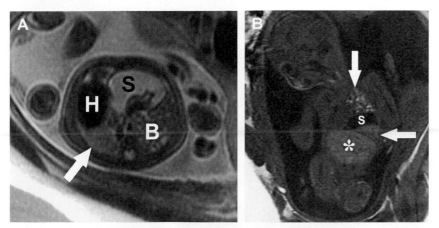

Fig. 18. (*A*) Axial ssFSE T2-weighted image of a fetus at 24 week's gestation with a left-sided congenital diaphragmatic hernia. The heart (H) and right lung (*arrow*) are displaced to the right. The left lung is not visible, and instead the left chest contains herniated stomach (S) and bowel (B). (*B*) Sagittal spoiled gradient-echo T1-weighted MRI shows the stomach (S) in the left chest. Note the liver (*asterisk*) is of relatively high signal intensity, facilitating the identification of the herniated left lobe (*horizontal arrow*) in the left chest. The herniated bowel loops (*vertical arrow*) in the left chest are also of relatively high signal intensity.

ultrasound, whereas subdiaphragmatic extra lobar pulmonary sequestration is typically easily identified at MRI as a mass of uniformly high T2-signal intensity (**Fig. 19**).

Gastrointestinal tract anomalies

Gastrointestinal-tract anomalies may also be encountered. Normal appearances of the fetal bowel have been described.[120] After 33 weeks the jejunum typically contains ingested amniotic fluid exhibiting low signal on T1 and high signal on T2. The signal intensity of distal small bowel is more variable and is dependent on meconium content and gestational age. Before 32 weeks the bowel is T1 hyperintense in greater than half of cases which reduces with gestation to 40% thereafter. Large bowel containing meconium is typically T1 hyperintense and T2 hypointense, with buildup of meconium after 20 weeks facilitating identification of the rectum. The left colon is frequently identified after 24 weeks with only 50% of transverse and ascending colon seen at 31 weeks. In duodenal atresia, stomach and duodenum contents are T2 hyperintense to the level of obstruction.[121] In the largest study to date, nine cases of small bowel atresia demonstrated dilated proximal small bowel (13–30 mm) at the level of the obstruction with variable signal intensity within the dilated small bowel. In cases of meconium peritonitis MRI allows for demonstration of associated small bowel obstruction with meconium pseudocysts having an intermediate signal on T1 and high signal on T2 with these signal characteristics allowing differentiation from other abdominal cystic collections including the bladder.[121] Enteric duplication cysts are secondary to failure of the lumen to recanalize during embryogenesis. These cysts are of similar signal to the bladder on all sequences, lacking typical meconium signal on T1-weighted sequences.

Genitourinary Abnormalities

Genitourinary anomalies account for 14% to 40% of anomalies detected on ultrasound examination.[122] Although ultrasound is the primary imaging modality in

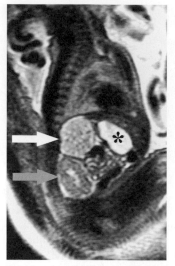

Fig. 19. Sagittal ssFSE T2-weighted image of a fetus at 22 week's gestation with a left-sided subdiaphragmatic extra lobar pulmonary sequestration (*white arrow*). Note the mass is of uniformly high T2-signal intensity and lies above the left kidney (*gray arrow*) and posterior to the stomach (*asterisk*). (*From* Hill BJ, Joe BN, Qayyum A, et al. Supplemental value of MRI in fetal abdominal disease detected on prenatal sonography: preliminary experience. AJR Am J Roentgenol 2005;184(3):993–8; with permission.)

detection of genitourinary abnormalities, oligohydramnios may be present in up to 50% of cases and can limit evaluation.[123] In these cases, MRI can provide additional information. The ability of the radiologist to make a correct diagnosis can have major management decisions as urinary tract anomalies may vary from minor abnormalities to fatal conditions.[124] Single-shot fast spin-echo sequences have been predominately used in the assessment of the genitourinary system,[123,125] because this T2-weighted sequence delineates fluid filled structures, such as amniotic fluid and urine. Uretero-pelvic junction obstruction is the commonest cause of hydronephrosis detected prenatally.[126] It appears that MRI and ultrasound are similar in the detection and characterization of hydronephrosis.[123] MRI may, however, have a role to play in assessing the fetal pelvic anatomy in technically difficult cases where images are obscured secondary to the boney fetal pelvis. To date cases of duplicated collecting systems have been imaged with MRI facilitating characterization of pelvic anatomy and identifying the insertion of duplicated ectopic ureters.[127] MRI has also correctly identified dilated posterior urethras in four cases of posterior urethral valves; none of these cases had hydroureter.[125] In the same series, two fetuses with prune belly syndrome were correctly characterized by MRI, although in our experience complex congenital genitourinary anomalies can be difficult to characterize (**Fig. 20**). In evaluating suspected genitourinary anomalies at prenatal MRI, it is important to assess both the urinary tract and the amniotic fluid volume. Axial T2-weighted imaging of the normal fetal abdomen typically demonstrates the kidneys at the same level as the gallbladder. The absence of bright signal on T2-weighted sequences from the renal pelvic urine at the level of the gallbladder would indirectly indicate renal agenesis. Caire and colleagues have defined normal amniotic fluid on MRI examination as three pockets greater than 2 cm in depth.[125] Polycystic kidneys appear to be adequately imaged with ultrasound as demonstrated in a study of 24 fetuses with severe oligohydramnios

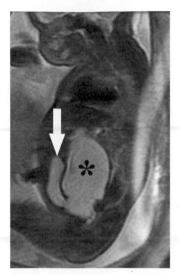

Fig. 20. Sagittal ssFSE T2-weighted image in a fetus at 30 week's gestation with a complex cystic abdominal mass seen at ultrasound The mass has two components, one anterior (*arrow*) and one posterior (*asterisk*). Prospectively, the anterior component was thought to be a urachal diverticulum and the posterior component a dilated bladder, possibly secondary to posterior urethral valves. Surgery performed after birth demonstrated that the anterior component was the bladder and the posterior component was a grossly dilated seminal vesicle secondary to ectopic insertion of the ipsilateral ureter. (*From* Hill BJ, Joe BN, Qayyum A, et al. Supplemental value of MRI in fetal abdominal disease detected on prenatal sonography: preliminary experience. AJR Am J Roentgenol 2005;184(3):993–8; with permission.)

or ultrasonographically suspected urinary tract abnormalities where MRI did not provide additional information.[123] In a series of seven cases of multicystic dysplastic kidneys imaged with MRI,[125] the typical appearance of multiple cysts within the kidneys was well demonstrated. Amniotic fluid was assessed and in cases of anhydramnios a lethal outcome was predicted secondary to pulmonary hypoplasia. In summary, MRI is equivalent to ultrasound in detecting renal anomalies and the role of MRI may be in the detection of associated extra-renal anomalies, or to confirm ultrasound findings when diagnostic certainty may be lowered by confounding oligohydramnios.

SUMMARY

Fetal MRI is being increasingly used to assess for fetal abnormalities. Although significant progress in the field of fetal MRI has occurred during the past 20 years, continued technical advances will likely contribute to significant growth of the field. Moreover, with continued hardware and software improvements, additional MRI sequences, which are rapid and therefore feasible to use in clinical practice, will likely become available. Prenatal MRI complements ultrasound because of larger field-of-view, superior soft tissue contrast, easier and more precise volumetric measurement, and greater accuracy in the demonstration of intracranial and spinal abnormalities. While ultrasound remains the primary modality for fetal imaging, these advantages of MRI make it a valuable adjunct to fetal surgery. Prenatal MRI can be used to assess the anomaly, exclude other defects that might preclude surgery, and to follow response and evaluate complications. Specific indications and guidelines are likely to remain in flux, because of the rapidly developing nature of both fetal surgery and prenatal MRI.

Because fetal MRI involves many disciplines, including obstetrics, perinatology, genetics, pediatric surgery, and pediatric neurology, the future promise of fetal MRI will likely best be achieved through multidisciplinary collaborative efforts.

REFERENCES

1. Coakley FV, Glenn O, Qayyum A, et al. A developing technique for the developing patient. AJR Am J Roentgenol 2004;182:243–52.
2. Raybaud C, Levrier O, Brunel H, et al. MR imaging of fetal brain malformations. Childs Nerv Syst 2003;19:455–70.
3. Filly RA, Goldstein RB, Callen PW. Fetal ventricle: importance in routine obstetric sonography. Radiology 1991;181:1–7.
4. Aubry MC, Aubry JP, Dommergues M. Sonographic prenatal diagnosis of central nervous system abnormalities. Childs Nerv Syst 2003;19:391–402.
5. Baker P, Johnson I, Harvey R, et al. A three-year follow-up of children imaged in utero with echo-planar magnetic resonance. Am J Obstet Gynecol 1994;170:32–3.
6. Chew S, Ahmadi A, Goh PS, et al. The effects of 1.5T magnetic resonance imaging on early murine in-vitro embryo development. J Magn Reson Imaging 2001;13:417–20.
7. Clements H, Duncan KR, Fielding K, et al. Infants exposed to MRI in utero have a normal paediatric assessment at 9 months of age. Br J Radiol 2000;73:190–4.
8. Glover P, Hykin J, Gowland PA, et al. An assessment of the intrauterine sound intensity level during obstetric echo-planar magnetic resonance imaging. Br J Radiol 1995;68:1090–4.
9. Kanal E, Barkovich AJ, Bell C, et al. ACR guidance document for safe MR practices: 2007. AJR Am J Roentgenol 2007;188:1447–74.
10. Kanal E, Borgstede JP, Barkovich AJ, et al. American College of Radiology white paper on MR safety. AJR Am J Roentgenol 2002;178:1335–47.
11. Kok RD, de Vries MM, Heerschap A, et al. Absence of harmful effects of magnetic resonance exposure aat 1.5T in utero during the third trimester of pregnancy: a follow-up study. Magn Reson Imaging 2004;22:851–4.
12. Myers C, Duncan KR, Gowland PA, et al. Failure to detect intrauterine growth restriction following in utero exposure to MRI. Br J Radiol 1998;71:549–51.
13. Chung HW, Chen CY, Zimmerman RA, et al. T2-Weighted fast MR imaging with true FISP versus HASTE: comparative efficacy in the evaluation of normal fetal brain maturation. AJR Am J Roentgenol 2000;175:1375–80.
14. Coakley FV, Hricak H, Filly RA, et al. Complex fetal disorders: effect of MR imaging on management - preliminary clinical experience. Radiology 1999;213:691–6.
15. Gandon Y, Guyeder D, Heautot JF. Hemochromatosis: diagnosis and quantification of liver iron with gradient - echo MR imaging. Radiology 1994;193:533–8.
16. Righini A, Bianchini E, Parazzini C, et al. Apparent diffusion coefficient determination in normal fetal brain: a prenatal MR imaging study. AJNR Am J Neuroradiol 2003;24:799–804.
17. Prayer D, Brugger P, Mittermayer C, et al. Diffusion-weighted imaging in intrauterine fetal brain development. Washington, DC: American Society of Neuroradiology; 2003.

18. Kok RD, van den Berg PP, van den Bergh AJ, et al. Maturation of the human fetal brain as observed by 1H MR spectroscopy. Magn Reson Med 2002;48:611–6.
19. McKenzie CA, Levine D, Morrin M, et al. ASSET enhanced SSFSE imaging of the fetus. Kyoto, Japan: International Society for Magnetic Resonance in Medicine; 2004.
20. Schneider MM, Berman JI, Baumer FM, et al. Normative ADC values in the developing fetal brain. Am J Neuroradiol, in press.
21. Busse R, Carrillo A, Brittain J, et al. On-demand real-time imaging: interactive multislice acquisition applied to prostate and fetal imaging. Honolulu (HI): International Society for Magnetic Resonance in Medicine; 2002.
22. Jiang S, Xue H, Glover A, et al. MRI of moving subjects using multislice snapshot images with volume reconstruction (SVR): application to fetal, neonatal, and adult brain studies. IEEE Trans Med Imaging 2007;26:967–80.
23. Rousseau F, Glenn O, Iordanova B, et al. A novel approach to high resolution fetal brain MR imaging. Med Image Comput Comput Assist Interv Int Conf Med Image Comput Comput Assist Interv 2005;8:548–55.
24. Baker PN, Johnson IR, Gowland PA. Fetal weight estimation by echo-planar magnetic resonance imaging. Lancet 1994;343:644–5.
25. Baker PN, Johnson IR, Gowland PA. Measurement of fetal liver, brain, and placental volumes with echo-planar magnetic resonance imaging. Br J Obstet Gynaecol 1995;102:35–9.
26. Baker PN, Johnson IR, Gowland PA, et al. Estimation of fetal lung volume using echo-planar magnetic resonance imaging. Obstet Gynecol 1994;83:951–4.
27. Coakley FV, Lopoo JB, Lu Y. Volumetric assessment of normal and hypoplastic fetal lungs by prenatal single-shot RARE MR imaging. Radiology 2000;216: 107–11.
28. Paek BW, Coakley FV, Lu Y. Prenatal evaluation of congenital diaphragmatic hernia by MR lung volumetry - preliminary experience. Radiology 2001;220:63–7.
29. Williams G, Coakley FV, Qayyum A, et al. Fetal relative lung volume: quantification by using prenatal MR imgaging lung volumetry. Radiology 2004;233:457–62.
30. Garel C. MRI of the fetal brain: normal development and cerebral pathologies. Berlin: Springer; 2004.
31. Garel C, Chantrel E, Elmaleh M, et al. normal gestational landmarks for cerebral biometry, gyration and myelination. Childs Nerv Syst 2003;19:422–5.
32. Girard N, Raybaud C, Poncet M. In vivo MR study of brain maturation in normal fetuses. AJNR Am J Neuroradiol 1995;16:407–13.
33. Glenn OA, Barkovich AJ. Magnetic resonance imaging of the fetal brain and spine: an increasingly important tool in prenatal diagnosis, part 1. AJNR Am J Neuroradiol 2006;27:1604–11.
34. Kostovic I, Judas M, Rados M, et al. Laminar organization of the human fetal cerebrum revealed by histochemical markers and magnetic resonance imaging. Cereb Cortex 2002;12:536–44.
35. Prayer D, Kasprian G, Krampl E, et al. MRI of normal fetal brain development. Eur J Radiol 2006;57:199–216.
36. Goldstein RB, La Pidus AS, Filly RA, et al. Mild lateral cerebral ventricular dilatation in utero: clinical significance and prognosis. Radiology 1990;176:237–42.
37. Levine D, Trop I, Mehta TS, et al. MR imaging appearance of fetal cerebral ventricular morphology. Radiology 2002;223:652–60.
38. Parazzini C, Righini A, Rustico M, et al. Prenatal magnetic resonance imaging: brain normal linear biometric values below 24 gestational weeks. Neuroradiology 2008;50:877–83.

39. Twickler DM, Reichel T, McIntire DD, et al. Fetal central nervous system ventricle and cisterna magna measurements by magnetic resonance imaging. Am J Obstet Gynecol 2002;187:927–31.
40. Garel C, Alberti C. Coronal measurement of the fetal lateral ventricles: comparison between ulrasonography and magnetic resonance imaging. Ultrasound Obstet Gynecol 2006;27:23–7.
41. Pretorius DH, Davis K, Manco-Johnson ML, et al. Clinical course of fetal hydrocephalus: 40 cases. AJR Am J Roentgenol 1985;144:827–31.
42. Nyberg DA, Mack LA, Hirsch J, et al. Fetal hydrocephalus: sonographic detection and clinical significance of associated anomalies. Radiology 1987;163: 187–91.
43. Vintzileos AM, Campbell WA, Weinbaum PJ, et al. Perinatal management and outcome of fetal ventriculomegaly. Obstet Gynecol 1987;69:5–11.
44. Chervenak FA, Duncan C, Ment LR, et al. Outcome of fetal ventriculomegaly. Lancet 1984;2:179–81.
45. Cochrane DD, Myles ST, Nimrod C, et al. Intrauterine hydrocephalus and ventriculomegaly: associated abnormalities and fetal outcome. Can J Neurol Sci 1985;12:51–9.
46. Morris JE, Rickard S, Paley MN, et al. The value of in-utero magnetic resonance imaging in ultrasound diagnosed fetal isolated cerebral ventriculomegaly. Clin Radiol 2007;62:140–4.
47. Salomon LJ, Ouahba J, Delezoide AL, et al. Third-trimester fetal MRI in isolated 10- to 12-mm ventriculomegaly: is it worth it? BJOG 2006;113:942–7.
48. Wagenvoort AM, Bekker MN, Go AT, et al. Ultrafast scan magnetic resonance in prenatal diagnosis. Fetal Diagn Ther 2000;15:364–72.
49. Levine D, Barnes PD, Madsen JR, et al. Central nervous system abnormalities assessed with prenatal magnetic resonance imaging. Obstet Gynecol 1999;94: 1011–9.
50. Simon EM, Goldstein RB, Coakley FV, et al. Fast MR imaging of fetal CNS anomalies in utero. AJNR Am J Neuroradiol 2000;21:1688–98.
51. de Laveaucoupet J, Audibert F, Guis F, et al. Fetal magnetic resonance imaging (MRI) of ischemic brain injury. Prenat Diagn 2001;21:729–36.
52. D'Ercole CD, Girard N, Boubli L, et al. Prenatal diagnosis of fetal cerebral abnormalities by ultrasonography and magnetic resonance imaging. Eur J Obstet Gynecol Reprod Biol 1993;50:177–84.
53. Gupta JK, Bryce FC, Lilford RJ. Management of apparently isolated fetal ventriculomegaly. Obstet Gynecol Surv 1994;49:716–21.
54. Bromley B, Frigoletto FD, Benacerraf BR. Mild fetal lateral cerebral ventriculomegaly: clinical course and outcome. Am J Obstet Gynecol 1991;164:863–7.
55. Greco P, Laforgia N, Vimercati A, et al. Mild ventriculomegaly as a counseling challenge. Fetal Diagn Ther 2001;16:398–401.
56. Arora A, Bannister CM, Russell S, et al. Outcome and clinical course of prenatally diagnosed cerebral ventriculomegaly. Eur J Pediatr Surg 1998;8: 198–9.
57. Patel MD, Filly RA, Hersch DR, et al. Isolated mild fetal cerebral ventriculomegaly: clinical course and outcome. Radiology 1994;192:759–64.
58. Pilu G, Falco P, Gabrielli S, et al. The clinical significance of fetal isolated cerebral borderline ventriculomegaly: report of 31 cases and review of the literature. Ultrasound Obstet Gynecol 1999;14:320–6.
59. Vergani P, Locatelli A, Strobelt N, et al. Clinical outcome of mild fetal ventriculomegaly. Am J Obstet Gynecol 1998;178:218–22.

60. Bloom SL, Bloom DD, Dellanebbia C, et al. The developmental outcome of children with antenatal mild isolated ventriculomegaly. Obstet Gynecol 1997;90: 93–7.
61. Mercier A, Eurin D, Mercier PY, et al. Isolated mild fetal cerebral ventriculomegaly: a retrospective analysis of 26 cases. Prenat Diagn 2001;21:589–95.
62. Gaglioti P, Danelon D, Bontempo S, et al. Fetal cerebral ventriculomegaly: outcome in 176 cases. Ultrasound Obstet Gynecol 2005;25:372–7.
63. Breeze A, Dey P, Lees C, et al. Obstetric and neonatal outcomes in apparently isolated mild fetal ventriculomegaly. J Perinat Med 2005;33:236–40.
64. Falip C, Blanc N, Maes E, et al. Postnatal clinical and imaging follow-up of infants with prenatal isolated mild ventriculomegaly: a series of 101 cases. Pediatr Radiol 2007;37:981–9.
65. Glenn O, Goldstein R, Li K, et al. Fetal MRI in the evaluation of fetuses referred for sonographically suspected abnormalities of the corpus callosum. J Ultrasound Med 2005;24:791–804.
66. Sonigo PC, Rypens FF, Carteret M, et al. MR imaging of fetal cerebral anomalies. Pediatr Radiol 1998;28:212–22.
67. Garel C, Brisse H, Sebag G, et al. Magnetic resonance imaging of the fetus. Pediatr Radiol 1998;28:201–11.
68. Levine D, Barnes PD, Madsen JR, et al. Fetal central nervous system anomalies: MR imaging augments sonographic diagnosis. Radiology 1997;204:635–42.
69. d'Ercole C, Girard N, Cravello L, et al. Prenatal diagnosis of fetal corpus callosum agenesis by ultrasonography and magnetic resonance imaging. Prenat Diagn 1998;18:247–53.
70. Rapp B, Perrotin F, Marret H, et al. Interet de l'IRM cerebrale foetale pour le diagnostic et le pronostic prenatal des agenesies du corps calleux. J Gynecol Obstet Biol Reprod (Paris) 2002;31:173–82.
71. Tang PH, Bartha AI, Norton ME, et al. Agenesis of the corpus callosum: an MR imaging analysis of associated abnormalities in the fetus. AJNR Am J Neuroradiol 2009;30:257–63.
72. Bajoria R, Wee LY, Anwar S, et al. Outcome of twin pregnancies complicated by single intrauterine death in relation to vascular anatomy of the monochorionic placenta. Humanit Rep 1999;14:2124–30.
73. Hack KEA, Derks JB, Elias SG, et al. Increased perinatal mortality and morbidity in monochorionic versus dichorionic twin pregnancies: clinical implications of a large Dutch cohort study. BJOG 2008;115.
74. Lopriore E, Stroeken H, Sueters M, et al. Term perinatal mortality and morbidity in monochorionic and dichorionic twin pregnancies: a retrosective study. Acta Obstet Gynecol Scand 2008;87:541–5.
75. van Heteren CF, Nijhuis JG, Semmekrot BA, et al. Risk for surviving twin after fetal death of co-twin in twin-twin transfusion syndrome. Obstet Gynecol 1998; 92:215–9.
76. Glenn O, Norton M, Goldstein RB, et al. Prenatal diagnosis of polymicrogyria by fetal magnetic resonance imaging in monochorionic co-twin death. J Ultrasound Med 2005;24:711–6.
77. Jelin AC, Norton ME, Bartha AI, et al. Intracranial magnetic resonance imaging findings in the surviving fetus after spontaneous monochorionic co-twin demise. Am J Obstet Gynecol 2008;199(398):e391–5.
78. Righini A, Salmona S, Bianchini E, et al. Prenatal magnetic resonance imaging evaluation of ischemic brain lesions in the survivors of monochorionic twin pregnancies: report of 3 cases. J Comput Assist Tomogr 2004;28:87–92.

79. Righini A, Kustermann A, Parazzini C, et al. Diffusion-weighted magnetic resonance imaging of acute hypoxic-ischemic cerebral lesions in the survivor of a monochorionic twin pregnancy: case report. Ultrasound Obstet Gynecol 2007;29:453–6.

80. Feldstein VA. Understanding twin-twin transfusion syndrome: role of Doppler ultrasound. Ultrasound Q 2002;18:247–54.

81. Graef C, Ellenrieder B, Hecher K, et al. Long-term neurodevelopmental outcome of 167 children after intrauterin laser treatment for severe twin-twin transfusion syndrome. Am J Obstet Gynecol 2006;194:303–8.

82. Haverkamp F, Lex C, Hanisch C, et al. Neurodevelopmental risks in twin-to-twin transfusion syndrome: preliminary findings. Europ J Paediatr Neurol 2001;5: 21–7.

83. Lenclen R, Paupe A, Ciarlo G, et al. Neonatal outcome in preterm monochorionic twins with twin-to-twin transfusion syndrome after intrauterine treatment with amnioreduction or fetoscopic laser surgery: comparison with dichorionic twins. Am J Obstet Gynecol 2007;196:450.e1–7.

84. Lopriore E, Middeldorp JM, Sueters M, et al. Long-term neurodevelopmental outcome in twin-to-twin transfusion syndrome treated with fetoscopic laser surgery. Am J Obstet Gynecol 2007;196:231.e1–4.

85. Pharoah PO, Price TS, Plomin R. Cerebral palsy in twins: a national study. Arch Dis Child Fetal Neonatal Ed 2002;87:F122–4.

86. Quarello E, Molho M, Ville Y. Incidence, mechanisms, and pattern of fetal cerebral lesions in twin-to-twin transfusion syndrome. J Matern Fetal Neonatal Med 2007;20:589–97.

87. Rossi AC, D'Addario V. Laser therapy and serial amnioreduction as treatment for twin-twin transfusion syndrome: a meta-analysis and review of literature. Am J Obstet Gynecol 2008;198:147–52.

88. Hikino S, Ohga S, Kanda T, et al. Long-term outcome of infants with twin-to-twin transfusion syndrome. Fetal Diagn Ther 2007;22:68–74.

89. Hu LS, Caire JT, Twickler DM. MR findings of complicated mulifetal gestations. Pediatr Radiol 2006;36:76–81.

90. Kline-Fath BM, Calvo-Garcia MA, O'Hara SM, et al. Twin-twin transfusion syndrome: cerebral ischemia is not the only fetal MR imaging finding. Pediatr Radiol 2007;37:47–56.

91. Miller E, Widjaja E, Blaser S, et al. The old and the new: supratentorial MR findings in chiari II malformation. Childs Nerv Syst 2008;24:563–75.

92. Gilbert JN, Jones KL, Rorke LB, et al. Central nervous system anomalies associated with meningomyelocele, hydrocephalus and the arnold-chiari malformation: reappraisal of theories regarding the pathogenesis of posterior neural tube closure defects. Neurosurgery 1986;18:559–64.

93. Wolpert S, Anderson M, Scott R, et al. Chiari II malformation: MR imaging evaluation. AJR Am J Roentgenol 1987;149:1033–42.

94. Sutton LN, Adzick NS, Bilaniuk LT, et al. Improvement in hindbrain herniation demonstrated by serial fetal magnetic resonance imaging following fetal surgery for myelomeningocele. JAMA 1999;282:1826–31.

95. von Koch CS, Glenn OA, Goldstein RB, et al. Fetal magnetic resonance imaging enhances detection of spinal cord anomalies in patients with sonographically detected bony anomalies of the spine. J Ultrasound Med 2005;24:781–9.

96. Appasamy M, Roberts D, Pilling D, et al. Antenatal ultrasound and magnetic resonance imaging in localizing the level of lesion in spina bifida and correlation with postnatal outcome. Ultrasound Obstet Gynecol 2006;27:530–6.

97. Robson CD, Barnewolt CE. MR imaging of fetal head and neck anomalies. Neuroimaging Clin N Am 2004;14:273–91, viii.

98. Hubbard AM, Crombleholme TM, Adzick NS. Prenatal MRI evaluation of giant neck masses in preparation for the fetal exit procedure. Am J Perinatol 1998; 15:253–7.

99. Kathary N, Bulas DI, Newman KD, et al. MRI imaging of fetal neck masses with airway compromise: utility in delivery planning. Pediatr Radiol 2001;31:727–31.

100. Knox EM, Muamar B, Thompson PJ, et al. The use of high resolution magnetic resonance imaging in the prenatal diagnosis of fetal nuchal tumors. Ultrasound Obstet Gynecol 2005;26:672–5.

101. Mota R, Ramalho C, Monteiro J, et al. Evolving indications for the EXIT procedure: the usefulness of combining ultrasound and fetal MRI. Fetal Diagn Ther 2007;22:107–11.

102. Ogamo M, Sugiyama T, Maeda Y, et al. The ex utero intrapartum treatment (EXIT) procedure in giant fetal neck masses. Fetal Diagn Ther 2005;20:214–8.

103. Quinn TM, Hubbard AM, Adzick NS. Prenatal magnetic resonance imaging enhances fetal diagnosis. J Pediatr Surg 1998;33:553–8.

104. Hedrick MH, Ferro MM, Filly RA, et al. Congential high airway obstruction syndrome (CHAOS): a potential for perinatal intervention. J Pediatr Surg 1994; 29:271–4.

105. Hubbard AM, Adzick NS, Crombleholme TM. Congenital chest lesions: diagnosis and characterization with prenatal MR imaging. Radiology 1999;212:43–8.

106. Quinn TM, Adzick NS. Fetal surgery. Obstet Gynecol Clin North Am 1997;24: 143–57.

107. Shimabukuro F, Sakumoto K, Masamoto H, et al. A case of congenital high airway obstruction syndrome managed by ex utero intrapartum treatment: case report and review of the literature. Am J Perinatol 2007;24:197–201.

108. Adzick NS, Harrison MR, Crombleholme TM, et al. Fetal lung lesions: management and outcome. Am J Obstet Gynecol 1998;179:884–9.

109. Dhingsa R, Coakley FV, Albanese CT, et al. Prenatal sonography and MR imaging of pulmonary sequestration. AJR Am J Roentgenol 2003;180:433–7.

110. Flake AW, Harrison MR. Fetal surgery. Annu Rev Med 1995;46:67–78.

111. Adzick SN, Harrison MR, Glick PL, et al. Diaphragmatic hernia in the fetus: prenatal diagnosis and outcome in 94 cases. J Pediatr Surg 1985;20:357–61.

112. Metkus AP, Filly RA, Stringer MD, et al. Sonographic predictors of survival in fetal diaphragmatic hernia. J Pediatr Surg 1996;31:148–52.

113. Leung JWT, Coakley FV, Hricak H. Prenatal MRI of congenital diaphragmatic hernia. AJR Am J Roentgenol 2000;174:1607–12.

114. Granata C, Fagnani AM, Gambini C, et al. Features and outcome of neuroblastoma detected before birth. J Pediatr Surg 2000;35:88–91.

115. Mittermayer C, Blaicher W, Grassauer D, et al. Fetal ovarian cysts: development and neonatal outcome. Ultraschall Med 2003;24:21–6.

116. Walsh DS, Adzick NS. Fetal surgical intervention. Am J Perinatol 2000;17:277–83.

117. Levine D. Ultrasound versus magnetic resonance imaging in fetal evaluation. Top Magn Reson Imaging 2001;12:25–38.

118. Hill BJ, Joe BN, Qayyum A, et al. Supplemental value of MRI in fetal abdominal disease detected on prenatal sonography: preliminary experience. AJR Am J Roentgenol 2005;184:993–8.

119. Curtis MR, Mooney DP, Vacarro TJ. Prenatal ultrasound characterization of the suprarenal mass: distinction between neuroblastoma and subdiaphragmatic extralobar pulmonary sequestration. J Ultrasound Med 1997;16:75–83.

120. Saguintaah M, Couture A, Veyrac C. MRI of the fetal gastrointestinal tract. Pediatr Radiol 2002;32:395–404.
121. Veyrac C, Couture A, Saguintaah M, et al. MRI of fetal GI tract abnormalities. Abdom Imaging 2004;29:411–20.
122. Filly RA, Feldstein VA. Fetal genitourinary tract. In: Callen PW, editor. Ultrasonography in obstetrics and gynecology. Philadelphia: Saunders; 2000. p. 515–50.
123. Poutamo J, Vanninen R, Partanen K, et al. Diagnosing fetal urinary tract abnormalities: benefits of MRI compared to ultrasonography. Acta Obstet Gynecol Scand 2000;79:65–71.
124. Rapola J. The kidneys and urinary tract. In: Wigglesworth JS, Singer DB, editors. Textbook of fetal and perinatal pathology. Boston: Blackwell Scientific Publications; 1991. p. 1109–43.
125. Caire JT, Ramus RM, Magee KP, et al. MRI of fetal genitourinary anomalies. AJR Am J Roentgenol 2003;181:1381–5.
126. Guys JM, Borella F, Monfort G. Ureteropelvic junction obstructions: prenatal diagnosis and neonatal surgery in 47 cases. J Pediatr Surg 1988;23:156–8.
127. Shinmoto H, Kashima K, Yuasa Y, et al. MR imaging of non CNS fetal abnormalities: a pictorial essay. Radiographics 2000;20:1227–43.

The Role of Fetal Echocardiography in Fetal Intervention: A Symbiotic Relationship

Priya Sekar, MD, MPH[a,b], Lisa K. Hornberger, MD[a,b,*]

KEYWORDS

- Fetal echocardiography • Congenital heart disease
- Twin-twin transfusion syndrome • Aortic valve stenosis
- Atrioventricular block • Supraventricular tachycardia
- Diaphragmatic hernia

The field of fetal cardiology has seen rapid growth in the past 10 years as a consequence of advances in ultrasound technology and increasing experience with structural, functional, and rhythm-related fetal heart disease. An accurate detailed definition of most structural heart defects is now possible in utero,[1–3] and serial assessment has provided a better understanding of their natural history and predictors of clinical outcome.[4] This has resulted in increased interest in the development of invasive therapies for structural heart disease, for instance, to prevent the evolution of more severe secondary pathologic conditions. Improved delineation of fetal arrhythmia mechanism has led to more appropriate and successful treatment strategies. Observations at fetal echocardiography have provided insight into what cardiovascular conditions are and are not tolerated by the fetal circulation, have led to more accurate prenatal counseling regarding prognosis, and have prompted the development of more aggressive perinatal management strategies resulting in improved survival. Fetal echocardiography has played an increasingly important role in risk stratification for noncardiac fetal interventions, such as congenital diaphragmatic hernia, twin-twin transfusion syndrome (TTTS), and arteriovenous malformations.[5] In addition to ruling out fetal cardiac structural pathologic findings, fetal echocardiography has provided insight into the pathophysiology of several noncardiac lesions,

[a] Department of Pediatrics, Division of Cardiology, Fetal and Neonatal Cardiology Program, WCMC 4C2 Stollery Children's Hospital, 8440 112th Street, Edmonton, Alberta T6G 2B7, Canada
[b] Department of Obstetrics and Gynecology, University of Alberta, Edmonton, Alberta T5H 3V9, Canada
* Corresponding author. Department of Pediatrics, Division of Cardiology, Fetal and Neonatal Cardiology Program, WCMC 4C2 Stollery Children's Hospital, 8440 112th Street, Edmonton, Alberta T6G 2B7, Canada.
E-mail address: lisa.hornberger@capitalhealth.ca (L.K. Hornberger).

Clin Perinatol 36 (2009) 301–327
doi:10.1016/j.clp.2009.03.013
0095-5108/09/$ – see front matter © 2009 Elsevier Inc. All rights reserved.

perinatology.theclinics.com

particularly those that alter the normal fetal hemodynamic load. Additionally, fetal echocardiography has been effectively used to monitor the fetal cardiovascular response during invasive fetal procedures for noncardiac pathologic findings.[6]

In this review, the authors explore the role of noninvasive and invasive fetal interventions in fetal cardiovascular disease guided by observations at fetal echocardiography (**Table 1**). They first review fetal cardiac lesions that may be ameliorated by fetal intervention and then review noncardiac fetal pathologic findings for which fetal echocardiography can provide important insight into the pathophysiology and aid in patient selection for and timing of intervention and postintervention surveillance.

FETAL CARDIAC INTERVENTION

Two general types of congenital heart pathologic conditions have been suggested as reasonable targets for in utero intervention[7]: (1) cardiac defects associated with the evolution of fetal heart failure or hydrops or that place the fetus at risk for spontaneous intrauterine death and (2) cardiac lesions associated with the development of severe secondary pathologic findings, ultimately necessitating numerous palliative procedures after birth, that carry a guarded prognosis long term. Intrauterine demise occurs in about 6% of fetuses with a cardiac diagnosis.[8,9] Although chromosomal abnormalities and extracardiac malformations play a role in the demise of some affected fetuses, cardiac pathologic findings in isolation may result in hemodynamic instability and the development of heart failure, which frequently leads to fetal and perinatal demise.[10] Cardiac lesions more commonly associated with fetal heart failure, in addition to spontaneous demise in the absence of heart failure, include persistent fetal tachycardias and bradycardias[11,12] and primary myocardial pathologic findings, particularly with diastolic dysfunction.[13] Structural heart defects that influence the function of both ventricles (eg, Ebstein's anomaly of the tricuspid valve, tetralogy of Fallot with absent pulmonary valve syndrome) or are associated with bilateral inflow or outflow tract obstruction (eg, tricuspid atresia with restrictive atrial septum, truncal valve stenosis) may also be associated with evolution of hydrops and sudden fetal demise.[14–16] In all cardiovascular lesions associated with the evolution of heart failure or hydrops, increased central venous pressure as a consequence of altered biventricular filling, often reflected in abnormal systemic venous Doppler patterns,[17] is believed to be the most important mechanism. Identifying these lesions before birth is imperative for close monitoring, fetal intervention when available, and early delivery with appropriate postnatal intervention if indicated. Preventing the evolution of hydrops in these lesions should be the goal for in utero therapy. This has been best demonstrated by the management of fetal supraventricular tachycardias through mechanism-appropriate maternal or transplacental antiarrhythmic therapy, which can be successful in 80% to 90% of pregnancies.[18] Even when affected fetuses present hydropic, successful intrauterine therapy has led to improved survival in from 50% to greater than 90% of treated cases.[19] For many structural and primary functional fetal heart pathologic findings associated with heart failure, however, the best strategies to achieve survival are still evolving.

Congenital Atrioventricular Block

Atrioventricular block (AVB) is one arrhythmia for which the best intrauterine treatment strategies are still unclear. Untreated fetal AVB is associated with significant mortality.[19] Observations at fetal echocardiography have identified ventricular rates of less than 55 beats per minutes,[12,20,21] which is associated with minimal to no beat-beat variability,[22] hydrops,[23] concomitant myocardial disease, and major structural heart disease[24] as risk factors for poor outcomes. Fetal AVB is most commonly attributable to the maternal autoantibodies anti-Ro and anti-La,[24] or it is associated with structural heart disease, most commonly left atrial isomerism or polysplenia syndrome.[25,26]

In maternal autoantibody-induced AVB, the autoantibodies anti-Ro and anti-La are believed to cross the placenta after 16 to 17 weeks of gestation and to be deposited on the fetal myocardium, most often the conduction system, leading to inflammation and eventual fibrosis.[27,28] Maternal-transplacental administration of dexamethasone and β-adrenergic stimulation for heart rates less than 55 beats per minute have been associated with moderate success in reducing mortality;[19] however, there continues to be a small proportion of fetuses evolving to more diffuse myocardial disease or having extremely low ventricular escape rates despite therapy and having a grim prognosis (**Fig. 1**). Intravenous γ-globulin, administered to the mother or intra-umbilically to the fetus,[29] and direct fetal pacing[30,31] have been explored as possible adjunctive therapies that may ultimately lead to improved survival.

Although several groups have documented attempts at direct fetal ventricular pacing in maternal autoantibody-induced AVB and in AVB associated with structural heart disease, long-term pacing has not been achieved and fetal demise has largely occurred with or shortly after the procedure.[30–32] Many affected fetuses with maternal autoantibody-induced AVB and extremely slow rates have more diffuse myocardial disease, which may necessitate more aggressive anti-inflammatory strategies and the use of sequential intrauterine atrial and ventricular pacing, not as yet attempted, to augment cardiac output and keep atrial and ventricular filling pressures at a minimum. The same is true for AVB associated with left atrial isomerism, in which noncompaction cardiomyopathy is usually observed.[25] Although fetal pacing has not yet achieved success, early neonatal pacing (<24 hours) of the affected high-risk newborns, even if premature, may result in improved survival.[33] Finally, with respect to maternal autoantibody-induced fetal AVB, greater knowledge of the pathogenic mechanism responsible for its evolution may lead to novel therapies to prevent this antenatally acquired condition.

Fetal Cardiac Catheter Intervention

Many structural heart lesions encountered prenatally are associated with the evolution of more severe structural and functional heart pathologic conditions, resulting in worse morbidity and mortality for the affected fetus and infant.[4,34] Two lesions that best exemplify this natural history are critical aortic and pulmonary valve stenosis (**Fig. 2**). In critical ventricular outflow tract obstruction that manifests in the first or second trimester, dysfunction of the ipsilateral ventricle leads to increased ventricular diastolic pressure, reduced forward flow through the ipsilateral ventricle, and a redistribution of flow toward the other ventricle through the foramen ovale. As long as the ventricle contralateral to the obstruction is able to maintain the equivalent of the combined ventricular output without significant changes in ventricular filling pressure, the fetus can thrive. With time, however, fetal echocardiography has demonstrated progressive hypoplasia of the ventricle with the obstructed outflow,[35–37] which is ultimately unable to sustain a normal systemic (critical aortic stenosis) or pulmonary (critical pulmonary stenosis) output after birth. Less commonly, severe ventricular dilation or atrioventricular valve insufficiency may occur ipsilateral to the outflow tract obstruction, which alters the filling of the contralateral ventricle, leading to increasing central venous pressures and fetal hydrops.

Fetal Aortic Valvuloplasty

Knowledge of the antenatal evolution of the simpler valve lesions, as documented at serial fetal echocardiography, has prompted the development of catheter-based

Table 1
Summary of primary cardiac and noncardiac fetal pathologic findings with potential for invasive fetal intervention

	Pathologic Findings	Outcome Without Fetal Intervention	Proposed Fetal Intervention	Role of Fetal Echocardiography
Primary cardiac lesions	Aortic stenosis	Potential for progression to HLHS Progressive left ventricular dilation, mitral insufficiency, fetal hydrops	Catheter-based balloon aortic valvuloplasty	Diagnosis/patient selection, intraprocedural guidance, postintervention serial assessment of left-sided structure growth and hemodynamics
	Pulmonary stenosis	Potential for progressive right heart hypoplasia Progressive tricuspid insufficiency, right ventricular dilation and fetal hydrops	Catheter-based balloon pulmonary valvuloplasty	Diagnosis, intraprocedural guidance, postintervention serial assessment of RV and RVOT
	HLHS and intact atrial septum	Critically ill neonate who has severe cyanosis and pulmonary congestion, high perioperative mortality attributable to pulmonary vascular changes	Catheter-based atrial septostomy and potential stenting of atrial septum	Diagnosis, intraprocedural guidance, postintervention of pulmonary venous Doppler scans and atrial septal anatomy and flow
	TGA with intact atrial septum	Critically ill, severely cyanotic neonate with high risk for mortality without emergent balloon atrial septostomy	Catheter-based atrial septostomy*	Diagnosis, intraprocedural guidance
	Congenital complete heart block	Evolution of hydrops and intrauterine fetal demise	Medical therapy: dexamethasone in autoantibody-positive mothers, intravenous γ-globulin Invasive therapy: direct fetal ventricular ± atrial pacing	Diagnosis, follow-up for ventricular rate, AV association, and surveillance for evolution of diffuse myocardial disease and hydrops

Extracardiac pathologic findings known to alter fetal ventricular loading condition	Twin-twin transfusion syndrome	Recipient twin with cardiac diastolic and then systolic dysfunction and development of hydrops with potential demise of one or both twins	Amnioreduction or laser therapy	Systolic and diastolic function assessment, exclusion/inclusion of pulmonary outflow pathology, cardiovascular response of recipient twin to intervention, ongoing follow-up of pulmonary valve anatomy and ventricular function
	Twin reversed arterial perfusion sequence	High-output cardiac failure in pump twin with potential demise	Selective (acardiac) feticide	Systolic and diastolic ventricular function assessment, cardiac output assessment, cardiovascular response to intervention
	Arteriovenous malformations	High-output cardiac failure with potential demise	Fetal surgery (debulking or less invasive occlusion of feeding vessels)	Combined cardiac output quantification before and after intervention; systolic and diastolic ventricular function assessment before and after therapy
Extracardiac pathologic findings associated with cardiopulmonary compression	CCAM	Direct cardiac compression with impaired filling, documentation of cardiac output and diastolic function parameters, (particularly ventricular inflows), systemic venous Doppler scans	Fetal surgery (debulking)	Pre- and postintervention assessment for compression
	Congenital diaphragmatic hernia	Severe cases associated with significant pulmonary hypoplasia, rarely associated with altered ventricular filling/compression and hydrops	Fetal surgery (tracheal occlusion)	Pulmonary artery size and Doppler assessment serially and before and after intervention to delivery

* Not performed to date in this condition.
Abbreviations: AV, atrioventricular; CCAM, congenital cystic adenomatous malformation; HLHS, hypoplastic left heart syndrome; RV, right ventricle; RVOT, right ventricular outflow tract; TGA, transposition of the great arteries.

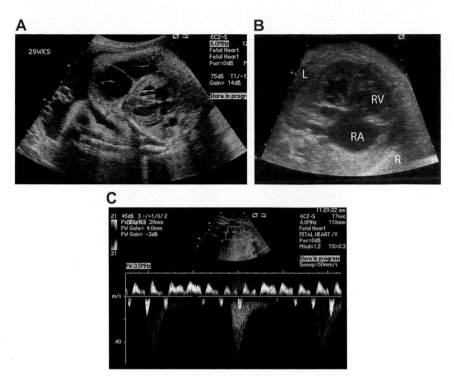

Fig.1. (A) Image obtained in a fetus with a gestational age of 29 weeks with maternal auto-immune-mediated AVB; there was myocardial thickening and systolic and diastolic dysfunction with evolving hydrops, as suggested by the presence of ascites. (B) Four-chamber view in another fetus with complete AVB associated with left atrial isomerism and a noncompaction type of cardiomyopathy. Note the extremely trabeculated ventricles. L, left; R, right; RA, right atrium; RV, right ventricle. (C) Simultaneous pulsed Doppler interrogation of the superior vena cava with its a-wave reversal correlating with atrial systole. The atrial rate is 140 to 150 beats per minute and the ventricular rate is 40 beats per minute with no relationship between atrial and ventricular systoles in a fetus with complete AVB.

intrauterine strategies to promote forward flow through the valve and more normal growth and function of the ipsilateral ventricle. Most reported cases have described achieving access to the fetal ventricle and valve through a transmaternal-transuterine approach with echocardiographic guidance.[8,35–37] To date, the largest proportion of fetal catheter-based interventions has been in critical aortic stenosis (**Fig. 3**).[36,38] Technical success of the procedure, which demands adequate positioning of the fetus for access to the apex of the left ventricle and the aortic valve, has been well described, with low risk for maternal morbidity and relatively low fetal mortality rates.[36,39] Fetal hemodynamic instability, characterized by fetal bradycardia and ventricular dysfunction, is not unusual during transventricular access, and pericardial effusion occasionally evolves.[40] In the largest recently reported experience, Selamet-Tierney and colleagues[39] documented fetal aortic balloon valvuloplasty in 42 pregnancies considered to be at high risk for developing fetal hypoplastic left heart syndrome (HLHS). Of 37 cases with uninterrupted pregnancies and known outcomes, 6 (16%) had fetal demise after the procedure, and of the remaining, even with clear hemodynamic improvement, only 8 (21%) had achieved two-ventricle circulation after birth, the ultimate goal of the procedure. Despite a more than doubling in the number of

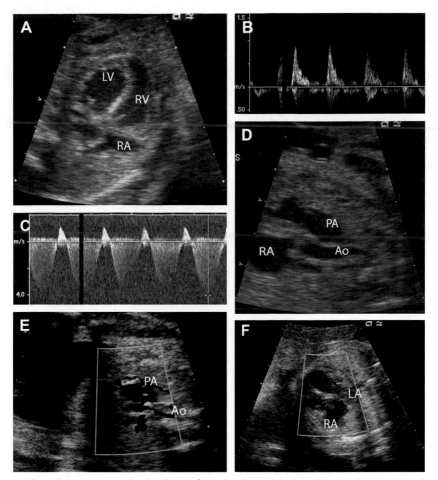

Fig. 2. These images were obtained in a fetus having critical aortic stenosis at a gestational age of 25 weeks. (*A*) Four-chamber view demonstrates a dilated and echogenic left ventricle. Features of critical aortic stenosis and potential for progression to hypoplastic left heart syndrome are shown in *B* through *F*. LV, left ventricle; RV, right ventricle; RA, right atrium. (*B*) Left ventricular inflow Doppler scan has a uniphasic flow pattern of short duration representing flow in atrial systole only. (*C*) Based on the Doppler interrogation of a small amount of mitral insufficiency, the velocity of 4 m/s corresponds to a left ventricular systolic pressure of at least 64 mm Hg plus a left atrial pressure that is far higher than the 25- to 30-mm Hg systolic systemic blood pressure of a normal fetus with a gestational age of 25 weeks. (*D*) Three-vessel sweep to the arches shows a smaller aortic arch (Ao) compared with ductal arch and pulmonary artery (PA). (*E*) There is retrograde flow in the distal Ao (red color flow map). (*F*) Reversed atrial level shunting, from left atrial (LA) to right atrial (RA) flow, is demonstrated (the reverse of normal foramen ovale shunting in utero).

cases and technical success that approaches 87%,[39] these outcomes did not differ significantly from the initial experience reported by the same group in 2003.[37]

The challenge in fetal valvuloplasty for critical aortic stenosis remains patient selection for borderline left ventricles. Trying to identify the small number of fetuses with borderline left ventricles that can be "salvaged" by this technique is still somewhat

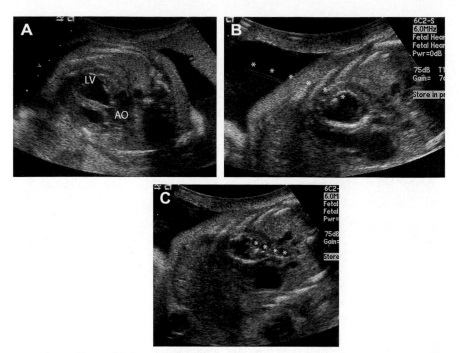

Fig. 3. Echocardiographic images obtained at the time of transuterine, transthoracic, fetal aortic valvuloplasty. (*A*) Image of the necessary orientation of the fetal left ventricular apex toward the anterior aspect of the uterus to have a direct path to the aortic valve. AO, aorta; LV, left ventricle. (*B*) Introduction of the needle with the bright tip demonstrated in the left ventricular cavity. (*C*) After a wire is introduced through the stylet across the aortic valve, a balloon-tipped catheter is positioned across the valve. The course of the stylet and catheter are both demonstrated in *B* and *C* by asterisks (*).

subjective. Although echocardiographic features, including retrograde flow in the transverse arch, left-to-right flow across the foramen ovale, and a monophasic mitral inflow, are observed in most midtrimester fetuses developing HLHS by term,[41] and may even be improved with technical success of the valvuloplasty,[39] the lack of significant improvement in the number of fetuses in which a biventricular repair has been achieved despite greater experience suggests that other factors may be involved in "salvaging" the left ventricle. More recent fetal echocardiographic observations among successful fetal aortic valvuloplasties include the presence of an apex-forming left ventricle and increased left ventricular pressure as assessed by the mitral insufficiency jet.[42] Further work in this area needs to include prospective multicenter randomized trials in the hands of experienced fetal treatment centers and may demand the development of animal models of the disease.

Prevention of left heart hypoplasia may be achieved in a group of these patients, but it is important to proceed with caution when making claims about prevention of HLHS. Children who have HLHS are known to have neurocognitive deficits.[43,44] In the past, these deficits have been attributed to chronic cyanosis and multiple exposures to cardiopulmonary bypass. Recent literature suggests that a portion of fetuses and neonates having HLHS are microcephalic, and although ascending aorta size may correlate with small head circumference, it is still unknown whether fetal aortic valvuloplasty has the potential to improve the neurocognitive outcomes for this patient population.[45,46] Furthermore, success of the fetal intervention must be measured against the improving postnatal outcomes for HLHS, with 2-year survival recently reported by the authors' center as high as 81% in the current surgical era.[47] The improvement in postnatal surgical outcomes is particularly important to consider, because fetal interventions place two lives at risk, the first of whom has no disease.

Fetal Pulmonary Valvuloplasty

Although prenatal intervention for critical pulmonary outflow tract obstruction has received much less attention, several isolated case reports have documented occasional technical success in fetal pulmonary valvuloplasty.[48,49] Recent publications have begun to define fetal echocardiographic predictors of postnatal outcome better, particularly size of the right ventricle and need for single-ventricle palliation. Gardiner and colleagues[50] recently derived scores to facilitate early prediction of postnatal univentricular or biventricular circulation based on fetal cardiac measurements in a retrospective review of 24 patients diagnosed before birth with pulmonary atresia and an intact ventricular septum or critical pulmonary stenosis. The most predictive variables were pulmonary valve z score (<23 weeks), median tricuspid valve z score (<26 weeks), and the combination of median pulmonary valve z score and median tricuspid valve/mitral valve ratio. They also introduced the so-called "right atrial pressure" (RAP) score, composed of the tricuspid valve, foramen ovale, and ductus venosus Doppler findings; a RAP score greater than 3 predicted biventricular repair with statistical significance, and the fetal detection of coronary fistulae usually predicted a univentricular route in that sample of patients. Roman and colleagues[51] have reported similar findings; in addition to a tricuspid/mitral valve ratio of less than 0.7, tricuspid valve inflow duration less than 31.5% of cardiac cycle length, and presence of right ventricular sinusoids, they identified another variable of right-to-left ventricular length ratio less than 0.6 as a potential predictor of non-biventricular outcome.

The rationale for fetal intervention in critical pulmonary stenosis is similar to that in critical aortic stenosis: to promote right ventricular growth and biventricular neonatal circulation. There is significant postnatal morbidity for this lesion, with biventricular circulation achieved after birth in only 32% to 55% of cases.[52,53] Enthusiasm for fetal pulmonary valvuloplasty has not reached the proportion of that for fetal aortic valvuloplasty for critical aortic stenosis, however, which may be attributable to several reasons. Postnatally, even small right ventricles may achieve a biventricular or 1.5 ventricle palliation, making right ventricular size an inconsistent predictor of outcome and perhaps making fetal intervention less critical. Affected babies may have a right ventricle-dependent coronary circulation, which demands high right ventricular pressures to maintain coronary perfusion in general. Although coronary fistulae can be identified by fetal echocardiography, the more important proximal coronary artery stenoses cannot, limiting the ability to predict outcomes even further and adding greater risk to fetal intervention. Of the reported cases with fetal pulmonary valvuloplasty, technical success rates have been high,[48,49] but the outcomes have remained similar to the natural history,[54] suggesting, again, the presence of additional factors that have an impact on ventricular growth in this disease and on ultimate postnatal hemodynamic outcome. Nevertheless, pulmonary valvuloplasty may be beneficial in cases of imminent hydrops, identified on fetal echocardiography by increased cardiothoracic ratio, pericardial effusion, holosystolic tricuspid regurgitation, and abnormal systemic venous Doppler findings. One small series reported technically successful fetal pulmonary valvuloplasty, with a subsequent decrease in central venous pressure and resolution of pericardial effusion with documented antegrade flow across the pulmonary valve.[49] Analogous to critical aortic stenosis, careful patient selection is required for optimal use of this technique, which has yet to be prospectively challenged.

Fetal Atrial Septoplasty

One final fetal catheter-based intervention strategy has been in the creation and dilation of atrial level communications for critical left heart obstruction, largely in HLHS. HLHS and simple transposition of the great arteries are associated with thickening and potential restriction of interatrial communication, which is deleterious to postnatal physiology in these lesions. A nonrestrictive atrial septal defect is necessary after birth for infants with HLHS to permit egress of blood from the left atrium and to avoid pulmonary congestion attributable to left atrial hypertension and consequent medial thickening of the pulmonary veins. Neonates who have HLHS and a restrictive atrial septum are known to have higher mortality compared with their counterparts with nonrestrictive interatrial communication.[33,55] The interatrial communication is necessary for infants with simple transposition of the great arteries for adequate mixing of the parallel systemic and pulmonary circulations in this lesion.

A recent report of 21 attempted percutaneous cardiac punctures for atrial septal defect creation in neonates found that an atrial septal defect measuring at least 3 mm was associated with higher postnatal oxygen saturation and less need for intervention before stage I single-ventricle palliation.[55] Two (9.5%) of the 21 neonates died within 24 hours of the procedure, and the remaining 19 underwent a stage I procedure with a surgical survival rate of 58%. Among the neonates who required urgent left atrial decompression, the surgical survival rate was lower (5 [48%] of 12) compared with those who had a routine stage I procedure (5 [86%] of 7). Survival in the prenatally diagnosed group was 52% (11 of 21), compared with reported survival rates of postnatally diagnosed neonates with a restrictive atrial septum, ranging from as low as 28%[56] to as high as 69%.[57] Although stenting of the atrial septum in the human fetus has been proposed to alter the evolution of left atrial hypertension, pulmonary venous thickening, and the subsequent pulmonary venous "arterialization" thought to be responsible for the significant postnatal morbidity in this population, this technique has only been reported in fetal sheep to date.[58]

Evaluation of the atrial septal defect anatomically by two-dimensional imaging and by Doppler interrogation across the atrial septum in severe left heart obstruction is not consistently feasible, and it is not an accurate indicator of significant atrial level restriction.[59] Indirect assessment of left atrial pressure at fetal echocardiography through the evaluation of pulmonary venous Doppler findings,[59,60] however, has been shown to be a significantly more reliable tool (**Fig. 4**). The pulmonary vein flow pattern and the ratio of the forward and reverse velocity-time integral (VTI) are predictive of left atrial hypertension and significant atrial level restriction after birth in babies who have HLHS, and therefore are useful in identifying the fetus in which atrial septoplasty may be necessary. The hemodynamics of atrial level restriction are typically well tolerated by fetuses having HLHS in utero, but ultrasound-guided fetal atrial septoplasty has been attempted in an effort to decompress the left atrium to facilitate the neonatal resuscitation of affected infants and reduce the secondary pulmonary vascular changes that occur in the context of long-term high left atrial pressure.[55] The future success of this intervention depends on determining optimal timing of left atrial decompression to prevent the development of long-standing pulmonary vascular hypertension.

High-intensity focused ultrasound (HIFU) is a newer modality that may provide less invasive means of creating and enlarging atrial level communications.[61] This technique does not involve percutaneous entry into the maternal abdomen but rather uses

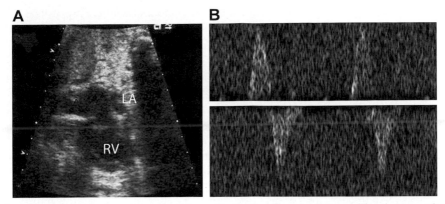

Fig. 4. (*A*) Four-chamber view of a fetus with HLHS and restrictive atrial level communication. The left atrium (LA) is diminutive. RV, right ventricle. (*B*) Definitive pulmonary venous flow pattern consistent with high left atrial pressures with to and fro blood flow.

ultrasound frequencies ranging from 500 kHz to 10 MHz to cause localized tissue hyperthermia and damage remotely at predictable depths without injuring adjacent tissue.[61,62] Although the use of HIFU in human fetuses having HLHS or transposition with restrictive atrial septum seems promising, it has not yet been attempted or reported in humans for this specific clinical scenario.

Prenatal Detection Rates

Finally, the potential impact of fetal cardiac intervention is and should continue to be significantly influenced by rate of prenatal detection. Despite the fact that more than 95% of major structural heart disease can be diagnosed before birth, current rates of prenatal detection range from 10% to 40% in North America, with a paucity of recent data,[63] to 20% in Japan in 2004[64] and 40% in Australia in 2003.[65] Although HLHS is one of the more commonly diagnosed lesions before birth, with prenatal detection rates reported from 40% to 91% across the world,[56,66–68] critical aortic stenosis with a dilated or more normal-sized ventricle is significantly less common. Thus, the subset of affected fetuses is quite small, limiting the exposure and experience of most centers that offer fetal catheter interventions. Without drastic improvements in prenatal detection rates of congenital heart disease, including earlier disease recognition, efforts at fetal cardiac intervention are never likely to achieve their full impact.

Improved perinatal and neonatal intervention in fetal cardiac disease

In addition to the development of fetal cardiac intervention, the development of improved, often more aggressive, perinatal and neonatal management strategies for critical fetal and neonatal cardiac pathologic findings has been of greater interest with the evolution of multidisciplinary fetal treatment and fetal cardiology programs. For instance, although severe tricuspid insufficiency is poorly tolerated by the fetal circulation, at least in part as a consequence of altered biventricular function,[69] early delivery with restriction of patency of the ductus arteriosus, followed by measures to reduce pulmonary vascular resistance, has significantly reduced the mortality of even more severe disease.[70] Given the extreme difficulty of resuscitation of the newborn who has HLHS and an intact atrial septum, let alone need to support the newborn through a cardiac catheter-based atrial septoplasty, some centers have chosen to place these prenatally identified neonates on extracorporeal membrane oxygen support immediately with or without an ex utero intrapartum treatment procedure.[71,72] As eluded to previously, even early ventricular pacing shortly after delivery has been identified as a newer strategy that may result in less morbidity and mortality among the highest risk fetuses with AVB.[33]

FETAL ECHOCARDIOGRAPHY IN NONCARDIAC PATHOLOGIC FINDINGS

Many noncardiac fetal pathologic findings have the potential to alter fetal ventricular loading conditions that predispose the fetus to cardiovascular compromise signifi-cantly, including TTTS, pregnancies complicated by acardiac twins, arteriovenous malformations, and intrathoracic pathologic findings that cause compression. Fetal echocardiography has played and should continue to play a critical role in the devel-opment of noninvasive and invasive treatment strategies for these conditions. It has also been used to define lung mass in noncardiac conditions associated with pulmo-nary hypoplasia, including congenital diaphragmatic hernia.

Twin-Twin Transfusion Syndrome

Severe TTTS, which occurs as a consequence of abnormal placental vascular connec-tions between twins, complicates 15% to 20% of monochorionic twin pregnancies.[73] Until recently, the clinical pathologic findings of the recipient twin was thought to reflect a simple transfusion and increased preload to that twin. Detailed echocardiographic evaluations of fetal heart function and structure performed serially, however, have led to new insight into the evolution of this pathologic condition, which is responsible for the morbidity and mortality associated with TTTS.[74] Early studies documented myocar-dial hypertrophy and reduced ventricular systolic function in recipient twins.[75,76] In addition to the ventricular hypertrophy, the authors have subsequently shown the ventricular chamber size to be reduced, rather than increased, in recipient twins who have TTTS with associated diastolic dysfunction, similar to what they observed in other forms of fetal hypertrophic cardiomyopathy,[77] suggesting that increased preload and a high-output state were not components of the disease. The authors further docu-mented early development of high ventricular systolic, and thus systemic blood pres-sures and myocardial diastolic or filling pathologic findings in the recipient twins, with uniphasic ventricular inflows, increased left ventricular isovolumic relaxation times, and increased reversal of flow in systemic veins during atrial systole (**Fig. 5**).[78,79] Indeed, ventricular diastolic dysfunction was present in two thirds of the recipient twins on initial assessment in the authors' initial series, with systolic dysfunction only evolving late in some twins; when it did develop, it mostly affected the right ventricle.[79] Others have subsequently documented similar observations at fetal echocardiography.[80–82] Clues to the pathogenesis of the recipient twin pathologic findings have also been provided by older histopathologic observations that have included myocyte hyperplasia and increased medial thickening secondary to the increased number of vascular smooth muscle cells diffusely demonstrated in systemic and pulmonary vascular beds of recip-ient twins only.[83] These preintervention clinical findings, fetal echocardiography obser-vations after successful laser therapy, and the documentation of high levels of endothelin-1 in the umbilical venous blood of recipient twins[84] have suggested a critical role of vasoactive peptides produced by the recipient twin placenta in response to these vascular connections in the pathogenesis of the recipient disease.[85] Elucidating these pathogenetic mechanisms is critical because they may provide clues to potentially effective less invasive therapies for this disease.

Fetal echocardiography plays an important role in the diagnosis and monitoring of patients who have TTTS. In the absence of successful laser therapy[86] or with late

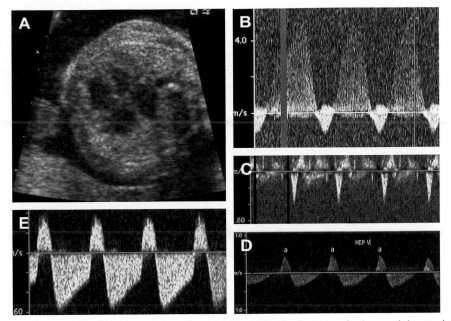

Fig. 5. (*A*) Four-chamber image demonstrates biventricular hypertrophy in a recipient twin at a gestational age of 20 weeks. (*B*) Doppler interrogation of the tricuspid insufficiency indicates a velocity of nearly 5 m/s, suggesting a right ventricular systolic pressure of greater than 100 mmHg plus the right atrial pressure. (*C*) Later in the disease with progressive right ventricular dysfunction, there is an extremely short-duration uniphasic right ventricular inflow Doppler flow pattern. Abnormal hepatic venous (*D*) and ductus venosus (*E*) Doppler flow pattern. scans with significant a-wave reversal are in keeping with high right ventricular filling and central venous pressures.

intervention,[76] recipient twins have a roughly 10% incidence of anatomic pulmonary outflow tract obstruction and a significantly lower incidence of other structural heart defects.[87] These pathologic findings may significantly influence the short- and long-term outcomes of affected recipient twins. Second, fetal echocardiography provides useful fetal cardiovascular functional information, which can define the extent of the pathologic findings, be correlated with the clinically applied Quintero stages,[78] and later be used to follow the response to intervention.[79] Routine evaluation of the fetal heart in TTTS includes documentation of (1) left and right ventricular wall thickness; (2) presence or absence of atrioventricular valve insufficiency; (3) documentation of ventricular systolic pressures if atrioventricular valve insufficiency is present by standard Doppler techniques; (4) evaluation of the pulmonary outflow tract for anatomic obstruction or pseudopulmonary atresia with or without pulmonary insufficiency and direction of ductus arteriosus flow; (5) diastolic function parameters of left ventricular isovolumic relaxation time; left and right ventricular inflow Doppler findings; and Doppler interrogation of the inferior vena cava, ductus venosus, and umbilical vein; (6) systolic and global ventricular function parameters (including shortening fractions and Tei indices [isovolumic relaxation time + isovolumic contraction time/ejection time]); and (7) presence or absence of fetal hydrops.[79]

Invasive therapies offered to ameliorate TTTS have included amnioreduction and fetoscopic laser therapy. Although some experts propose that therapeutic amnioreduction may lead to a better prognosis by reducing the risk for preterm labor, and thus significant prematurity, it does not improve the cardiovascular pathologic condition, which continues to evolve in the recipient twin.[79] In contrast, the authors showed an acute improvement in right ventricular systolic function and gradual resolution of the ventricular hypertrophy and diastolic dysfunction after successful laser therapy (**Fig. 6**). Interestingly, despite acute improvement in fetal ventricular systolic function, in a couple of cases in which the data were available, the authors did not observe an acute change in the high ventricular systolic pressure based on Doppler interrogation of the atrioventricular valve regurgitation, suggesting that vascular remodeling of the histopathologic findings may require additional time.[79]

High Cardiac Output States

Fetal echocardiography can be used to monitor the hemodynamic influence of extracardiac abnormalities associated with increased cardiac output, including such conditions as twin pregnancies complicated by an acardiac twin; arteriovenous malformations, including vein of Galen aneurysm and sacrococcygeal teratoma; agenesis of the ductus venosus; and fetal anemia.[88–98] In addition to the fetal ventricular systolic and diastolic function assessment as described in TTTS, fetal echocardiography can permit the calculation of left and right ventricular stroke volumes through pulsed Doppler interrogation of the semilunar valves with measurement of the VTI of the spectral tracing multiplied by the cross-sectional area of the semilunar valve, which is calculated by πr^2, where r is the radius of the valve. The ventricular output is then calculated by the stroke volume multiplied by the fetal heart rate at the time of measurement (**Fig. 7**). Trends in fetal left and right ventricular stroke volume and

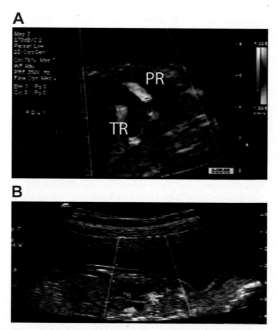

Fig. 6. (*A*) Severe right ventricular dysfunction in this recipient fetus with a gestational age of 24 weeks was associated with severe tricuspid regurgitation (TR) and even systolic pulmonary regurgitation (PR) with no forward right ventricular outflow. (*B*) Within 24 hours of a successful laser procedure, forward right ventricular outflow and minimal tricuspid regurgitation was observed.

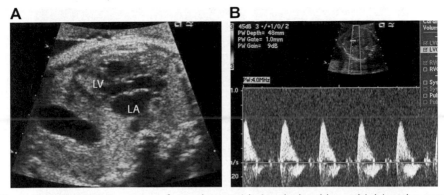

Fig. 7. Stroke volume assessment for each ventricle is calculated by multiplying the cross-sectional area of the semilunar valve and the VTI of the spectral tracing acquired through Doppler interrogation across the same semilunar valve. (*A*) To calculate left ventricular output, the aortic valve annulus is measured in a cardiac long axis, as shown in this image. LA, left atrium; LV, left ventricle. (*B*) Depicted here is the pulsed Doppler signal obtained by interrogation of the aortic valve. Tracing this waveform yields the VTI. Cardiac output is then calculated by multiplying the stroke volume by the fetal heart rate at the time of the Doppler interrogation.

output, in addition to the combined cardiac output with gestational age, have been documented in normal human pregnancies.[99,100] Because increases in ventricular stroke volume and cardiac output are usually the cause of fetal heart failure in most affected pregnancies, as described previously, monitoring changes in fetal output can be useful in anticipating the potential for the evolution of fetal hydrops. Once an increased cardiac output is present, close fetal echocardiographic surveillance of fetal myocardial function, including systolic and diastolic function parameters, and assessment for cardiomegaly and atrioventricular valve insufficiency can assist in determining the best timing of fetal intervention, if clearly indicated.

Two of the most studied high cardiac output states that have led to the development of invasive fetal therapies include monochorionic pregnancies complicated by an acardiac twin, or so-called "twin reversed arterial perfusion" (TRAP) sequence, and sacrococcygeal teratomas. The TRAP sequence, a rare condition that complicates approximately 1% of monochorionic twin gestations, occurs when one twin has no functional heart and is perfused in reverse through vascular connections within the placenta by a healthy pump twin.[101] The acardiac mass is usually somewhat amorphous and cystic but can have a trunk and extremities. Rarely, recognizable but nonfunctioning cardiac structures can be demonstrated (**Fig. 8**). The perinatal mortality rate for the pump twin, without intervention, is reported to range from 50% to 75% and is mainly a result of polyhydramnios, preterm labor, and congestive heart failure attributable to the high cardiac output state to the acardiac mass.[96,102,103] Not surprisingly, in one review of fetal echocardiographic features of the disease, the umbilical arterial pulsatility index of the acardiac twin was lower than that of the pump twin, reflecting a lower vascular resistance in the acardiac twin or greater run-off from the pump twin; these hemodynamics correlated with worse outcome.[104] Interestingly, the pump twin's cardiothoracic ratio, a gross measure of changes in ventricular preload, did not correlate with clinical outcome of the pregnancy. Thus, perhaps factors other than altered cardiac output contribute to a worse clinical outcome. The authors have observed stable but increased combined cardiac output

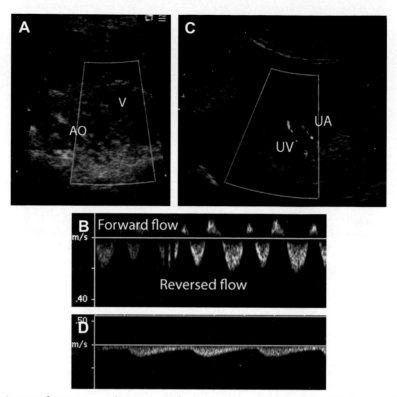

Fig. 8. Images from an acardiac twin with a substantial cardiac mass. (A) A recognizable single ventricle (V) that was nearly akinetic with a single atrioventricular valve and great artery; a presumptive aorta (AO) could be visualized. There was retrograde descending aortic flow, severe semilunar valve insufficiency that was in systole (shown) and diastole, and severe atrioventricular valve insufficiency. (B) Bidirectional but predominantly retrograde inferior vena cava flow was observed. (C) Classic pulsatile forward flow to the acardiac twin (blue color flow map) with laminar low-velocity flow through the umbilical vein (UV) of the acardiac twin away from this twin toward the pump twin. UA, umbilical artery. (D) UA Doppler flow signal to the acardiac twin is shown. Fetal echocardiography observations provided insight into the evolution of the "acardiac" twin, which likely evolved secondary to severe structural heart disease with progressive dysfunction.

in some affected pump twins without intervention and without evolution of hydrops (**Fig. 9**). In one pregnancy, however, they observed an acute increase in cardiac output associated with acute changes in flow to the acardiac twin and increased cardiac output with evolution of myocardial dysfunction and hydrops in the pump twin. In the latter, cord ligation of the acardiac twin resulted in an acute normalization of cardiac output and function of the pump twin. Such variable natural history warrants further fetal echocardiographic evaluation and a reassessment of the need for routine fetal intervention in all affected pregnancies, at least on the basis of risk for the evolution of fetal hydrops.[105] The rarity of the disease and common application of invasive intervention for this condition have made serial evaluation of the change in fetal cardiovascular output that occurs as part of the natural history and its influence on fetal heart function increasingly more difficult. Finally, with newer invasive interventions, including laser coagulation of the vascular connections and the common placenta,[106] potential

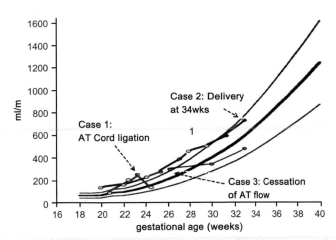

Fig. 9. Graph of serially assessed right ventricular outputs for three pump twins in acardiac pregnancies superimposed on normal right ventricular output curves. One (case 1) had an acute decrease in acardiac umbilical arterial resistance, which was accompanied by an acute increase in cardiac output of the pump and evolution of high central venous pressures. Acute normalization of the cardiac output followed cord ligation of the acardiac twin. The baby was delivered at 35 weeks of gestation with no significant sequelae. In case 2, because of technical limitations preventing invasive intervention, the pregnancy was followed expectantly from 20 weeks of gestation. Despite a mildly increased combined ventricular output, no evidence of ventricular dysfunction occurred and the baby was successfully delivered at 34 weeks. In case 3, abdominal ascites had developed earlier in the pregnancy associated with mildly increased cardiac output. The pump twin's combined cardiac output normalized, however, and the ascites spontaneously resolved concomitant with spontaneous loss of flow to the acardiac twin.

for residual flow to the acardiac twin may warrant ongoing assessment of the pump twin by fetal echocardiography.

Large vascular sacrococcygeal teratomas are known to lead to a high fetal cardiac output state, and this has been well documented. In 1989, Schmidt and colleagues[107] and, more recently, Rychik and colleagues[6] reported combined fetal cardiac outputs as determined by fetal echocardiography to exceed twofold normal for gestational age when fetal hydrops has evolved. As with acardiac twin pregnancies, evaluation of changes in fetal cardiac output and their influence on fetal heart function should be an integral part of the ongoing management of these pregnancies.

Lesions Associated with Cardiac Compression

Several fetal pathologic findings are associated with potential for compression of the fetal heart or systemic veins, leading to inadequate filling and consequent reduced cardiac output in addition to increasing central venous pressures and fetal hydrops. Fetal echocardiographic features of cardiac compression and reduced ventricular preload include reduced ventricular output and an increased ventricular inflow Doppler-derived E/A-wave ratio as demonstrated with Doppler interrogation (**Fig. 10**). This has been best demonstrated for congenital cystic adenomatous malformations,[98,108] large pleural effusions,[109,110] and large pericardial teratomas with or without a massive pericardial effusion.[107,111,112] Although cardiac compression with altered systemic venous return has been considered the primary cause of fetal hydrops in such conditions, in some cases, on Doppler interrogation, altered ventricular

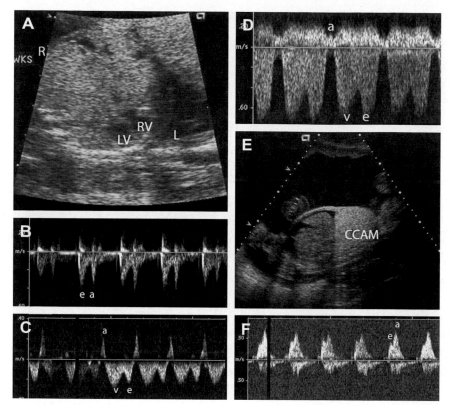

Fig. 10. These fetal echocardiography images were obtained from two pregnancies with abdominal ascites. (*A*) The fetal heart was clearly compressed by a massive congenital cystic adenomatous malformation. L, left; LV, left ventricle; R, right; RV, right ventricle. (*B*) There were ventricular inflow Doppler findings consistent with compression with an increased velocity during early ventricular diastole, the so-called "e-wave," compared with the a-wave during atrial contraction. In keeping with compression, the inferior vena cava (large a-wave reversal) (*C*) and ductus venosus (presence of a-wave reversal) (*D*) Doppler flow patterns suggested high central venous pressures. V, forward flow during ventricular systole and e-flow during early ventricular diastole. In a second fetus with evolving ascites and a flattened diaphragm as a consequence of a large cystic adenomatous malformation (*E*), the ventricular inflow Doppler interrogations (*F*) were normal, as were the systemic venous Doppler interrogations, suggesting a different mechanism for the ascites. CCAM, congenital cystic adenomatous malformation.

inflow has not been consistently observed in the presence of fetal ascites (**Fig. 10**). This could suggest a different pathophysiology and pathogenic mechanism of the ascites, such as a more direct influence of the mass or altered diaphragm position on lymphatic flow.[113] Further delineation of the different pathophysiologic findings and their associated clinical outcome may assist in identifying the fetus for which invasive intervention is warranted, and the timing of such interventions.

Fetal Echocardiography in the Evaluation of Congenital Diaphragmatic Hernia

Many fetal pathologic findings are associated with the evolution of pulmonary hypoplasia. Congenital diaphragmatic hernia is one such entity that has received significant

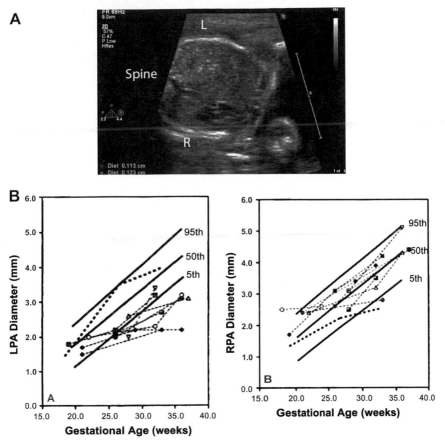

Fig. 11. (A) Two-dimensional image obtained in a 19-week gestational age fetus with left congenital diaphragmatic hernia. There is significant dextroposition of the cardiac structures, as shown in this modified three-vessel view that demonstrates the diameter measurement of both branch pulmonary arteries. The left pulmonary artery course is extremely distorted because of compression by the abdominal contents in the chest. L, left; R, right. Graphs demonstrating growth of the left pulmonary artery (A, LPA) and right pulmonary artery (B, RPA) in fetuses with a diagnosis of left (*light dashed line*) or right (*dark dashed line*) diaphragmatic hernia. The bold solid lines represent normal growth curves for branch pulmonary artery diameters as documented in 55 healthy pregnancies without fetal anomalies. (*From* Sokol J, Bohn D, Lacro RV, et al. Fetal pulmonary artery diameters and their association with lung hypoplasia and postnatal outcome in congenital diaphragmatic hernia. Am J Obstet Gynecol 2002;186:1085; with permission.)

attention in the field of fetal intervention, beginning in the early 1990s through the efforts of Harrison and colleagues.[114] Accurate definition of the severity of pulmonary hypoplasia, including correlation with clinical outcome and the potential for progression, has become a critical focus in the counseling of affected pregnancies and the development of invasive fetal therapies to improve pulmonary growth. Lung-to-head ratio as estimated by fetal ultrasound and MRI-determined fetal lung volumes have been used with some success.[115–117]

Fetal echocardiography is important in all affected pregnancies for the exclusion of structural fetal cardiac pathologic findings, which occur in up to 10% of affected fetuses and infants and significantly worsen the prognosis.[118] More recently, echo-cardiography has been used to define lung mass better through measurement of branchpulmonary artery diameters before[119,120] and after[121] birth and documenta-tion of fetal pulmonary arterial flow patterns.[114,122] The authors had previously shown branch pulmonary artery diameters measured at fetal echocardiography to correlate positively with lung weights at fetal autopsy.[119] They subsequently found smaller left pulmonary arteries in left diaphragmatic hernia to correlate with worse postnatal respiratory morbidity, including length of ventilation and length of supple-mental oxygen therapy.[120] Serial branch pulmonary artery diameter growth confirmed the progressive nature of the pulmonary hypoplasia in many affected fetuses, which most commonly involved the lung ipsilateral to the defect but included progressive bilateral lung hypoplasia in more severe disease (eg, bilateral diaphragmatic hernia) (**Fig. 11**).[119,120] Although in the authors' experience, inter- and intraobserver variability for branch pulmonary artery measurements was low,[119] this may not be observed in other centers with less experience and less uniformity in measuring such diminutive structures. Furthermore, branch pulmonary artery diameters may best be used in conjunction with other ultrasound- or MRI-based techniques, and their utility in assessment of lung mass in other conditions associated with pulmonary hypoplasia has not as yet been documented.

Pulmonary blood flow Doppler velocimetry may be an additional useful tool to predict the degree of pulmonary hypoplasia before and after birth.[122,123] Before birth, the normal branch pulmonary artery Doppler waveform shows a "spike-and-dome" pattern, and there is some evidence that the ratio of pulmonary artery acceleration time (time from onset to peak of flow) to ejection time (onset to end of systole) (AT/ET) is diminished in fetuses having congenital diaphragmatic hernia and pulmo-nary hypoplasia compared with gestational-age matched normal fetuses,[122] which may reflect an increase in pulmonary vascular resistance or anatomic distortion of the pulmonary arteries. A normal AT/ET ratio in at least one branch pulmonary artery is associated with survival, whereas a low AT/ET ratio from both pulmonary arteries, or from one pulmonary artery with the ratio from the other side not attainable, was asso-ciated with pulmonary hypoplasia.[122] Accurate assessment of lung growth with predictors of postnatal mortality and morbidity is critical for identification of the fetus in which fetal intervention is warranted, and for subsequent assessment of pulmonary growth and flow as measures of success of the intervention.

SUMMARY

Rapid advances in ultrasound technology afford early and accurate prenatal cardiac imaging and hemodynamic data. Coupled with the plethora of exciting new fetal inter-ventional techniques, fetal echocardiography and fetal intervention together are entering exciting scientific frontiers. Maternal-fetal specialists are currently poised to acquire fresh insight into cardiac and extracardiac lesions that result in hemodynamic compromise to the fetal patient, with fetal echocardiography affording the opportunity to gain an improved understanding of the natural history of cardiac lesions and with the prospect of altering the natural history of lesions with a guarded or dismal prog-nosis. Additionally, fetal echocardiography is likely to continue to play an important role in elucidating the pathogenesis and hemodynamic effects of noncardiac lesions, such as TTTS or cystic adenomatous malformations. Detailed hemodynamic assess-ment of the fetus has already opened doors to creative solutions beyond our postnatal experience and should allow the opportunity for the application of molecular scientific knowledge to practice "bench to bedside" medicine. As we proceed into adopting fetal intervention into routine practice, however, researchers and clinicians involved in the care of these patients need to be absolutely certain that the benefit is worth the risk, given the presence of two patients and the vulnerability of the "healthy" mother. As the concept of the fetus as a patient becomes widely accepted, prospective multicenter collaborative efforts are imperative to proceed in an evidence-based manner and identify the patients who can truly benefit from these exciting new technologies.[124]

REFERENCES

1. Gottliebson WM, Border WL, Franklin CM, et al. Accuracy of fetal echocardiography: a cardiac segment-specific analysis. Ultrasound Obstet Gynecol 2006; 28:15–21.
2. Taketazu M, Lougheed J, Yoo SJ, et al. Spectrum of cardiovascular disease, accuracy of diagnosis, and outcome in fetal heterotaxy syndrome. Am J Cardiol 2006;97:720–4.
3. Tometzki AJ, Suda K, Kohl T, et al. Accuracy of prenatal echocardiographic diagnosis and prognosis of fetuses with conotruncal anomalies. J Am Coll Cardiol 1999;33:1696–701.
4. Trines J, Hornberger LK. Evolution of heart disease in utero. Pediatr Cardiol 2004;25:287–98.
5. Kunisaki SM, Jennings RW. Fetal surgery. J Intensive Care Med 2008;23:33–51.
6. Rychik J, Tian Z, Cohen MS, et al. Acute cardiovascular effects of fetal surgery in the human. Circulation 2004;110:1549–56.
7. Verrier ED, Vlahakes GJ, Hanley FL, et al. Experimental fetal cardiac surgery. In: Harrison G, Filly, editors. The unborn patient: prenatal diagnosis and treatment. 2nd edition. Philadelphia: WB Saunders Company; 1991. p. 548.
8. Gardiner HM. In-utero intervention for severe congenital heart disease. Best Pract Res Clin Obstet Gynaecol 2008;22:49–61.
9. Hoffman JI. Incidence of congenital heart disease: II. Prenatal incidence. Pediatr Cardiol 1995;16:155–65.
10. Wieczorek A, Hernandez-Robles J, Ewing L, et al. Prediction of outcome of fetal congenital heart disease using a cardiovascular profile score. Ultrasound Obstet Gynecol 2008;31:284–8.
11. Jaeggi ET, Hamilton RM, Silverman ED, et al. Outcome of children with fetal, neonatal or childhood diagnosis of isolated congenital atrioventricular block. A single institution's experience of 30 years. J Am Coll Cardiol 2002;39:130–7.
12. Schmidt KG, Ulmer HE, Silverman NH, et al. Perinatal outcome of fetal complete atrioventricular block: a multicenter experience. J Am Coll Cardiol 1991;17: 1360–6.
13. Ellis C, Pymar H, Windrim R, et al. A puzzling intrauterine death: non-compaction of the fetal ventricular myocardium presenting with reversed end-diastolic flow velocity in the umbilical arteries. J Obstet Gynaecol Can 2005;27:695–8.
14. Allan LD, Sharland GK, Milburn A, et al. Prospective diagnosis of 1,006 consecutive cases of congenital heart disease in the fetus. J Am Coll Cardiol 1994;23: 1452–8.
15. Hornberger LK, Sahn DJ, Kleinman CS, et al. Tricuspid valve disease with significant tricuspid insufficiency in the fetus: diagnosis and outcome. J Am Coll Cardiol 1991;17:167–73.
16. Moon-Grady AJ, Tacy TA, Brook MM, et al. Value of clinical and echocardiographic features in predicting outcome in the fetus, infant, and child with

tetralogy of Fallot with absent pulmonary valve complex. Am J Cardiol 2002;89: 1280–5.

17. Tulzer G, Gudmundsson S, Wood DC, et al. Doppler in non-immune hydrops fetalis. Ultrasound Obstet Gynecol 1994;4:279–83.

18. Simpson JM, Sharland GK. Fetal tachycardias: management and outcome of 127 consecutive cases. Heart 1998;79:576–81.

19. Jaeggi ET, Fouron JC, Silverman ED, et al. Transplacental fetal treatment improves the outcome of prenatally diagnosed complete atrioventricular block without structural heart disease. Circulation 2004;110:1542–8.

20. Eronen M, Heikkila P, Teramo K. Congenital complete heart block in the fetus: hemodynamic features, antenatal treatment, and outcome in six cases. Pediatr Cardiol 2001;22:385–92.

21. Groves AM, Allan LD, Rosenthal E. Outcome of isolated congenital complete heart block diagnosed in utero. Heart 1996;75:190–4.

22. Hornberger LK, Collins K. New insights into fetal atrioventricular block using fetal magnetocardiography. J Am Coll Cardiol 2008;51:85–6.

23. Eronen M. Long-term outcome of children with complete heart block diagnosed after the newborn period. Pediatr Cardiol 2001;22:133–7.

24. Buyon JP, Hiebert R, Copel J, et al. Autoimmune-associated congenital heart block: demographics, mortality, morbidity and recurrence rates obtained from a national neonatal lupus registry. J Am Coll Cardiol 1998; 31:1658–66.

25. Jaeggi ET, Hornberger LK, Smallhorn JF, et al. Prenatal diagnosis of complete atrioventricular block associated with structural heart disease: combined experience of two tertiary care centers and review of the literature. Ultrasound Obstet Gynecol 2005;26:16–21.

26. Lim JS, McCrindle BW, Smallhorn JF, et al. Clinical features, management, and outcome of children with fetal and postnatal diagnoses of isomerism syndromes. Circulation 2005;112:2454–61.

27. Krishnan AN, Sable CA, Donofrio MT. Spectrum of fetal echocardiographic findings in fetuses of women with clinical or serologic evidence of systemic lupus erythematosus. J Matern Fetal Neonatal Med 2008;21:776–82.

28. Salomonsson S, Sonesson SE, Ottosson L, et al. Ro/SSA autoantibodies directly bind cardiomyocytes, disturb calcium homeostasis, and mediate congenital heart block. J Exp Med 2005;201:11–7.

29. Trucco S, Jaeggi E, Cuneo B, et al. Use of intravenous gamma-globulin and steroids in the treatment of maternal autoantibody mediated cardiomyopathy. Presented at the Pediatric Academic Societies' Annual Meeting, Honolulu, Hawaii, May 2–6, 2008.

30. Assad RS, Zielinsky P, Kalil R, et al. New lead for in utero pacing for fetal congenital heart block. J Thorac Cardiovasc Surg 2003;126:300–2.

31. Walkinshaw SA, Welch CR, McCormack J, et al. In utero pacing for fetal congenital heart block. Fetal Diagn Ther 1994;9:183–5.

32. Carpenter RJ Jr, Strasburger JF, Garson A Jr, et al. Fetal ventricular pacing for hydrops secondary to complete atrioventricular block. J Am Coll Cardiol 1986; 8:1434–56.

33. Glatz AC, Gaynor JW, Rhodes LA, et al. Outcome of high-risk neonates with congenital complete heart block paced in the first 24 hours after birth. J Thorac Cardiovasc Surg 2008;136:767–73.

34. Acharya G, Archer N, Huhta JC. Functional assessment of the evolution of congenital heart disease in utero. Curr Opin Pediatr 2007;19:533–7.

35. Allan LD, Maxwell DJ, Carminati M, et al. Survival after fetal aortic balloon valvo-plasty. Ultrasound Obstet Gynecol 1995;5:90–1.
36. Marshall AC, Tworetzky W, Bergersen L, et al. Aortic valvuloplasty in the fetus: technical characteristics of successful balloon dilation. J Pediatr 2005;147:535–9.
37. Tworetzky W, Marshall AC. Fetal interventions for cardiac defects. Pediatr Clin North Am 2004;51:1503–13.
38. Wilkins-Haug LE, Tworetzky W, Benson CB, et al. Factors affecting technical success of fetal aortic valve dilation. Ultrasound Obstet Gynecol 2006;28:47–52.
39. Selamet-Tierney ES, Wald RM, McElhinney DB, et al. Changes in left heart hemodynamics after technically successful in-utero aortic valvuloplasty. Ultrasound Obstet Gynecol 2007;30:715–20.
40. Mizrahi-Arnaud A, Tworetzky W, Bulich LA, et al. Pathophysiology, management, and outcomes of fetal hemodynamic instability during prenatal cardiac interven-tion. Pediatr Res 2007;62:325–30.
41. Makikallio K, McElhinney DB, Levine JC, et al. Fetal aortic valve stenosis and the evolution of hypoplastic left heart syndrome: patient selection for fetal interven-tion. Circulation 2006;113:1401–5.
42. McElhinney DB, Tworetzky W. Anatomic predictors of technical success and postnatal biventricular outcome after in utero aortic valvuloplasty for aortic stenosis with evolving hypoplastic left heart syndrome. New Orleans (LA): American Heart Association Scientific Sessions; November 2008.
43. Tabbutt S, Nord AS, Jarvik GP, et al. Neurodevelopmental outcomes after staged palliation for hypoplastic left heart syndrome. Pediatrics 2008;121:476–83.
44. Wernovsky G. Current insights regarding neurological and developmental abnormalities in children and young adults with complex congenital cardiac disease. Cardiol Young 2006;16(Suppl 1):92–104.
45. Hinton RB, Andelfinger G, Sekar P, et al. Prenatal head growth and white matter injury in hypoplastic left heart syndrome. Pediatr Res 2008;64:364–9.
46. Shillingford AJ, Ittenbach RF, Marino BS, et al. Aortic morphometry and micro-cephaly in hypoplastic left heart syndrome. Cardiol Young 2007;17:189–95.
47. Atallah J, Dinu IA, Joffe AR, et al. Two-year survival and mental and psychomotor outcomes after the Norwood procedure: an analysis of the modified Blalock-Taussig shunt and right ventricle-to-pulmonary artery shunt surgical eras. Circulation 2008;118:1410–8.
48. Galindo A, Gutierrez-Larraya F, Velasco JM, et al. Pulmonary balloon valvulo-plasty in a fetus with critical pulmonary stenosis/atresia with intact ventricular septum and heart failure. Fetal Diagn Ther 2006;21:100–4.
49. Tulzer G, Arzt W, Franklin RC, et al. Fetal pulmonary valvuloplasty for critical pulmonary stenosis or atresia with intact septum. Lancet 2002;360:1567–8.
50. Gardiner HM, Belmar C, Tulzer G, et al. Morphologic and functional predictors of eventual circulation in the fetus with pulmonary atresia or critical pulmonary stenosis with intact septum. J Am Coll Cardiol 2008;51:1299–308.
51. Roman KS, Fouron JC, Nii M, et al. Determinants of outcome in fetal pulmonary valve stenosis or atresia with intact ventricular septum. Am J Cardiol 2007;99:699–703.
52. Daubeney PE, Wang D, Delany DJ, et al. Pulmonary atresia with intact ventric-ular septum: predictors of early and medium-term outcome in a population-based study. J Thorac Cardiovasc Surg 2005;130:1071–5.
53. Dyamenahalli U, McCrindle BW, McDonald C, et al. Pulmonary atresia with intact ventricular septum: management of, and outcomes for, a cohort of 210 consec-utive patients. Cardiol Young 2004;14:299–308.

54. Matsui H, Gardiner H. Fetal intervention for cardiac disease: the cutting edge of perinatal care. Semin Fetal Neonatal Med 2007;12:482–9.
55. Marshall AC, Levine J, Morash D, et al. Results of in utero atrial septoplasty in fetuses with hypoplastic left heart syndrome. Prenat Diagn 2008;28:1023–8.
56. Glatz JA, Tabbutt S, Gaynor JW, et al. Hypoplastic left heart syndrome with atrial level restriction in the era of prenatal diagnosis. Ann Thorac Surg 2007;84:1633–8.
57. Vida VL, Bacha EA, Larrazabal A, et al. Hypoplastic left heart syndrome with intact or highly restrictive atrial septum: surgical experience from a single center. Ann Thorac Surg 2007;84:581–5.
58. Schmidt M, Jaeggi E, Ryan G, et al. Percutaneous ultrasound-guided stenting of the atrial septum in fetal sheep. Ultrasound Obstet Gynecol 2008;32:923–8.
59. Taketazu M, Barrea C, Smallhorn JF, et al. Intrauterine pulmonary venous flow and restrictive foramen ovale in fetal hypoplastic left heart syndrome. J Am Coll Cardiol 2004;43:1902–7.
60. Michelfelder E, Gomez C, Border W, et al. Predictive value of fetal pulmonary venous flow patterns in identifying the need for atrial septoplasty in the newborn with hypoplastic left ventricle. Circulation 2005;112:2974–9.
61. Lee LA, Simon C, Bove EL, et al. High intensity focused ultrasound effect on cardiac tissues: potential for clinical application. Echocardiography 2000;17:563–6.
62. Kennedy JE, Ter Haar GR, Cranston D. High intensity focused ultrasound: surgery of the future? Br J Radiol 2003;76:590–9.
63. Friedberg M, Silverman NH, Moon-Grady AJ, et al. Prenatal detection of congenital heart disease: the experience of three fetal and pediatric heart centers in northern California. J Pediatr 2009, in press.
64. Shima Y, Shindoh F, Nakajima M, et al. Prenatal diagnosis of congenital heart disease: clinical experience and analysis. J Nippon Med Sch 2004;71:328–32.
65. Wong SF, Chan FY, Cincotta RB, et al. Factors influencing the prenatal detection of structural congenital heart diseases. Ultrasound Obstet Gynecol 2003;21:19.
66. Garne E. Prenatal diagnosis of six major cardiac malformations in Europe— a population based study. Acta Obstet Gynecol Scand 2001;80:224–8.
67. Garne E, Stoll C, Clementi M. Evaluation of prenatal diagnosis of congenital heart diseases by ultrasound: experience from 20 European registries. Ultrasound Obstet Gynecol 2001;17:386–91.
68. Tworetzky W, McElhinney DB, Reddy VM, et al. Improved surgical outcome after fetal diagnosis of hypoplastic left heart syndrome. Circulation 2001;103:1269–73.
69. Inamura N, Taketazu M, Smallhorn JF, et al. Left ventricular myocardial performance in the fetus with severe tricuspid valve disease and tricuspid insufficiency. Am J Perinatol 2005;22:91–7.
70. Wald RM, Adatia I, Van Arsdell GS, et al. Relation of limiting ductal patency to survival in neonatal Ebstein's anomaly. Am J Cardiol 2005;96:851–6.
71. Johnson BA, Ades A. Delivery room and early postnatal management of neonates who have prenatally diagnosed congenital heart disease. Clin Perinatol 2005;32:921–46.
72. Marwan A, Crombleholme TM. The EXIT procedure: principles, pitfalls, and progress. Semin Pediatr Surg 2006;15:107–15.
73. Sebire NJ, Snijders RJ, Hughes K, et al. The hidden mortality of monochorionic twin pregnancies. Br J Obstet Gynaecol 1997;104:1203–7.
74. Brennan JN, Diwan RV, Rosen MG, et al. Fetofetal transfusion syndrome: prenatal ultrasonographic diagnosis. Radiology 1982;143:535–6.

75. Paladini D, Vassallo M, Sglavo G, et al. Diagnosis and outcome of congenital heart disease in fetuses from multiple pregnancies. Prenat Diagn 2005;25: 403–6.
76. Zosmer N, Bajoria R, Weiner E, et al. Clinical and echographic features of in utero cardiac dysfunction in the recipient twin in twin-twin transfusion syndrome. Br Heart J 1994;72:74–9.
77. Pedra SR, Smallhorn JF, Ryan G, et al. Fetal cardiomyopathies: pathogenic mechanisms, hemodynamic findings, and clinical outcome. Circulation 2002; 106:585–91.
78. Barrea C, Alkazaleh F, Ryan G, et al. Prenatal cardiovascular manifestations in the twin-to-twin transfusion syndrome recipients and the impact of therapeutic amnioreduction. Am J Obstet Gynecol 2005;192:892–902.
79. Barrea C, Hornberger LK, Alkazaleh F, et al. Impact of selective laser ablation of placental anastomoses on the cardiovascular pathology of the recipient twin in severe twin-twin transfusion syndrome. Am J Obstet Gynecol 2006; 195:1388–95.
80. Bensouda B, Fouron JC, Raboisson MJ, et al. Relevance of measuring diastolic time intervals in the ductus venosus during the early stages of twin-twin transfusion syndrome. Ultrasound Obstet Gynecol 2007;30:983–7.
81. Michelfelder E, Gottliebson W, Border W, et al. Early manifestations and spectrum of recipient twin cardiomyopathy in twin-twin transfusion syndrome: relation to Quintero stage. Ultrasound Obstet Gynecol 2007;30:965–71.
82. Rychik J, Tian Z, Bebbington M, et al. The twin-twin transfusion syndrome: spectrum of cardiovascular abnormality and development of a cardiovascular score to assess severity of disease. Am J Obstet Gynecol 2007;197:392.e1–8.
83. Naeye RL. Human intrauterine parabiotic syndrome and its complications. N Engl J Med 1963;268:804–9.
84. Bajoria R, Sullivan M, Fisk NM. Endothelin concentrations in monochorionic twins with severe twin-twin transfusion syndrome. Humanit Rep 1999;14:1614–8.
85. Bajoria R, Ward S, Chatterjee R. Natriuretic peptides in the pathogenesis of cardiac dysfunction in the recipient fetus of twin-twin transfusion syndrome. Am J Obstet Gynecol 2002;186:121–7.
86. Lougheed J, Sinclair BG, Fung Kee Fung K, et al. Acquired right ventricular outflow tract obstruction in the recipient twin in twin-twin transfusion syndrome. J Am Coll Cardiol 2001;38:1533–8.
87. Lopriore E, Bokenkamp R, Rijlaarsdam M, et al. Congenital heart disease in twin-to-twin transfusion syndrome treated with fetoscopic laser surgery. Congenit Heart Dis 2007;2:38–43.
88. Bigras JL, Suda K, Dahdah NS, et al. Cardiovascular evaluation of fetal anemia due to alloimmunization. Fetal Diagn Ther 2008;24:197–202.
89. Bond SJ, Harrison MR, Schmidt KG, et al. Death due to high-output cardiac failure in fetal sacrococcygeal teratoma. J Pediatr Surg 1990;25:1287–91.
90. Jaeggi ET, Fouron JC, Hornberger LK, et al. Agenesis of the ductus venosus that is associated with extrahepatic umbilical vein drainage: prenatal features and clinical outcome. Am J Obstet Gynecol 2002;187:1031–7.
91. Jeanty P, Kepple D, Roussis P, et al. In utero detection of cardiac failure from an aneurysm of the vein of Galen. Am J Obstet Gynecol 1990;163:50–1.
92. Osborn P, Gross TL, Shah JJ, et al. Prenatal diagnosis of fetal heart failure in twin reversed arterial perfusion syndrome. Prenat Diagn 2000;20:615–7.
93. Paternoster DM, Manganelli F, Moroder W, et al. Prenatal diagnosis of vein of Galen aneurysmal malformations. Fetal Diagn Ther 2003;18:408–11.

94. Sepulveda W, Platt CC, Fisk NM. Prenatal diagnosis of cerebral arteriovenous malformation using color Doppler ultrasonography: case report and review of the literature. Ultrasound Obstet Gynecol 1995;6:282–6.

95. Silverman NH, Schmidt KG. Ventricular volume overload in the human fetus: observations from fetal echocardiography. J Am Soc Echocardiogr 1990;3:20–9.

96. Sogaard K, Skibsted L, Brocks V. Acardiac twins: pathophysiology, diagnosis, outcome and treatment. Six cases and review of the literature. Fetal Diagn Ther 1999;14:53–9.

97. Sydorak RM, Kelly T, Feldstein VA, et al. Prenatal resection of a fetal pericardial teratoma. Fetal Diagn Ther 2002;17:281–5.

98. Szwast A, Tian Z, McCann M, et al. Impact of altered loading conditions on ventricular performance in fetuses with congenital cystic adenomatoid malformation and twin-twin transfusion syndrome. Ultrasound Obstet Gynecol 2007; 30:40–6.

99. Allan LD, Chita SK, Al-Ghazali W, et al. Doppler echocardiographic evaluation of the normal human fetal heart. Br Heart J 1987;57:528–33.

100. Kenny JF, Plappert T, Doubilet P, et al. Changes in intracardiac blood flow velocities and right and left ventricular stroke volumes with gestational age in the normal human fetus: a prospective Doppler echocardiographic study. Circulation 1986;74:1208–16.

101. James WH. A note on the epidemiology of acardiac monsters. Teratology 1977; 16:211–6.

102. Moore TR, Gale S, Benirshke K. Perinatal outcome of 49 pregnancies complicated by a cardiac twinning. Am J Obstet Gynecol 1990;163:907–12.

103. Van Allen MI, Smith DW, Shepard TH. Twin reversed arterial perfusion (TRAP) sequence: a study of 14 twin pregnancies with acardius. Semin Perinatol 1983;7:285–93.

104. Brassard M, Fouron JC, Leduc L, et al. Prognostic markers in twin pregnancies with an acardiac fetus. Obstet Gynecol 1999;94:409–14.

105. Weisz B, Peltz R, Chayen B, et al. Tailored management of twin reversed arterial perfusion (TRAP) sequence. Ultrasound Obstet Gynecol 2004;23: 451–5.

106. Gul A, Gungorduk K, Yildirim G, et al. Fetal therapy in twin reversed arterial perfusion sequence pregnancies with alcohol ablation or bipolar cord coagulation. Arch Gynecol Obstet 2008;278:541–5.

107. Schmidt KG, Silverman NH, Harison MR, et al. High-output cardiac failure in fetuses with large sacrococcygeal teratoma: diagnosis by echocardiography and Doppler ultrasound. J Pediatr 1989;114:1023–8.

108. Mahle WT, Rychik J, Tian ZY, et al. Echocardiographic evaluation of the fetus with congenital cystic adenomatoid malformation. Ultrasound Obstet Gynecol 2000;16:620–4.

109. Klam S, Bigras JL, Hudon L. Predicting outcome in primary fetal hydrothorax. Fetal Diagn Ther 2005;20:366–70.

110. Longaker MT, Laberge JM, Dansereau J, et al. Primary fetal hydrothorax: natural history and management. J Pediatr Surg 1989;24:573–6.

111. Bader R, Hornberger LK, Nijmeh LJ, et al. Fetal pericardial teratoma: presentation of two cases and review of literature. Am J Perinatol 2006;23:53–8.

112. Liddle AD, Anderson DR, Mishra PK. Intrapericardial teratoma presenting in fetal life: intrauterine diagnosis and neonatal management. Congenit Heart Dis 2008;3:449–51.

113. Shum DJ, Clifton MS, Coakley FV, et al. Prenatal tracheal obstruction due to double aortic arch: a potential mimic of congenital high airway obstruction syndrome. AJR Am J Roentgenol 2007;188:W82–5.
114. Harrison MR, Adzick NS, Bullard KM, et al. Correction of congenital diaphragmatic hernia in utero VII: a prospective trial. J Pediatr Surg 1997;32:1637–42.
115. Ba'ath ME, Jesudason EC, Losty PD. How useful is the lung-to-head ratio in predicting outcome in the fetus with congenital diaphragmatic hernia? A systematic review and meta-analysis. Ultrasound Obstet Gynecol 2007;30:897–906.
116. Cannie M, Jani J, Meersschaert J, et al. Prenatal prediction of survival in isolated diaphragmatic hernia using observed to expected total fetal lung volume determined by magnetic resonance imaging based on either gestational age or fetal body volume. Ultrasound Obstet Gynecol 2008;32:633–9.
117. Kilian AK, Schaible T, Hofmann V, et al. Congenital diaphragmatic hernia: predictive value of MRI relative lung-to-head ratio compared with MRI fetal lung volume and sonographic lung-to-head ratio. AJR Am J Roentgenol 2009; 192:153–8.
118. Falkensammer CB, Ayres NA, Altman CA, et al. Fetal cardiac malposition: incidence and outcome of associated cardiac and extracardiac malformations. Am J Perinatol 2008;25:277–81.
119. Sokol J, Bohn D, Lacro RV, et al. Fetal pulmonary artery diameters and their association with lung hypoplasia and postnatal outcome in congenital diaphragmatic hernia. Am J Obstet Gynecol 2002;186:1085–90.
120. Sokol J, Shimizu N, Bohn D, et al. Fetal pulmonary artery diameter measurements as a predictor of morbidity in antenatally diagnosed congenital diaphragmatic hernia: a prospective study. Am J Obstet Gynecol 2006;195:470–7.
121. Suda K, Bigras JL, Bohn D, et al. Echocardiographic predictors of outcome in newborns with congenital diaphragmatic hernia. Pediatrics 2000;105:1106–9.
122. Fuke S, Kanzaki T, Mu J, et al. Antenatal prediction of pulmonary hypoplasia by acceleration time/ejection time ratio of fetal pulmonary arteries by Doppler blood flow velocimetry. Am J Obstet Gynecol 2003;188:228–33.
123. Okazaki T, Okawada M, Shiyanagi S, et al. Significance of pulmonary artery size and blood flow as a predictor of outcome in congenital diaphragmatic hernia. Pediatr Surg Int 2008;24:1369–73.
124. Kleinman CS. Fetal cardiac intervention: innovative therapy or a technique in search of an indication? Circulation 2006;113:1378–81.

Changing Perspectives on the Perinatal Management of Isolated Congenital Diaphragmatic Hernia in Europe

Jan A. Deprest, MD, PhD[a],*, Eduardo Gratacos, MD, PhD[b],
Kypros Nicolaides, MD, PhD[c], Elise Done, MD[a], Tim Van Mieghem, MD[a],
Leonardo Gucciardo, MD[a], Filip Claus, MD, PhD[d], Anne Debeer, MD[a],
Karel Allegaert, MD, PhD[a], Irwin Reiss, MD, PhD[e], Dick Tibboel, MD, PhD[e]

KEYWORDS

- Congenital diaphragmatic hernia • Prenatal diagnosis
- Fetal tracheal occlusion • Prediction of outcome
- Neonatal management

Congenital diaphragmatic hernia (CDH) occurs sporadically, with an incidence of 1 in 2500 to 1 in 5000 of newborns, depending on whether stillbirths are included. The embryology and molecular and genetic mechanisms behind this anomaly are beyond the scope of this article and can be found elsewhere.[1,2] CDH does not designate a single clinical entity, and outcomes are accordingly diverse. Most cases are left sided (LCDH); 13% are right sided (RCDH); and bilateral lesions, complete agenesis, and other rarities total up to less than 2% of cases. In around 40% of cases, there are associated anomalies, representing an independent predictor of neonatal death, with less than 15% of babies surviving in this group.[2,3] Most of these cases are thus apparently isolated, although they might still be part of a yet unidentified spectrum of a disease affecting multiple organs. Key to the problem is that CDH lungs display severe developmental arrest of airway and vessels, resulting in lung hypoplasia.[4,5]

---

[a] Woman and Child Division, Fetal Medicine Unit, University Hospital Gasthuisberg, Herestraat 49, B-3000 Leuven, Belgium
[b] Department of Obstetrics, Hospital Clinic, Barcelona, Spain
[c] Harris Birthright Center for Fetal Medicine, King's College Hospital, London, UK
[d] Division of Medical Imaging, University Hospital Gasthuisberg, Leuven, Belgium
[e] Neonatal Intensive Care, Departments of Intensive Care and Pediatric Surgery, Erasmus Medical Centre, Sophia Kinderziekenhuis, Rotterdam, The Netherlands
* Corresponding author.
E-mail address: jan.deprest@uzleuven.be (J.A. Deprest).

Clin Perinatol 36 (2009) 329–347
doi:10.1016/j.clp.2009.03.004
0095-5108/09/$ – see front matter © 2009 Elsevier Inc. All rights reserved.

perinatology.theclinics.com

There are fewer alveoli, thickened alveolar walls, increased interstitial tissue, and markedly diminished alveolar air space and gas exchange surface area. There are a reduced number of vessels, adventitial thickening, medial hyperplasia, and peripheral extension of the muscle layer into the smaller intra-acinar arterioles. Although both lungs are affected, the ipsilateral one is affected more so than the contralateral one. These morphologic changes only become obvious when the lung becomes functional at birth. They lead to variable degrees of respiratory insufficiency and pulmonary hypertension (PH). Reduced air space and vascular bed lead to hypoxia, hypercarbia, and PH. The abnormal vasculature is also more sensitive to pulmonary vasoconstriction, which worsens PH, further increasing the right-to-left shunt. This leads to a vicious cycle preventing gas exchange of the shunted blood in addition to increasing acidosis and hypoxia (Fig. 1).

Today, screening programs allow prenatal detection of the condition, at least in two of three cases.[6] In view of the consequences of a prenatal diagnosis, it is desirable that this rate be improved further.[7] Effective counseling consists of describing the typical postnatal course of a newborn who has CDH, together with the range of morbidities that might be encountered. Additionally, counseling should include individualized information derived from comprehensive prenatal assessment. The latter information has recently dramatically changed prenatal management. In mild or moderate cases (ie, with a predicted survival rate of >50%), arrangements for planned delivery at a referral center should be made in a timely fashion. In more severe cases, or those with associated serious anomalies (hence, with a poor prognosis), termination of pregnancy should be discussed with the parents. Another more recent advance is that prenatal therapy has been offered to severe but isolated cases. The recent changes in prenatal management have, as a consequence, increased interest in this condition and revived collaboration and research initiatives among prenatal and postnatal management specialists. In this article, the authors discuss in more detail what has been achieved recently in prenatal prediction of individual prognosis; describe fetal

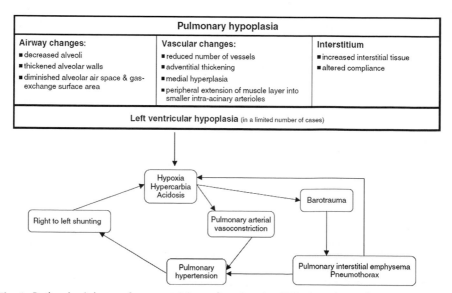

Fig. 1. Pathophysiology of neonatal lung function in CDH. (*From* Doné E, Gucciardo L, Van Mieghem T, et al. Prenatal diagnosis, prediction of outcome and in utero therapy of isolated congenital diaphragmatic hernia. Prenat Diagn 2008;28:583; with permission).

therapy for severe cases; and discuss the recently started clinical trial in moderate lung hypoplasia, which has included the establishment of consensus guidelines on standardized neonatal management. These changes have certainly altered in Europe perinatal management of the pregnant woman carrying a fetus who has CDH.

ANTENATAL PREDICTION OF OUTCOME
Two-Dimensional Ultrasound of the Contralateral Lung Area

The best validated prediction method is by two-dimensional (2D) measurement of the contralateral lung area assessed through the so-called "lung area-to-head circumference ratio" (LHR).[8] Different methods for measuring have been described, but the most reproducible and accurate method involves tracing the lung contours (**Fig. 2**).[9] The predictive value of the LHR was validated in the antenatal CDH registry on 184 consecutive cases of isolated LCDH managed at 10 tertiary centers, which were examined at 22 to 28 weeks of gestation and resulted in live births beyond 30 weeks.[10] In that study, the intrathoracic position of the liver was an independent predictor of outcome. Several additional studies have confirmed that the LHR and liver position relate to survival.[11–13]

Between 12 and 32 weeks, the normal lung area increases four times more than the head circumference, such that the LHR must be referenced to gestational age. The

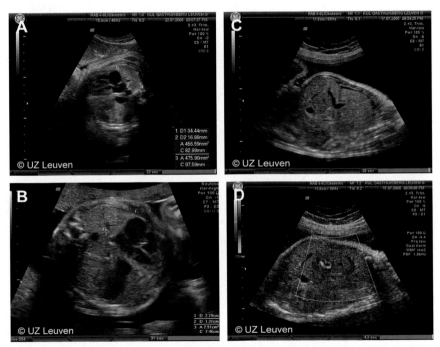

Fig. 2. Fetus with CDH on two-dimensional ultrasound. (A) Measurement of the lung in a section through the so-called "four-chamber view" with the so-called "longest axis method" and "tracing method." This is used to calculate the LHR. (B) Measurement of the lung 1 day after balloon insertion, with changed echogenicity visible. (C) Herniation of the liver. (D) Visualization of the major vessels help in identification of the liver. (From Deprest J, Flemmer A, Gratacos E, et al. Antenatal prediction of lung volume and in-utero treatment by fetal endoscopic tracheal occlusion in the severe isolated congenital diaphragmatic hernia. Semin Fetal Neonatal Med 2009;14:9; with permission.)

effect of gestational age on the LHR can be discounted by expressing the observed LHR as a ratio to the expected mean LHR for that gestational age. Normative curves for the LHR using different methods are available,[9] but an easy tool with which to calculate an individual observed/expected (O/E) LHR is available on the Total trial's Web site (www.totaltrial.eu), irrespective of the method used.[14] In a second study from the CDH antenatal registry, 354 fetuses with unilateral (left and right) isolated CDH were evaluated between 18 and 38 weeks.[15] The O/E LHR predicted outcome, with a trend for better prediction when the O/E LHR was determined at 32 to 33 weeks rather than at 22 to 23 weeks, as observed by others as well.[13,16] In that larger study, the liver position was no longer an independent predictor. Additionally, the O/E LHR correlates with short-term morbidity indicators, such as oxygen and ventilatory needs, in addition to the requirement for patch repair.[17]

Based on the consistency of these observations, the authors proposed a prenatal stratification according to expected outcome based on determination of the O/E LHR and the liver position (**Fig. 3**).[18–20] They included the position of the liver, because it remains uncertain whether liver and lung size are independent predictive factors. This empiric clinical classification ranges from extreme to mild, which reflects the severity as perceived by the parents, based on predicted postnatal survival rates. The numbers quoted here are from the antenatal CDH registry and apply to isolated LCDH.

- Fetuses with an O/E LHR less than 15% have virtually no chance to survive, such that the hypoplasia is extreme. The liver is typically up in these cases. Morbidity rates in these patients are unknown, given the few reported cases.
- Fetuses with an O/E LHR from 15% to 24.9% have severe pulmonary hypoplasia. Their predicted survival rate is less than 20%, less if the liver is up. The rate of bronchopulmonary dysplasia (BPD) in the (rare) survivors is greater than 75%.
- Fetuses with an O/E LHR between 26% and 35% (irrespective of the liver position) and those with an O/E LHR between 36% and 45% and liver up have

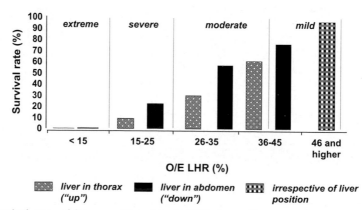

Fig. 3. Survival rates of fetuses with isolated LCDH, depending on measurement of the O/E LHR measurements and liver position as in the antenatal congenital diaphragmatic hernia registry. (*From* Deprest J, Flemmer A, Gratacos E, et al. Antenatal prediction of lung volume and in-utero treatment by fetal endoscopic tracheal occlusion in the severe isolated congenital diaphragmatic hernia. Semin Fetal Neonatal Med 2009;14:11; with permission.)

moderate hypoplasia. They have a predicted survival rate around 50% (range: 30%–60%). The rate of BPD is around 30%.

- Fetuses with an O/E LHR between 36% and 45% with liver down and those with an O/E LHR greater than 45% have mild hypoplasia and are likely (>75%) to survive. In the latter group, the rate of BPD is around 10%.

The antenatal CDH registry study is also one of the few prenatal studies reporting outcomes of right-sided lesions, which have poorer outcomes. The overall survival rate in 25 cases of RCDH was 44%, and a cutoff of the O/E LHR at less than 45% for lower viability chances seems to be present. As a consequence, this cutoff is currently used to define severe hypoplasia in that group.

2D ultrasound measurements have the advantage that most fetal medicine specialists are used to this imaging method, such that it can be widely applied. Protocols for antenatal clinical interventions were also based on this stratification, because most data are available with this method. There are certainly possible objections to this. It certainly needs practice and standardization. In addition, not all are convinced that this is the best predictor, or that outcome can be predicted at all.[21] The LHR is also, per definition, limited to measurement of one lung only because it relies on a cross section through one (contralateral) lung.

Volumetry of Lungs and the Degree of Liver Herniation

Three-dimensional (3D) ultrasound and MRI allow measurement in three dimensions, permitting quantification of bilateral (total) lung volume. In analogy to this, expressing observed measurements in comparison to those expected in a normal fetus is advocated. At this time, the superiority of 3D over 2D sonographic measurements has yet to be demonstrated.[22] The authors' experience with 3D ultrasound has been disappointing, because the ipsilateral lung could not be measured in 40% of cases, but this has been questioned by others.[22–24] Conversely, fetal MRI has a high spatial resolution, can be applied in obese patients, and, more importantly to CDH, the contralateral lung and the ipsilateral lung can be accurately measured. Expected lung volume can be predicted by comparison with a match, chosen on the basis of gestational age, liver volume, or, more accurately, fetal body volume, which discounts the effect of gestational age, in addition to differences in growth (**Fig. 4**).[12,25–27] The authors expect this method to become the method of choice when others validate the findings from a recent European study, which coincide with the relation of lung size and survival as determined by ultrasound.[28] MRI can also be used to quantify the degree of liver herniation. Making this a continuous rather than categoric variable has the potential to make prediction more accurate. Also, clear definition of landmarks may overcome the relatively ambiguity around what is considered as "intrathoracic" liver. Several reference points can be used, such as the distance between the most apical part of the liver and the dome of the chest. This can then be proportioned to the distance between the diaphragmatic remnant and the thoracic apex.[29] In a retrospective study on 40 patients from Lille and Leuven, the herniated liver volume was compared with the total lung volume. On transverse planes, the thoracic cavity, the lungs, and the liver were traced. Intrathoracic liver was considered to be what lies above a reference line from the lower tip of the xiphoid on a midsagittal view to the corresponding vertebral body (see **Fig. 4**).[30] Areas are added and multiplied by slice thickness so that volumes can be calculated. This results in a calculated liver-to-thorax ratio (LiTR) at that point in gestation. At first glance, LiTR and lung volume are inversely related; however, in reality, they are independent in cases with liver up (LiTR >0). In that study, both continuous variables were independent predictors of outcome. The superiority of these

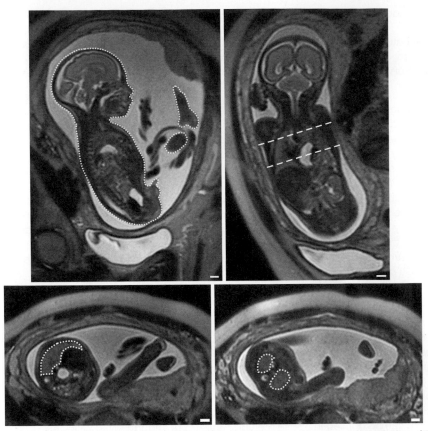

Fig. 4. T2-weighted images of fetus with LCDH at 26 weeks without liver herniation. (*Top left*) Sagittal section with tracing (*dotted lines*) of the body contours. (*Top right*) Coronal view of the fetus demonstrates the level (*dashed lines*) at which the two axial images are made. (*Bottom*) Lung tracing (*dotted lines*) on the two axial views. (Scale: white bar in right lower corner is 1 cm.)

volumetric rather than 2D techniques is difficult to demonstrate in view of the numbers needed for that.[31]

Prediction of Pulmonary Hypertension

Next to ventilatory insufficiency, PH is a major neonatal problem. It is believed to find its origins in structural vessel changes, which, in theory, might be documented during fetal life. One can measure the number of branches, vessel diameters, flow velocimetry, or flow volume with 2D or 3D techniques. There has recently been a lot of work done in this field, as recently summarized by Gucciardo and colleagues.[19] The validation status of these techniques is more limited at this time in terms of numbers and reproducibility among centers. In the authors' opinion, the most important work comes from Toronto and Paris, respectively. Hornberger and colleagues[32,33] demonstrated that the ipsilateral branch main pulmonary vessel diameter is related to outcome. Ruano and colleagues[34,35] established nomograms for branch main pulmonary artery diameters, but the Necker group (Paris) also used 3D power Doppler to assess the entire lung vasculature for the prediction of survival and the occurrence of PH. Recently, the authors studied the value of the peak early-diastolic reversed flow (PEDRF) and several other Doppler indices in proximal arterial branches in the contralateral lung, as well as ipsilateral lungs.[36] They observed a strong correlation of the PEDRF with the O/E LHR, but the added value of this parameter in prediction needs to be determined. The authors have further studied pulmonary artery reactivity after maternal hyperoxygenation. The so-called "hyperoxygenation" test involves Doppler measurements of the pulsatility index (PI) in the first branch of the contralateral pulmonary artery before and after maternal administration of 60% oxygen (O_2) by mask. A decrease of 20% or greater of the PI value after O_2 exposure is considered reactive.[37] In an initial study on 22 fetuses with severe CDH evaluated after 30 weeks, a reactive test result was predictive of survival, whereas a negative test result predicted an increased risk for severe pulmonary arterial hypertension and neonatal death.[38] Unfortunately, this test can only be done late in gestation, such that it may not be that useful for prenatal decision making unless, for instance, for referral to an extracorporeal membrane oxygenation (ECMO) center, once validated.

NEONATAL MANAGEMENT AND ACTUAL SURVIVAL RATES

Before the 1990s, the cornerstone of neonatal management was emergency repair of the defect, aggressive ventilation, and hyperoxygenation, together with other measures for controlling PH.[39] These two tenets have been questioned, and, today, "gentle ventilation," followed by delayed surgery, has improved results. Gentle ventilation protocols or "spontaneous breathing" without muscle paralysis and with permissive hypercapnia and minimal sedation reduces barotrauma and volutrauma.[40,41] The avoidance of PH seems key. Therefore, all efforts must be made to prevent postnatal hypoxia, and the presence of all identified risk factors for vasoconstriction (eg, low pH, hypercapnia, metabolic acidosis, pain, agitation, hypothermia) should be prevented. For that reason, ventilatory support is started immediately after birth.[42,43] When present, PH is most often treated by inhaled nitric oxide, although there is presently no evidence for this practice.[44–46] In approximately 30% of cases, a positive response (10% increase in arterial Pao_2) is observed. More recently, the use of prostaglandin (PG) E_1 has been suggested when there is severe secondary right ventricular cardiac dysfunction. PGE_1 keeps the ductus arteriosus patent.[47,48]

High-frequency oscillatory (HFO) ventilation has increasingly been used as a primary ventilation mode in cases of lung hypoplasia, but most centers consider it as rescue therapy in case of carbon dioxide retention before the institution of ECMO.[49–51] Some centers are proponents of the liberal use of ECMO.[52] The role of ECMO has been criticized because of its unproved benefits and its inherent complications and because it is not widely available. The only randomized trial on the use of ECMO (the UK collaborative trial) was underpowered to assess the place of ECMO in CDH. According to the ELSO registry, overall survival in ECMO-treated CDH cases is 40% (Source: Extra Corporeal Life Support (ELSO) registry, 2009).

For many years, it has been suggested that CDH is associated with a primary surfactant deficiency, but this has recently been refuted. In contrast, surfactant inactivation attributable to artificial ventilation and the presence of an inflammatory response in the hypoplastic lungs are suspected to underlie part of the respiratory insufficiency.[53] As a consequence, the use of surfactant has no proved benefit in the treatment of CDH, even in selected subgroups.[52,54] The same applies to infants on ECMO and preterm infants.[55]

With advances in neonatal therapy, one would expect to see increasing survival rates over time. In contrast, reported survival rates continue to vary widely for several reasons, however. Obvious reasons are that the case mix at each center may be different. Series might include isolated cases in addition to those with additional problems, in utero referred cases, and postnatal transfers. Further consideration needs to be given to termination of pregnancy. In the United Kingdom, termination rates range from 9% for isolated CDH to 51% in case of associated anomalies.[56] The mismatch between numbers reported by postnatal as opposed to fetal medicine specialists, who use different denominators, is referred to as "hidden mortality." Also included in the prenatal losses are the 1% to 2% of cases in which spontaneous demise occurs.[57] The simple practice of termination of pregnancy, particularly its increased use in cases that are considered to have poor prognostic indicators, may lead to an apparent increase in survival in postnatal series. Conversely, prenatal diagnosis may prompt in utero referral to a tertiary center, which, in return, also can increase survival. For example, in France, this policy significantly increased survival from 41% to 66% ($P = .03$).[57] Centralized management, with an increased case load and the use of consistent neonatal protocols, leads to increased survival rates. This was demonstrated by the Canadian Neonatal Network, which showed that high-volume centers (>12 CDH admissions over a 22-month period) had a 13% higher survival rate than low-volume centers.[58]

For these reasons, it has become difficult to define the natural history of CDH. Population-based statistics remain our best source of information.[59] Studies from France, Australia, and the United Kingdom report survival rates of between 50% and 70% for isolated CDH.[60–62] That this is a realistic estimate is confirmed by a comparable 60% to 70% survival rate reported by the CDH study group.[39] Certain centers quote rates in excess of 80% to 90% and claim that this is a result of their local neonatal management protocol, using one or another particular ventilation strategies, or ECMO, for example. It is, however, impossible to rule out bias in their statistics by prenatal selection or perinatal loss before referral.[63,64] In Europe, the most optimistic survival rates published by large referral centers, which have a caseload of more than 25 cases per year and offer ECMO, are 70% to 75%.[65]

Last but not least, fetal medicine specialists should not forget that survivors may have morbidity, including pulmonary, gastrointestinal (gastroesophagal reflux and feeding problems), orthopedic, hearing, and neurodevelopmental problems.[66] For that reason, survivors should remain in long-term (possibly for life) specialized multidisciplinary follow-up programs.[67,68] Around the world, more and more interdisciplinary follow-up teams have been set up for the evaluation and follow-up of the multiorgan morbidity associated with this anomaly. The American Academy of Pediatrics has recently proposed such a structured follow-up program.[69] Although not the primary goal, cost-effectiveness is also an important parameter. In the future, this should be a requirement when evaluating any suggested therapeutic approach.

TRACHEAL OCCLUSION IN EUROPE UNTIL 2008

Under the assumption that a population with a poor prognosis can be identified in a timely manner, one may attempt an antenatal intervention that accelerates lung development and restores lung function. In utero anatomic repair may do so but technically requires open fetal surgery.[70] In addition, it cannot be offered to fetuses with liver herniation. As an alternative, it was suggested to trigger lung growth by tracheal occlusion (TO).[71] The authors refer to some recent reviews on the experimental basis of TO.[72,73] In brief, the action mechanism takes advantage of a physiologic process through which lung growth and maturation are steered. During fetal life, the lung secretes fluid, stenting the fetal airways under pressure, as long as the glottis is closed. During fetal breathing, the glottis opens and the pressure gradient is leveled. These cyclic pressure changes are essential to balanced lung growth and maturation.[74] Prenatal TO prevents egress of lung fluid, which increases airway pressure, causing proliferation, increased alveolar air space, and maturation of pulmonary vasculature. TO also has a potentially deleterious effect; when sustained, it reduces the number of type II cells and surfactant expression. This can be alleviated by in utero release, a concept that was captured by the term *plug-unplug sequence*.[75] In brief, eventual pulmonary architecture, lung function, mechanics, and hemodynamics depend on a variety of factors that can be controlled, such as timing and duration of TO and its release and the use of antenatal steroids or postnatal surfactant, but also on other factors that are often beyond control, such as the severity of lung hypoplasia, gestational age at birth, and individual response.

Clinical TO was first achieved through maternal laparotomy, hysterotomy, neck dissection, and clipping.[76] Animal experience demonstrated the feasibility of endoluminal occlusion using a balloon, which was initially applied through hysterotomy and 5-mm equipment.[77,78] In Europe, the authors introduced percutaneous fetoscopic endoluminal tracheal occlusion (FETO) by means of a 3.3-mm cannula and under local or locoregional anesthesia (**Fig. 5**).[79] Purposefully designed 1.3-mm fiber endoscopes, blunted and curved sheaths, a puncture needle, and balloon retrieval forceps, developed with support from the European Union,[80] are used.[81] The detachable balloon is normally used in interventional radiology. Based on extrapolation of lung development stages in experiments on fetal lambs, the authors inserted the balloon at 26 to 28 weeks and reversed the occlusion at 34 weeks by fetoscopy or ultrasound-guided puncture.[18,75] Emergency peripartum removal by laryngotracheoscopy or an ex utero

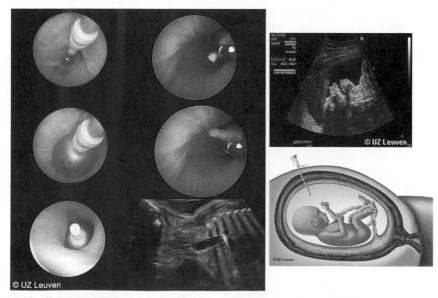

Fig. 5. (*Left*) Fetoscopic images of balloon insertion. (*Top to bottom, left to right*) Catheter loaded with the balloon is inserted; the balloon is inflated between the carina and vocal cords and is then detached. (*Bottom right*) Ultrasound image of the balloon in place. (*Right*) Schematic access to the uterus. (*From* Gucciardo L, Deprest J, Done E, et al. Prediction of outcome in isolated congenital diaphragmatic hernia and its consequences for fetal therapy. Best Pract Res Clin Obstet Gynaecol 2008;22:133; with permission.)

intrapartum treatment procedure must be available at all times in case of preterm labor. If not, dramatic situations arise, such as those the authors have witnessed in some patients who were locally managed by an unprepared team rather than being referred back to a FETO center.

To date, the European FETO consortium has offered fetal intervention to those who have liver herniation and an O/E LHR less than 27% to 28% (corresponding to an LHR <1.0 in the early third trimester). No maternal complications were observed in an experience now numbering more than 150 cases, but iatrogenic preterm rupture of membranes (iPPROMs), typically presenting as amniorrhexis but without immediate onset of labor, was more frequent than desired. In such cases, patients are admitted at the FETO center so that the tracheal balloon can be swiftly and safely removed once labor occurs or when infection mandates delivery. Thus far, more than 75% of patients have delivered beyond 34 weeks (mean gestational age at birth = 36 weeks). The neonatal survival rate was higher with prenatal versus perinatal balloon retrieval (83.3% versus 33.3%; P = .013), a trend persisting until discharge (67% versus 33%; not significant). The overall survival rate is greater than 50%, which is better than what is predicted for cases of the same severity.[82] The best predictors of survival are gestational age at delivery and lung size before FETO. Fetuses with the smallest lungs are less likely to respond than those with larger lungs.[83] Apart from that, the individual increase in lung area or volume after FETO is an independent predictor of survival.[84] Also, the pulmonary vascular reactivity changes after FETO are predictive of survival and occurrence of PH.[38]

Most newborns require surgical patching of the diaphragm, indicating the size of the defect in this selected group. Short-term morbidity in survivors is better than expected; it compares with that of cases with moderate pulmonary hypoplasia, which were managed after birth.[85] So far, the authors have not been able to report on long-term morbidity, partly because of the fact that most babies are not born at one of the FETO centers, making follow-up more difficult. Information by way of other tertiary centers is also less standardized. Based on the feedback from those centers, the nature of the morbidity in survivors is no different from that of those managed ex utero; however, whether it is less frequent than should be expected remains to be demonstrated. The Flemish government (Instituut voor Wetenschap en Technologie [IWT] 070715) is now partly supporting the recall of patients for such long-term evaluation in Belgium, and collaboration with Dutch and French centers should make evaluation of a reasonable number of patients possible.

2009 AND BEYOND: THE CURRENT PROGRAM AND TRIAL OF THE FETOSCOPIC ENDOLUMINAL TRACHEAL OCCLUSION CONSORTIUM
Fetoscopic Endoluminal Tracheal Occlusion for Severe Hypoplasia

Many have argued against fetal therapy for CDH, even for selected cases, but the FETO consortium has continued to provide therapy for fetuses with severe lung hypoplasia.[21,86] This is based on several observations. First, current neonatal management has still not dramatically changed the limits of viability. The published mortality rates remain virtually unchanged, with PH as a leading cause of death in up to 30% of patients.[11–13,65] This leaves some fetuses that can theoretically benefit from an (antenatal) intervention that reverses pulmonary hypoplasia. Second, a growing number of studies show that survival chances can be predicted based on lung size or liver position. This is a prerequisite for case selection when considering fetal intervention. Third, current instrumentation and experience have made FETO a reproducible procedure with acceptable invasiveness, without identified maternal risks to date. All these arguments have previously been discussed in detail in this article.

Another often-heard argument is that it has already been demonstrated in a randomized controlled trial by Harrison and colleagues[87] that there is no benefit from fetal therapy for this condition. The authors think, however, that this trial was not conclusive for the population that is treated at the current time in Europe. In that study, only three cases with an LHR less than 1.0 (O/E LHR = 27%) and liver up, matching the prenatal criteria of severe hypoplasia, were included, with one of these patients surviving. There are several other arguments why the current European program is not a mere duplication of that study (**Table 1**). The FETO procedure is a single 3.3-mm port and completely percutaneous procedure. The use of a balloon avoids neck dissection, accommodates tracheal growth, and makes reversal easier. iPPROMs indeed remains a problem. FETO is associated with a 20% iPPROM rate before 34 weeks; however, more than three quarters of patients deliver at 34 weeks or later. This compares favorably with the National Institutes of Health (NIH) trial (rupture rate = 100%), and may be attributable to the reduced diameter of instruments, growing experience, and short operation times.[88]

The authors' experience is fairly uncontrolled to date and can only be positioned versus historical or contemporary controls. Over the past years, the authors have attempted to set up a randomized trial. Apart from other more logistic and financial restrictions, they also experienced unexpected resistance from patients and physicians to a trial with an expectant management arm. Opponents of the trial found it difficult to accept that one of every two pregnant mothers carrying a fetus with an expected mortality as high as 80% and a pulmonary morbidity rate as high as 75% when managed in the postnatal period would get randomized to a treatment arm with exactly that poor perspective. Also, in view of the fact that FETO had been offered for exactly that same reason for all those years, opponents of the trial would perceive this as a "no therapy" arm. The authors admit that this objection is certainly debatable, because it is clear that the assumption of an extremely poor chance of survival may turn out afterward not to be necessarily true.[88] Outcomes may be better than

Table 1
Fetal surgery for congenital diaphragmatic hernia: trends in clinical experience

	Harrison et al (2003)	FETO Consortium (Ongoing)
Criteria for surgery	LHR <1.4 and liver "up"	LHR <1.0 and liver "up"
Anesthesia	General	Locoregional or local
Access through abdominal wall	Laparotomy	Percutaneous
Access diameter	5-mm cannula	3.3-mm cannula
Occlusive device	Clip or endoluminal balloon	Endoluminal balloon
Reversal of occlusion	EXIT delivery	In utero reversal
PPROMs <34 weeks	100%	20%
Mean gestational age at birth	30.8 (28–34) weeks	35 (27–38) weeks
Survival after TO (LHR <1.4)	73% (n = 11) (controls: 77%)	(not eligible)
Survival after TO (LHR <1.0)	33% (n = 3)	50%–55% (uncontrolled)[a]

Abbreviations: EXIT; ex utero intrapartum treatment; PPROMs, preterm rupture of membranes.
[a] In the antenatal CDH registry, survival in this group is less than 15%.

predicted by a trial effect or by questioning the validity of the used prenatal prediction methods. The validity of prenatal selection is obviously a condition sine qua non for a fetal therapy trial, and although that is still under debate, the authors' group has accepted the potential of appropriate prediction because of the high numbers currently available in their studies. Given that no consensus could be reached on the group with severe hypoplasia, FETO is still being offered to all fetuses, but the authors are considering a trial testing the hypothesis as to whether TO at different time points may increase survival.[18,20] At this time, however, the authors do not consider occlusion of the trachea in the saccular phase (>30 weeks of gestational age) of lung development in severe cases. Their experience is not encouraging in that perspective because they have shown that for severely hypoplastic lungs, later occlusion could be at the expense of lung growth.[18,89]

MODERATE HYPOPLASIA: THE TRACHEAL OCCLUSION TO ACCELERATE LUNG GROWTH TRIAL

The previously cited objections led the authors to reconsider a trial in case of moderate hypoplasia, corresponding to a predicted survival rate of 50% (range: 30%–60%) (see **Fig. 3**). They propose to randomize patients to expectant management during pregnancy or to insertion of a balloon at a FETO center at 30 to 32 weeks and its removal at 34 to 35 weeks, followed by standardized postnatal management (**Table 2**). Patients randomized to FETO are to be offered the opportunity to stay on campus for as long as the trachea is occluded, such that optimal facilities are available for balloon removal in an emergency. This is a multicenter trial in which mothers return to their tertiary referral center after removal of the balloon or when randomized to expectant management. The main outcome measure is to be a neonatal morbidity indicator. The authors hypothesize that fetal intervention decreases BPD (the need for O_2 supplementation at 28 days) by 20%. This is based on two independent observations. Keller and colleagues[90] demonstrated in survivors from the NIH trial that TO had several beneficial effects on pulmonary function, including an improvement in alveolar-arterial oxygen difference and lung compliance, and this despite premature birth at around 30 weeks. In the authors' experience, however, with more severe cases, the occurrence of BPD was around 30% lower than expected in the same severity controls.[86]

The current trial design should allay fears that studies have focused too long on mortality, whereas the morbidity in survivors is clinically even more relevant. Power calculations have demonstrated that such a study is realistic, such that all now depends on the disciplined attitude of the fetal medical community not to offer FETO outside this (or other) trials to allow sufficient patient recruitment. The first patients were recruited in October 2008 in Leuven and were later joined by the Barcelona group.[14] After the success of the Eurofoetus study on twin-twin transfusion syndrome, the authors are now defining criteria for trial participation in high-volume fetoscopy centers, which have meanwhile gained sufficient FETO experience and can ensure around-the-clock services of a team familiar with emergency balloon extraction and neonatal management of babies who have CDH. Although far from ideal, the multicenter setting accounts for a European reality, with limitations of national boundaries for certain patients or insurance companies but with the availability of a few pioneers with consistent experience in fetoscopy.[91]

STANDARDIZATION OF POSTNATAL MANAGEMENT

Such a trial would obviously be meaningless without standardization of postnatal management, which is done at a tertiary care center with a proved track record.

Table 2
Summary of the most important items in the postnatal treatment of patients who have congenital diaphragmatic hernia based on the consensus statement of the European congenital diaphragmatic hernia consortium

Treatment in the delivery room	No bag masking Immediate intubation Peak pressure <25 cm H_2O Nasogastric tube
Treatment on the NICU/PICU	Adapt ventilation to obtain preductal saturation between 85% and 95% pH >7.20, lactate 3–5 mmol/L CMV or HFOV maximum peak pressure of 25 to 28 cm H_2O in CMV and mean airway pressure of 17 cm H_2O in HFO Target blood pressure: normal value for gestational age Consider inotropic support
Treatment of PH	Perform echocardiography iNO is the first choice; in case of nonresponse, stop iNO In the chronic phase: phosphodiesterase inhibitors, endothelin antagonist, tyrosine kinase inhibitors
ECMO	Only start if the patient is able to achieve a preductal saturation >85% Inability to maintain preductal saturation >85% Respiratory acidosis Inadequate oxygen delivery (lactate >5 mmol/L) Therapy-resistant hypotension
Surgical repair	Fraction of inspired oxygen (Fio_2) <0.5 Mean blood pressure normal for gestational age Urine output >2 mL/kg/h No signs of persistent PH

Abbreviations: CMV, conventional mechanical ventilation; FiO_2, fraction of inspired oxygen; HFOV, high-frequency oscillation ventilation; H_2O, water; iNO, inhaled nitric oxide; NICU, neonatal intensive care unit; PICU, pediatric intensive care unit.

Ideally, these would be high-volume centers (≥ 7 admissions per year), based on the Canadian experience that using consistent neonatal protocols and experience improves infant survival.[58] Before entry in the trial at a postnatal treatment center, vital statistics of the past years would be documented and the center would have to adhere to written standardization guidelines, which were recently drafted by a European consortium of postnatal treatment centers, grouping 16 units in eight European countries. These centers have agreed on a consensus standardized postnatal protocol for the treatment of babies who have CDH from the moment of birth, including the period in the delivery room (see **Table 2**). The protocol covers such issues as ventilatory support, analgesia and sedation, fluid regimen, and adjustment of ventilation based on preductal arterial Pao_2 values. This protocol was drafted for reasons other than the prenatal trial, but it was a prerequisite for a successful multicenter trial. Needless to say that the level of evidence supporting these guidelines cannot be higher than a consensus document because of the absence of data based on properly designed (randomized) trials in any aspect of therapy in CDH. Over the years, this approach should provide solid morbidity data to fill in the gap of knowledge on injury and repair of these susceptible lungs and the relation between prenatal variables, postnatal management (with detailed knowledge of neonatal demographics), and outcome.

ACKNOWLEDGMENTS

The clinical studies on prenatal assessment and management have been supported, in part, by the European Commission (EuroSTEC, Sixth Framework, LSHC-CT-2006-037,409). The Flemish Community of Belgium supports the clinical trial (IWT 070,715) and J. Deprest as a "clinical researcher" by means of the Fonds voor Wetenschappelijk Onderzoek Vlaanderen (1.8.012.07.N.02). The authors are indebted to all their colleagues of the antenatal CDH registry, who brought together essential data on prenatal prediction, in addition to their colleagues from the Fetal Medicine Unit and Anesthesiology for permanent availability of perinatal care of the fetus with its trachea occluded.

REFERENCES

1. Ackerman KG, Pober BR. Congenital diaphragmatic hernia and pulmonary hypoplasia: new insights from developmental biology and genetics. Am J Med Genet C Semin Med Genet 2007;145:105–8.
2. Rottier R, Tibboel D. Fetal lung and diaphragm development in congenital diaphragmatic hernia. Semin Perinatol 2005;29:86–93.
3. Skari H, Bjornland K, Haugen G, et al. Congenital diaphragmatic hernia: a meta-analysis of mortality factors. J Pediatr Surg 2000;35:1187–97.
4. Heerema AE, Rabban JT, Sydorak RM, et al. Lung pathology in patients with congenital diaphragmatic hernia treated with fetal surgical intervention, including tracheal occlusion. Pediatr Dev Pathol 2003;6:536–46.
5. O'Toole SJ, Irish MS, Holm BA, et al. Pulmonary vascular abnormalities in congenital diaphragmatic hernia. Clin Perinatol 1996;23:781–94.
6. Garne E, Haeusler M, Barisic I, et al, for the Euroscan Study Group. Congenital diaphragmatic hernia: evaluation of prenatal diagnosis in 20 European regions. Ultrasound Obstet Gynecoll 2002;19:329–33.
7. Deprest J, Jani J, Van Schoubroeck D, et al. Current consequences of prenatal diagnosis of congenital diaphragmatic hernia. J Pediatr Surg 2006;41:423–30.
8. Metkus AP, Filly RA, Stringer MD, et al. Sonographic predictors of survival in fetal diaphragmatic hernia. J Pediatr Surg 1996;31:148–51 [discussion: 151–2].
9. Peralta CF, Cavoretto P, Csapo B, et al. Assessment of lung area in normal fetuses at 12–32 weeks. Ultrasound Obstet Gynecol 2005;26:718–24.
10. Jani J, Keller RL, Benachi A, et al. Prenatal prediction of survival in isolated left-sided diaphragmatic hernia. Ultrasound Obstet Gynecol 2006;27:18–22.
11. Hedrick HL, Danzer E, Merchant A, et al. Liver position and lung-to-head ratio for prediction of extracorporeal membrane oxygenation and survival in isolated left congenital diaphragmatic hernia. Am J Obstet Gynecol 2007;197:422, e1–4.
12. Datin-Dorriere V, Rouzies S, Taupin P, et al. Prenatal prognosis in isolated congenital diaphragmatic hernia. Am J Obstet Gynecol 2008;198:80, e1–5.
13. Yang SH, Nobuhara KK, Keller RL, et al. Reliability of the lung-to-head ratio as a predictor of outcome in fetuses with isolated left congenital diaphragmatic hernia at gestation outside 24–26 weeks. Am J Obstet Gynecol 2007;197:30, e1–7.
14. Congenital Diaphragmatic Hernia. Available at: www.totaltrial.eu.

15. Jani J, Nicolaides KH, Keller RL, et al. Observed to expected lung area to head circumference ratio in the prediction of survival in fetuses with isolated diaphragmatic hernia. Ultrasound Obstet Gynecol 2007;30:67–71.

16. Jani J, Nicolaides KH, Benachi A, et al. Timing of lung size assessment in the prediction of survival in fetuses with diaphragmatic hernia. Ultrasound Obstet Gynecol 2008;31:37–40.

17. Jani JC, Benachi A, Nicolaides KH, et al, for the Antenatal CDH Registry Group. Prenatal prediction of neonatal morbidity in survivors with congenital diaphragmatic hernia: a multicenter study. Ultrasound Obstet Gynecol 2009;33:64–9.

18. Deprest J, Jani J, Gratacos E, et al. Reply to a letter. J Pediatr Surg 2006;41: 1345–6.

19. Gucciardo L, Deprest J, Done E, et al. Prediction of outcome in isolated congenital diaphragmatic hernia and its consequences for fetal therapy. Best Pract Res Clin Obstet Gynaecol 2008;22:123–38.

20. Deprest J, Flemmer A, Gratacos E, et al. Antenatal prediction of lung volume and in-utero treatment by fetal endoscopic tracheal occlusion in the severe isolated congenital diaphragmatic hernia. Semin Fetal Neonatal Med 2009;14:8–13.

21. Deprest J, Hyett J, Flake A, et al. Current controversies in prenatal diagnosis 4: should fetal surgery be done in all cases of severe diaphragmatic hernia. Prenatal Diagnosis 2009;29:15–9.

22. Ruano R, Benachi A, Joubin L, et al. Three-dimensional ultrasonographic assessment of fetal lung volume as prognostic factor in isolated congenital diaphragmatic hernia. BJOG 2004;111:423–9.

23. Jani JC, Cannie M, Peralta CF, et al. Lung volumes in fetuses with congenital diaphragmatic hernia: comparison of 3D US and MR imaging assessments. Radiology 2007;244:575–82.

24. Ruano R, Aubry MC, Dumez Y, et al. Predicting neonatal deaths and pulmonary hypoplasia in isolated congenital diaphragmatic hernia using the sonographic fetal lung volume-body weight ratio. Am J Roentgenol 2008;190:1216–9.

25. Coakley FV, Lopoo JB, Lu Y, et al. Normal and hypoplastic fetal lungs: volumetric assessment with prenatal single-shot rapid acquisition with relaxation enhancement MR imaging. Radiology 2000;216:107–11.

26. Williams G, Coakley FV, Qayyum A, et al. Fetal relative lung volume: quantification by using prenatal MR imaging lung volumetry. Radiology 2004;233:457–62.

27. Cannie M, Jani JC, De Keyzer F, et al. Fetal body volume: use at MR imaging to quantify relative lung volume in fetuses suspected of having pulmonary hypoplasia. Radiology 2006;241:847–53.

28. Jani J, Cannie M, Sonigo P, et al. Value of prenatal magnetic resonance imaging in the prediction of postnatal outcome in fetuses with diaphragmatic hernia. Ultrasound Obstet Gynecol 2008;32:793–9.

29. Walsh DS, Hubbard AM, Olutoye OO, et al. Assessment of fetal lung volumes and liver herniation with magnetic resonance imaging in congenital diaphragmatic hernia. Am J Obstet Gynecol 2000;183:1067–9.

30. Cannie M, Jani J, Chaffiotte C, et al. Quantification of intrathoracic liver herniation by magnetic resonance imaging and prediction of postnatal survival in fetuses with congenital diaphragmatic hernia. Ultrasound Obstet Gynecol 2008;32: 627–32.

31. Cannie M, Jani J, Meersschaert J, et al. Prenatal prediction of survival in isolated diaphragmatic hernia using observed to expected total fetal lung volume determined by magnetic resonance imaging based on either gestational age or fetal body volume. Ultrasound Obstet Gynecol 2008;32:633–9.

32. Sokol J, Bohn D, Lacro RV, et al. Fetal pulmonary artery diameters and their association with lung hypoplasia and postnatal outcome in congenital diaphragmatic hernia. Am J Obstet Gynecol 2002;186:1085–90.

33. Sokol J, Shimizu N, Bohn D, et al. Fetal pulmonary artery diameter measurements as a predictor of morbidity in antenatally diagnosed congenital diaphragmatic hernia: a prospective study. Am J Obstet Gynecol 2006;195:470–7.

34. Ruano R, de Fatima Yukie Maeda M, Ikeda Niigaki J, et al. Pulmonary artery diameters in healthy fetuses from 19–40 weeks gestation. J Ultrasound Med 2007;26:309–16.

35. Ruano R, Aubry MC, Barthe B, et al. Quantitative analysis of pulmonary vasculature by 3D- power Doppler ultrasonography in isolated congenital diaphragmatic hernia. Am J Obstet Gynecol 2006;195:1720–8.

36. Moreno-Alvarez O, Hernandez-Andrade E, Oros D, et al. Association between intrapulmonary arterial Doppler parameters and degree of lung growth as measured by the lung-to-head ratio in fetuses with congenital diaphragmatic hernia. Ultrasound Obstet Gynecol 2008;31:164–70.

37. Broth RE, Wood DC, Rasanen J, et al. Prediction of lethal pulmonary hypoplasia: the hyperoxygenation test for pulmonary artery reactivity. Am J Obstet Gynecol 2002;187:940–5.

38. Doné E, Jani J, Van Schoubroeck D, et al. Maternal hyperoxygenation test in fetuses with prenatally treated severe diaphragmatic hernia: longitudinal observation study. Am J Obstet Gynecol 2006;195:45 (S21).

39. Moya FR, Lally KP. Evidence based management of infants with congenital diaphragmatic hernia. Semin Perinatol 2005;29:112–7.

40. Vitali A. Bench-to-bedside review: ventilator strategies to reduce lung injury—lessons from pediatric and neonatal intensive care. Crit Care 2005; 9:177–83.

41. Boloker J, Bateman D, Wung J, et al. Congenital diaphragmatic hernia in 120 infants treated consecutively with permissive hypercapnea/spontaneous respiration/elective repair. J Pediatr Surg 2002;37:357–66.

42. Logan JW, Cotten CM, Goldberg RN, et al. Mechanical ventilation strategies in the management of congenital diaphragmatic hernia. Semin Pediatr Surg 2007; 16:115–25.

43. Ng GY, Derry C, Marston L, et al. Reduction in ventilator-induced lung injury improves outcome in congenital diaphragmatic hernia? Pediatr Surg Int 2008; 24:145–50.

44. Kinsella J, Parker T, Dunbar I, et al. Noninvasive delivery of inhaled nitric oxide therapy for late pulmonary hypertension in newborn infants with congenital diaphragmatic hernia. J Pediatr 2003;142:397–401.

45. Clark RH, Kueser TJ, Walker MW, et al. Low-dose nitric oxide therapy for persistent pulmonary hypertension of the newborn. Clinical Inhaled Nitric Oxide Research Group. N Engl J Med 2000;342:469–74.

46. De Luca D, Zecca E, Vento G, et al. Transient effect of epoprostenol and sildenafil combined with iNO for pulmonary hypertension in congenital diaphragmatic hernia. Paediatr Anaesth 2006;16:597–8.

47. Kinsella J, Dunbar I, Abman S. Pulmonary vasodilator therapy in congenital diaphragmatic hernia: acute, late, and chronic pulmonary hypertension. Semin Perinatol 2005;29:123–8.

48. Inamura N, Kubota A, Nakajima T, et al. A proposal of new therapeutic strategy for antenatally diagnosed congenital diaphragmatic hernia. J Pediatr Surg 2005;40:1315–9.

49. Okuyama H, Kubota A, Oue T, et al. Inhaled nitric oxide with early surgery improves the outcome of antenatally diagnosed congenital diaphragmatic hernia. J Pediatr Surg 2002;37:1188–90.

50. Smith N, Jesudason E, Featherstone N, et al. Recent advances in congenital diaphragmatic hernia. Arch Dis Child 2005;90:426–8.

51. Migliazza L, Bellan C, Alberti D, et al. Retrospective study of 111 cases of congenital diaphragmatic hernia treated with early high-frequency oscillatory ventilation and presurgical stabilization. J Pediatr Surg 2007;42:1526–32.

52. Khan A, Lally K. The role of extracorporeal membrane oxygenation in the management of infants with congenital diaphragmatic hernia. Semin Perinatol 2005;29:118–22.

53. Boucherat O, Benachi A, Chailley-Heu B, et al. Surfactant maturation is not delayed in human fetuses with diaphragmatic hernia. PLoS Med 2007;4:e237.

54. Van Meurs K, Congenital Diaphragmatic Hernia Study Group. Is surfactant therapy beneficial in the treatment of the term newborn infant with congenital diaphragmatic hernia? J Pediatr 2004;145:312–6.

55. Colby C, Lally K, Hintz S, et al. Surfactant replacement therapy on ECMO does not improve outcome in neonates with congenital diaphragmatic hernia. J Pediatr Surg 2004;39:1632–7.

56. Tonks A, Wyldes M, Somerset DA, et al. Congenital malformations of the diaphragm: findings of the West Midlands Congenital Anomaly Register 1995 to 2000. Prenat Diagn 2004;24:596–604.

57. Gallot D, Boda C, Ughetto S, et al. Prenatal detection and outcome of congenital diaphragmatic hernia: a French registry-based study. Ultrasound Obstet Gynecol 2007;29:276–83.

58. Javid P, Jaksic T, Skarsgard E, et al, for the Canadian Neonatal Network. Survival rate in congenital diaphragmatic hernia: the experience of the Canadian Neonatal Network. J Pediatr Surg 2004;39:657–60.

59. Ontario Congenital Anomalies Study Group. Apparent truth about congenital diaphragmatic hernia: a population-based database is needed to establish benchmarking for clinical outcomes for CDH. J Pediatr Surg 2004;39:661–5.

60. Stege G, Fenton A, Jaffray B. Nihilism in the 1990s. The true mortality of CDH. Pediatrics 2003;112:532–5.

61. Gallot D, Coste K, Francannet C, et al. Antenatal detection and impact on outcome of congenital diaphragmatic hernia: a 12-year experience in Auvergne (France). Eur J Obstet Gynecol Reprod Biol 2005;125:202–5.

62. Colvin J, Bower C, Dickinson J, et al. Outcomes of congenital diaphragmatic hernia: a population-based study in Western Australia. Pediatrics 2005;116:356–63.

63. Bagolan P, Casaccia G, Crescenzi F, et al. Impact of a current treatment protocol on outcome of high-risk congenital diaphragmatic hernia. J Pediatr Surg 2004;39:313–8.

64. Downard C, Jaksic T, Garza JJ, et al. Analysis of an improved survival rate for congenital diaphragmatic hernia. J Pediatr Surg 2003;38:729–32.

65. Sartoris J, Varnholt V, Dahlheim D, et al. CDH in Mannheim—algorithm and results. Monatschr Kinderheilkd 2006;153:717.

66. Muratore C, Kharasch V, Lund D, et al. Pulmonary morbidity in 100 survivors of congenital diaphragmatic hernia monitored in a multidisciplinary clinic. J Pediatr Surg 2001;36:133–40.

67. West SD, Wilson JM. Follow up of infants with congenital diaphragmatic hernia. Semin Perinatol 2005;29:129–33.

68. Bagolan P, Morini F. Long-term follow up of infants with congenital diaphragmatic hernia. Semin Pediatr Surg 2007;16:134–44.
69. Lally KP, Engle W. Postdischarge follow-up of infants with congenital diaphragmatic hernia. Pediatrics 2008;121:627–32.
70. Harrison MR, Adzick NS, Flake AW, et al. Correction of congenital diaphragmatic hernia in utero. VI. Hard-earned lessons. J Pediatr Surg 1993;28:1411–7 [discussion: 1417–8].
71. DiFiore JW, Fauza DO, Slavin R, et al. Experimental fetal tracheal ligation reverses the structural and physiological effects of pulmonary hypoplasia in congenital diaphragmatic hernia. J Pediatr Surg 1994;29:248–56 [discussion: 256–7].
72. Nelson SC, Cameron AD, Deprest J. Fetoscopic surgery for in utero management of congenital diaphragmatic hernia. Fet Mat Medicine Rev 2006;17:69–104.
73. Khan PA, Cloutier M, Piedboeuf B. Tracheal occlusion: a review of obstructing fetal lungs to make them grow and mature. Am J Med Genet C Semin Med Genet 2007;145:125–38.
74. Nelson SM, Hajivassiliou CA, Haddock G, et al. Rescue of the hypoplastic lung by prenatal cyclical strain. Am J Respir Crit Care Med 2005;171:1395–402.
75. Flageole H, Evrard VA, Piedboeuf B, et al. The plug-unplug sequence: an important step to achieve type II pneumocyte maturation in the fetal lamb model. J Pediatr Surg 1998;33:299–303.
76. Flake AW, Crombleholme TM, Johnson MP, et al. Treatment of severe congenital diaphragmatic hernia by fetal tracheal occlusion: clinical experience with fifteen cases. Am J Obstet Gynecol 2000;183:1059–66.
77. Flageole H, Evrard V, Vandenberghe K, et al. Tracheoscopic tracheal occlusion in the ovine model: possible application in congenital diaphragmatic hernia. J Pediatr Surg 1997;32:1328–32.
78. Harrison MR, Sydorak RM, Farrell JA, et al. Fetoscopic temporary tracheal occlusion for congenital diaphragmatic hernia: prelude to a randomized, controlled trial. J Pediatr Surg 2003;38:1012–20.
79. Deprest J, Gratacos E, Nicolaides KH. Fetoscopic tracheal occlusion (FETO) for severe congenital diaphragmatic hernia: evolution of a technique and preliminary results. Ultrasound Obstet Gynecol 2004;24:121–6.
80. EuroSTEC. Available at: www.eurostec.eu. Accessed June 17, 2009.
81. Klaritsch P, Albert K, Van Mieghem T, et al. Instrumental requirements for minimal invasive fetal surgery. BJOG 2009;116:188–97.
82. Jani J, Gratacos E, Greenough A, et al. Percutaneous fetal endoscopic tracheal occlusion (FETO) for severe left-sided congenital diaphragmatic hernia. Clin Obstet Gynecol 2005;48:910–22.
83. Jani JC, Nicolaides KH, Gratacos E, et al. Fetal lung-to-head ratio in the prediction of survival in severe left-sided diaphragmatic hernia treated by fetal endoscopic tracheal occlusion (FETO). Am J Obstet Gynecol 2006;195:1646–50.
84. Peralta CF, Jani JC, Van Schoubroeck D, et al. Fetal lung volume after endoscopic tracheal occlusion in the prediction of postnatal outcome. Am J Obstet Gynecol 2008;198:60, e1–5.
85. Jani JC, Benachi A, Nicolaides KH, et al. (Antenatal-CDH-Registry group). Prenatal prediction of neonatal morbidity in survivors with congenital diaphragmatic hernia: a multicenter study. Ultrasound Obstet Gynecol 2009;33:64–9.
86. Willyard C. Tinkering within the womb: the future of fetal surgery. Nature Medicine 2008;14:1176–7.

87. Harrison MR, Keller RL, Hawgood SB, et al. A randomized trial of fetal endo-scopic tracheal occlusion for severe fetal congenital diaphragmatic hernia. N Engl J Med 2003;349:1916–24.
88. Deprest J, Jani J, Gratacos E, et al. Fetal intervention for congenital diaphrag-matic hernia: the European experience. Semin Perinatol 2005;29:94–103.
89. Cannie M, Jani J, Dekeyzer F, et al. Lung response to fetal tracheal occlusion is better prior to 29 weeks than after [abstract 554 SMFM 2008]. Am J Obstet Gynecol 2007;197:S161.
90. Keller R, Hawgood S, Neuhaus J, et al. Infant pulmonary function in a randomized trial of fetal tracheal occlusion for severe congenital diaphragmatic hernia. Pediatr Res 2004;56:818–25.
91. Deprest J, Jani J, Lewi L, et al. Fetoscopic surgery: encouraged by clinical expe-rience and boosted by instrument innovation. Semin Fetal Neonatal Med 2006;11: 398–412.

Tracheal Occlusion for Fetal Congenital Diaphragmatic Hernia: The US Experience

Eric Jelin, MD, Hanmin Lee, MD*

KEYWORDS

- Congenital diaphragmatic hernia • Fetal tracheal occlusion
- Fetal surgery • Lung hypoplasia • Pulmonary hypertension

Congenital diaphragmatic hernia (CDH) occurs in approximately 1 in 2400 live births[1] and is characterized by a defect in the diaphragm that permits abdominal viscera to herniate into the chest. These herniated viscera are thought to compress the growing lung and cause lung parenchymal and vascular hypoplasia. The genetic defects that cause the diaphragmatic defect may also contribute primarily to lung hypoplasia.[2] Postnatal reduction of the herniated abdominal viscera and correction of the diaphragmatic defect are easily achievable, but the lung hypoplasia persists, often leading to persistent fetal circulation and respiratory failure.

The severity of CDH is highly variable and seems to be related to the timing and amount of herniated viscera.[3] Some infants who have mild lung hypoplasia do well with advanced neonatal care, whereas those who have severe lung hypoplasia are often unsalvageable. Several prognostic indicators have been developed to determine where on the spectrum a fetus that has CDH lies, but the most reliable have been the presence or absence of liver herniation and sonographic estimation of the lung-to-head ratio (LHR). Fetal intervention for CDH in the United States originally gained interest because high-risk fetuses were found to have dismal prognoses. The aim of intervention was to promote lung growth in the fetus that had severe CDH before it was born to enhance postnatal survival. Open fetal repair of the diaphragmatic defect was successful in large animals but proved technically impossible in human fetuses with liver herniation into the chest. More recently, the strategy of temporary tracheal occlusion (TO) to induce lung growth was developed as a viable therapy for severe CDH.

Refinement of TO has been accompanied by improvements in postnatal therapy for CDH in the United States, and gentle ventilatory strategies have dramatically

Division of Pediatric Surgery, Department of Surgery, Fetal Treatment Center, University of California, San Francisco, 513 Parnassus Avenue, HSW-1601, San Francisco, CA 94143–0570, USA
* Corresponding author.
E-mail address: hanmin.lee@ucsfmedctr.org (H. Lee).

Clin Perinatol 36 (2009) 349–361
doi:10.1016/j.clp.2009.03.011
0095-5108/09/$ – see front matter © 2009 Elsevier Inc. All rights reserved.

increased survival for infants who have severe CDH. Thus far, TO has not been shown to improve survival or postnatal morbidity for fetuses that have CDH in the United States. This article reviews the experimental basis of fetal therapy for CDH and the US clinical experience with TO.

NATURAL HISTORY OF CONGENITAL DIAPHRAGMATIC HERNIA AND PRENATAL PROGNOSIS

A critical aspect in the development of fetal therapy for CDH has been to understand the natural history of the disease. Effective treatment can only be delivered in utero if patients who are likely to have poor outcomes can be identified. To understand the natural history of fetuses that have CDH better, the University of California, San Francisco (UCSF) conducted a prospective study of outcome in patients diagnosed with fetal CDH between 1989 and 1993. In that study, 83 fetuses that had isolated CDH (ie, no associated anomalies) identified before 24 weeks of gestation were followed prospectively.[4] The mortality rate in these patients was 58%. Of the 48 patients that did not survive, 7 died in utero and 16 died of respiratory distress before extracorporeal membranous oxygenation (ECMO) therapy could be initiated. The remaining nonsurvivors died despite ECMO support that lasted from 2 to 30 days.

The 42% survival rate in this study was considerably lower than that in previous studies from neonatal tertiary referral centers with ECMO therapy, which reported survival rates of 70% to 76%.[5,6] This discrepancy in survival has been attributed to the "hidden mortality" of prenatally diagnosed CDH. Without prenatal diagnosis, the cause of death in the fetuses that died in utero or shortly after birth would not have been attributed to CDH unless an autopsy had been performed. Studies that have examined outcomes in postnatally diagnosed CDH likely miss this subset of patients with early mortality, and therefore report inflated survival rates. The results of the UCSF study are not applicable to all patients who have prenatal CDH, however, because fetuses that were diagnosed with CDH after 24 weeks (all 10 survived) and fetuses with associated anomalies were excluded.[4]

An important finding of studies of prenatally and postnatally diagnosed CDH is that the clinical spectrum of the disease is broad. Some infants are minimally affected and do well with high-quality prenatal care, whereas other infants succumb to their disease despite all interventions. To select appropriate candidates for fetal intervention, the ability to determine where the fetus is on the clinical spectrum of severity is essential.

Several prenatal prognostic indicators have been associated with poor outcome, including early gestational age at diagnosis,[4] polyhydramnios,[7] presence of an intrathoracic stomach,[8,9] small lung/thorax area,[10,11] and underdevelopment of the left heart.[12] The most reliable and consistent prognostic indicators of outcome, however, have been the presence or absence of liver herniation ("liver-up" versus "liver-down" CDH) and the sonographic measurement of the LHR. Several studies have found an association between liver position and outcome, and the current survival rate for liver-up CDH is thought to be less than 50%.[13–17] The LHR is obtained by sonographically measuring the right lung area at the level of the cardiac atria (measured in square millimeters) and dividing that measurement by the head circumference (measured in millimeters). A recent retrospective multicenter analysis of the use of the LHR as a stratifying variable confirmed the utility of the LHR in fetuses with liver herniation into the chest.[14] One hundred eighty-four patients had ultrasound scans between 22 and 28 weeks of gestation at 10 centers (9 European centers and UCSF). This study demonstrated that the LHR only has utility when coupled with liver herniation into the chest and that a higher LHR in fetuses with liver herniation is associated with higher survival rates.

The validity of the LHR measurement as a prognostic indicator has been questioned by some. A recent retrospective study from Columbia University concluded that the fetal LHR was not related to outcome for prenatally diagnosed CDH.[18] There were several significant problems with that study, however. First, the conclusions of the study were not supported by the data: survival for an LHR less than 1.0 was 73% versus 94% for an LHR greater than 1.0. Although this difference was not statistically significant ($P = .114$), survival was more than 20% higher in the group with an LHR greater than 1.0. Second, it was a small study (n = 28), in addition to being the center's first experience with LHR evaluation. The LHR has been noted by many ultrasound experts to be a challenging measurement and one that requires validation by those experienced in its measurement. Third, the Columbia University investigators did not exclude patients without liver herniation. UCSF has previously reported that the LHR does not correlate with survival in patients without liver herniation[17]; regardless of the LHR, survival in this group is nearly 100% at UCSF. When patients without liver herniation are excluded from the Columbia University study's analysis (n = 12), survival drops to 75%. In their even smaller cohort of patients with liver herniation and an LHR less than 1.0 (n = 6), survival was 67%. Again, although this is not statistically significant, survival trends are lower when the LHR and liver herniation are incorporated into the analysis.

The emergence of liver position and the LHR as prognostic indicators for CDH has permitted targeting of fetal therapy to only those patients unlikely to survive without intervention. Patients without liver herniation have a favorable prognosis regardless of their LHR, with an overall survival rate of approximately 80%.[14] Prenatal intervention is thus not indicated in this group. For patients with liver herniation, overall survival is significantly decreased to approximately 50% and the LHR is useful in predicting outcome. For patients with liver up and an LHR greater than 1.4, survival is near 100%, and prenatal therapy is thus not indicated. Ideal therapy for patients with liver up and an LHR between 1.0 and 1.4 historically has been ambiguous because of the high morbidity of the intensive care techniques (prolonged intubation, high frequency ventilation, and ECMO) that are required in this population. Recently, advances in neonatal care strategies, most notably permissive hypercapnia, seem to have significantly increased survival and improved morbidity in this group.[19] These improved outcomes have led investigators in the United States to discontinue fetal therapy in this subset of patients.

For patients with liver up and an LHR less than 1.0, morbidity and mortality are high and may warrant experimental therapies, such as prenatal TO, to improve outcome. In this group, the LHR continues to be useful in predicting outcome and guiding therapy. In their recent analysis of the antenatal CDH registry, Jani and colleagues[14] found that survival in the group with an LHR from 0.8 to 0.9 was approximately 16%. They found 0% survival for fetuses with an LHR from 0.4 to 0.8 (n = 8). Unpublished data of a larger group of patients from UCSF indicate a survival rate of 25% for patients with an LHR less than 0.8 (n = 36).

REVERSING CONGENITAL DIAPHRAGMATIC HERNIA-INDUCED LUNG HYPOPLASIA

The first step in developing fetal therapy for CDH was to demonstrate that CDH-induced lung hypoplasia could be reversed in utero. In a landmark 1980 study, Harrison and colleagues[20] placed silicone rubber balloons in the thoracic cavity of fetal lambs during the third trimester. These balloons were progressively inflated to simulate the space-occupying lesion of herniated viscera. At delivery, these lambs (n = 4) developed severe respiratory distress and, despite maximal therapy, died within 2 hours. Pathologic examination of the lungs of these lambs revealed severe hypoplasia. To examine whether this process was reversible, balloons in another group of lambs that had been inflated were subsequently deflated after 20 days.[21] Five of these five lambs survived the neonatal period and had normal pulmonary function. Subsequent pathologic examination revealed that the lambs that had undergone "simulated repair" of CDH by balloon deflation had increased lung weight air capacity, compliance, and pulmonary vascularity when compared with controls that had not been deflated. This balloon model of CDH was limited, however, because, in vivo, the diaphragmatic defect is present in the first trimester.

To mimic human CDH better, another round of experiments in fetal lambs was conducted surgically to create a defect in the fetal lamb's diaphragm in the first trimester.[22] A cohort of the lambs underwent open fetal repair of the defect in the second trimester, whereas a control cohort was left unrepaired. The repaired cohort had significantly less lung hypoplasia when compared with the control cohort. The control cohort exhibited characteristic findings of CDH, including decreased lung vascularity and increased muscularity of the vascular bed.

OPEN REPAIR IN HUMANS

The success of large animal studies in demonstrating that CDH-induced lung hypoplasia could be reversed in utero led to fetal therapy for CDH in humans. Although neonates who had mild to moderate CDH were able to survive with intensive neonatal therapy, those who had severe CDH nearly always died. This group of neonates became candidates for the same kind of open repair that had been done in the lamb. The initial 1993 report of this experience, however, was disappointing; of the 14 attempted fetal repairs for isolated severe left CDH, only four fetuses survived beyond birth.[23] The key difficulty was the inability to reduce the herniated liver into the abdomen without kinking the umbilical vein and causing subsequent fetal demise. After this experience, investigators concluded that open fetal CDH repair was not technically feasible in the subgroup of fetuses with the worst prognosis, that is, those with liver herniation.

These early studies did show that open repair could be done successfully in fetuses without liver herniation, however. To test the efficacy of open fetal surgery in this subset of patients, a prospective trial was conducted and the results were published in 1997.[24] Eleven fetuses with liver-down CDH were recruited into the trial. Four underwent open fetal repair, and 7 were treated conventionally. Survival in the two groups was equivalent (75% in the surgery group and 86% in the conventional group), but gestational age at delivery was significantly decreased in the open fetal repair group (32 versus 38 weeks of gestation). Secondary outcome variables, including length of hospital stay, length of ventilatory support, and requirement for ECMO, did not differ between the two groups. The study reinforced the feasibility of open fetal CDH repair but failed to show improved outcomes for fetuses without liver herniation.

Overall survival in this study was substantially higher than that reported for CDH in general (75% and 86%, respectively, in the two groups versus 40% for fetal CDH in general).[4] Fetuses with liver down, however, have a much better prognosis those with liver up and demonstrate high rates of survival regardless of fetal intervention. The increased overall survival rates in this study highlight the importance of directing fetal intervention to the fetuses that stand to benefit the most (ie, those with liver herniation at high risk for severe pulmonary hypoplasia and death). Frustratingly, the results of nearly 2 decades of work up to this point exploring fetal therapy for CDH had demonstrated that open repair was only technically achievable in a subset of patients for whom the procedure was not beneficial.

TRACHEAL OCCLUSION: RATIONALE AND BASIC SCIENCE

The failure of open CDH repair in fetuses with liver herniation prompted exploration into alternative techniques to stimulate in utero lung growth. The reversibility of CDH-related lung hypoplasia had been established, but a technique to accomplish hypoplasia reversal safely in high-risk fetuses was lacking. The observations that fetuses with congenital high airway obstruction develop hyperplastic lungs and fetuses that have oligohydramnios develop hypoplastic lungs[25] led to the idea that TO could be used to stimulate lung growth in fetuses that had CDH. Fetal lungs actively secrete fluid, which escapes through the trachea and mixes with the amniotic fluid. Lung distention is maintained by a closed glottis and the dynamic relation between the pressure inside the lungs and in the amniotic cavity. By blocking the egress of lung fluid, TO attempts to mimic the situation observed in fetuses with congenital high airway obstruction and produces lung hyperplasia.[26–28]

To take advantage of TO-induced lung hyperplasia in infants who had CDH, the technique and its effects required extensive study. Several investigators once again turned to the fetal lamb model of surgically created CDH. These investigators found that TO in fetal lambs with surgically created CDH caused lung expansion, reduction of herniated viscera into the abdomen, and improved postnatal respiratory function.[28–30] Further work in large and small animals demonstrated that the increase in lung growth after TO results from greater numbers of alveoli and capillaries.[29,31,32] Moreover, the increased numbers of arterioles in fetal lungs after TO undergo significant remodeling and seem less prone to pulmonary hypertension.[33–37] TO, however, is not without negative consequences. Type II pneumocytes, which secrete surfactant, decrease in number after TO. Discontinuation of TO before birth may ameliorate this effect.[38–41] The underlying mechanism of TO remains elusive, but it seems that stretch within the lung induces mechanotransduction pathways that result in lung growth.[42–44]

TRACHEAL OCCLUSION IN HUMANS

After the efficacy of TO in animals was established, the strategy was applied to human fetuses that had severe isolated CDH and liver herniation (**Table 1**). Open repair had proved technically impossible, but the rationale for in utero intervention for severe CDH was still compelling. The first human interventions were performed at UCSF in 1996 through maternal laparotomy and hysterotomy, followed by fetal neck dissection and occlusion of the trachea with an internal plug or external clip.[45] In the first case, a water-impermeable foam plug was used and the fetus's lungs responded well. Removal of the plug was difficult, however, and the neonate developed tracheomalacia. A smaller gelatin-coated plug was used in the second case, but this smaller plug failed to induce lung hyperplasia and the patient did not survive. Subsequently, an approach using external clips was undertaken; however, this too failed because the clips could not be removed or were too leaky. The first true success came with use of two large opposing hemoclips with a suture attached to facilitate removal.

During the initial UCSF series, a special technique had to be developed to remove the tracheal occlusive device at birth and establish an airway. The typical technique for a cesarean section was modified to allow for extended maternofetal circulation so that an airway could be established while fetal gas exchange was still being performed by the placenta. During this procedure, which was named the ex utero intrapartum

Table 1
Summary of US experience with tracheal occlusion

Author	Harrison et al	Flake et al	Harrison et al	Harrison et al
Year	1998	2000	2001	2003
Study period	1994–1997	1995–1999	2000	1999–2001
Study design	Prospective case series	Prospective case series	Case report	Randomized controlled trial
Inclusion criteria	Left, liver up, LHR <1.4	Left, liver up, LHR <1.0 or right, liver up without left lung visualization	Right, liver up	Left, liver up, LHR <1.4
No. patients	21	15	2	11
TO method(s)	Open (13), FETENDO surgical clip (8)	Open	FETENDO surgical balloon	FETENDO surgical clip (2), FETENDO surgical balloon (9)
Survival (%)	Open 15%, FETENDO surgical clip 75%	33	100%	73%

treatment (EXIT) procedure, the mother is administered general anesthesia and a uterine relaxant. The fetal upper body is delivered through a hysterotomy leaving the lower body in the womb. A bronchoscope is then passed into the trachea to monitor in real time as the internal plug or external clip is dislodged and removed. If necessary, the trachea is then repaired. The last step is to secure the airway with an endotracheal tube or a tracheostomy.[46]

Overall results from this first series were discouraging. In the 13 fetuses that underwent open TO (liver up, average LHR: 1.1 ± 0.2), survival was 15%.[47] Survival was significantly higher, at 38%, in 13 comparable fetuses (liver up, average LHR: 1.1 ± 0.1) that received standard postnatal therapy. The average gestational age at delivery in the TO group was 30 ± 0.6 weeks compared with 37.5 ± 0.5 weeks in the control group. The low survival in this series was largely thought to be attributable to complications secondary to the evolution of the technique and to the preterm labor incurred from the large uterine incision.

A second series examining open TO was performed at the Children's Hospital of Pennsylvania and reported in 2000.[48] Fifteen fetuses with isolated liver-up CDH with an LHR less than 1.0 underwent open TO with two hemoclips in alternating directions. The first 9 patients underwent TO at 27 to 28 weeks of gestation, whereas the subsequent 6 underwent the procedure at 25 to 26 weeks of gestation. Delivery was performed by means of the EXIT procedure. Survival in this series was 30%. Causes of fetal and prenatal death included multiorgan failure after prolonged intensive care in 6 patients, preterm birth less than 1 week after TO in 2 patients, atrial perforation from a central line in 1 patient, and inadequate lung growth in 1 patient. An important finding in this study was that in contrast to the fetal lambs with surgically created CDH, TO in human fetuses that had CDH did not consistently improve lung function;

furthermore, the researchers note that even the enlarged lungs in the fetuses that survived were significantly functionally impaired.

MINIMALLY INVASIVE TRACHEAL OCCLUSION

The poor results with open TO seen in these first series led investigators at UCSF to pursue a less invasive approach. Advances in laparoscopy and endoscopy allowed investigators to perform TO successfully in the fetal lamb model using fetoscopy and miniaturized instruments (**Fig. 1**).[49] This innovation, the fetal endoscopic (FETENDO) surgical procedure, was then applied to fetuses with liver herniation and an LHR less than 1.4 between 1995 and 1998.[47] In the first few cases, several challenges were encountered, including variable placental location, a mobile fetus, tenuously attached fetal membranes, and a cramped fluid-filled operative field. These early challenges were incrementally overcome, but, initially, required conversion to an open procedure. In the later patients, successful FETENDO surgery was achieved by means of maternal laparotomy and sonographically guided insertion of trocars. The fetal trachea was then dissected fetoscopically, and a tracheal clip was placed. The EXIT procedure was used for delivery.

The results of this FETENDO surgical clip series were encouraging. Survival in the eight patients who successfully underwent the FETENDO surgical clip procedure was 75% compared with 38% in a comparable group of controls that did not undergo fetal intervention. Despite the success in this series, several new and unexpected problems emerged. Of the six survivors, two had vocal cord paralysis, and the expected decrease in preterm labor with a more minimally invasive approach was not seen. This finding that less invasive FETENDO surgery did not significantly reduce

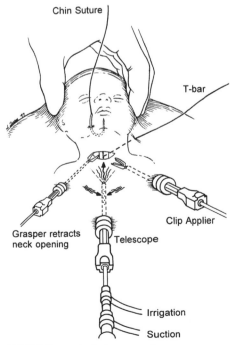

Fig. 1. Schematic of the FETENDO surgical clip procedure.

several important measures of maternal morbidity was confirmed in a large retrospective study at UCSF examining FETENDO versus open fetal surgery for all indications. The study found that although FETENDO surgery decreased the incidence of cesarean section (58.8% versus 94.8%), requirement for maternal intensive care unit stay (1.4% versus 26.4%), length of hospital stay (7.9 versus 11.9 days), and requirement for blood transfusion (2.9% versus 12.6%), there was no significant difference between the incidence of premature rupture of membranes, maternal pulmonary edema, placental abruption, or preterm delivery.[50]

The laryngeal nerve complications encountered in the FETENDO surgical clip series led to further attempts to make the TO procedure less invasive. Work with fetal lambs and ex vivo human tracheas demonstrated that a balloon designed to occlude cerebral aneurysms could also be used successfully to occlude the fetal trachea.[51–53] Advances in detachable balloon technology and the development of small continuous perfusion fetoscopes permitted these balloons to be inserted by means of one-port FETENDO surgery (**Fig. 2**).[54] Encouragingly, the FETENDO surgical balloon technique was found to be effective at stimulating lung growth without damaging the trachea.

A RANDOMIZED CONTROLLED TRIAL

The success of the FETENDO surgical clip series led to the design of a National Institutes of Health (NIH)-sponsored prospective randomized trial to compare endoscopic TO with standard postnatal therapy in fetuses that had severe CDH. The study was performed between 1999 and 2001, and inclusion criteria were the presence of isolated left-sided liver-up CDH with an LHR less than 1.4. The primary outcome measure was survival to 90 days of life. Secondary outcomes included need for ECMO, need for ventilatory support, and other measures of gastrointestinal and neurologic morbidity. The first two patients randomized to intervention in the trial underwent TO by means of the FETENDO surgical clip technique. Successful demonstration of the FETENDO surgical balloon technique[54] led to protocol modification to use this procedure for the rest of the trial. All fetuses were delivered by means of the EXIT procedure after TO.

Early results showed equivalent survival at 90 days between the TO and postnatal therapy groups (73% and 77%, respectively) and led to early cessation of the trial. In all, 11 patients underwent TO (2 by means of the FETENDO surgical clip and 9 by means of the FETENDO surgical balloon) and 13 were treated with standard postnatal care. The unexpectedly high survival in the control group was thought to reflect

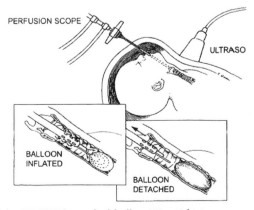

Fig. 2. Schematic of the FETENDO surgical balloon procedure.

advances in prenatal care, including permissive hypercapnia. Preterm birth was significantly increased in the TO group, with an average gestational age at delivery of 30.8 ± 2 weeks versus 37.0 ± 1.5 weeks in the control group. Secondary outcomes, including need for ECMO, chronic lung disease, hernia recurrence, gastroesophageal reflux disease, and growth retardation, did not differ between the two groups. Despite the dramatic differences in rates of preterm birth, the equivalent survival and postnatal morbidity seen in the two groups were argued to highlight the physiologic success of TO.

A criticism of the trial was that its inclusion criterion of an LHR less than 1.4 was too broad to uncover a survival benefit for TO. Outcomes for fetuses with an LHR between 1.0 and 1.4 had been variable, with some reports indicating relatively high survival. Subgroup analysis of the trial's results further reinforces this point. Survival for fetuses with an LHR greater than 1.06 in the TO and standard postnatal care groups was 100%. Conversely, survival in fetuses with an LHR less than 1.06 was not significantly different between the two groups. Of the 7 patients in the TO group with an LHR less than 1.06, 5 (71%) survived, and of the 11 patients in the control group, 8 (73%) survived.

EUROPEAN EXPERIENCE

The development of smaller fetoscopes and mounting experience with TO technique led Deprest and colleagues[51] to pioneer the strategy of completely percutaneous TO with reversal of the occlusion before delivery. The encouraging initial results from their work and the ongoing prospective trial are discussed in a separate article in this issue.

CURRENT STATE OF TRACHEAL OCCLUSION IN THE UNITED STATES

The European success with minimally invasive reversible TO has rekindled enthusiasm for TO in the United States. A US Food and Drug Administration (FDA)-approved trial to test percutaneous and reversible TO is underway at UCSF. The inclusion criteria for the trial are isolated CDH with liver up and an LHR less than 1.0. The aim is to recruit 20 patients so as to evaluate the feasibility, safety, and preliminary efficacy of the minimally invasive reversible TO procedure for severe CDH. A similar trial is being conducted at Brown University.

FUTURE DIRECTIONS FOR TRACHEAL OCCLUSION

The driving force in treatment for CDH over the past 20 years has been the advancement of neonatal ventilatory strategies to improve outcome. Although outcomes have indeed improved, there is still a subset of patients for whom mortality is extremely high. TO has matured significantly as a possible technique to treat this subset of patients. If centers in the United States are able to confirm the promising results in Europe, the next step is randomized control trials that directly compare percutaneous reversible TO in severely affected patients who have CDH with standard postnatal care.

Another important consideration for the future of TO is the postnatal morbidity of CDH. Fetuses that have severe CDH and survive the neonatal period are at high risk for chronic disorders, such as chronic lung disease, neurodevelopmental delay, gastroesophageal reflux disease, hearing loss, and failure to thrive.[55] Because survival has improved so dramatically with advanced neonatal care, the focus of TO may now shift to reducing postnatal morbidity. If the current trend, only seen in Europe thus far, toward decreased preterm birth after TO continues and can be replicated in the United States, TO may become a viable strategy for reducing the morbidity of severe CDH.

In terms of technical innovations for TO, several laboratories are investigating different modifications of the technique, including TO by ultrasound guidance alone,[56] TO with in-tracheal delivery of a rapidly polymerizing gel for balloon stabilization,[57] and TO with simultaneous surfactant or corticosteroid administration.[58] A more complete understanding of the molecular and cellular mechanisms of TO is also actively being pursued.

REFERENCES

1. Butler N, Claireaux AE. Congenital diaphragmatic hernia as a cause of perinatal mortality. Lancet 1962;1:659–63.
2. Guilbert TW, Gebb SA, Shannon JM. Lung hypoplasia in the nitrofen model of congenital diaphragmatic hernia occurs early in development. Am J Physiol Lung Cell Mol Physiol 2000;279:L1159–71.
3. Harrison MR. The unborn patient: the art and science of fetal therapy. 3rd edition. Philadelphia: WB Saunders; 2001. p. xv, 709.
4. Harrison MR, Adzick NS, Estes JM, et al. A prospective study of the outcome for fetuses with diaphragmatic hernia. JAMA 1994;271:382–4.
5. Sharland GK, Lockhart SM, Heward AJ, et al. Prognosis in fetal diaphragmatic hernia. Am J Obstet Gynecol 1992;166:9–13.
6. Adzick NS, Harrison MR, Glick PL, et al. Diaphragmatic hernia in the fetus: prenatal diagnosis and outcome in 94 cases. J Pediatr Surg 1985;20:357–61.
7. Stringer MD, Goldstein RB, Filly RA, et al. Fetal diaphragmatic hernia without visceral herniation. J Pediatr Surg 1995;30:1264–6.
8. Hatch EI Jr, Kendall J, Blumhagen J. Stomach position as an in utero predictor of neonatal outcome in left-sided diaphragmatic hernia. J Pediatr Surg 1992;27:778–9.
9. Burge DM, Atwell JD, Freeman NV. Could the stomach site help predict outcome in babies with left sided congenital diaphragmatic hernia diagnosed antenatally? J Pediatr Surg 1989;24:567–9.
10. Teixeira J, Sepulveda W, Hassan J, et al. Abdominal circumference in fetuses with congenital diaphragmatic hernia: correlation with hernia content and pregnancy outcome. J Ultrasound Med 1997;16:407–10.
11. Hasegawa T, Kamata S, Imura K, et al. Use of lung-thorax transverse area ratio in the antenatal evaluation of lung hypoplasia in congenital diaphragmatic hernia. J Clin Ultrasound 1990;18:705–9.
12. Crawford DC, Wright VM, Drake DP, et al. Fetal diaphragmatic hernia: the value of fetal echocardiography in the prediction of postnatal outcome. Br J Obstet Gynaecol 1989;96:705–10.
13. Metkus AP, Filly RA, Stringer MD, et al. Sonographic predictors of survival in fetal diaphragmatic hernia. J Pediatr Surg 1996;31:148–51.
14. Jani J, Keller RL, Benachi A, et al. Prenatal prediction of survival in isolated left-sided diaphragmatic hernia. Ultrasound Obstet Gynecol 2006;27:18–22.
15. Kitano Y, Nakagawa S, Kuroda T, et al. Liver position in fetal congenital diaphragmatic hernia retains a prognostic value in the era of lung-protective strategy. J Pediatr Surg 2005;40:1827–32.
16. Walsh DS, Hubbard AM, Olutoye OO, et al. Assessment of fetal lung volumes and liver herniation with magnetic resonance imaging in congenital diaphragmatic hernia. Am J Obstet Gynecol 2000;183:1067–9.

17. Albanese CT, Lopoo J, Goldstein RB, et al. Fetal liver position and perinatal outcome for congenital diaphragmatic hernia. Prenat Diagn 1998;18:1138–42.
18. Arkovitz MS, Russo M, Devine P, et al. Fetal lung-head ratio is not related to outcome for antenatal diagnosed congenital diaphragmatic hernia. J Pediatr Surg 2007;42:107–10.
19. Harrison MR, Sydorak RM, Farrell JA, et al. Fetoscopic temporary tracheal occlusion for congenital diaphragmatic hernia: prelude to a randomized, controlled trial. J Pediatr Surg 2003;38:1012–20.
20. Harrison MR, Jester JA, Ross NA. Correction of congenital diaphragmatic hernia in utero. I. The model: intrathoracic balloon produces fatal pulmonary hypoplasia. Surgery 1980;88:174–82.
21. Harrison MR, Bressack MA, Churg AM, et al. Correction of congenital diaphragmatic hernia in utero. II. Simulated correction permits fetal lung growth with survival at birth. Surgery 1980;88:260–8.
22. Adzick NS, Outwater KM, Harrison MR, et al. Correction of congenital diaphragmatic hernia in utero. IV. An early gestational fetal lamb model for pulmonary vascular morphometric analysis. J Pediatr Surg 1985;20:673–80.
23. Harrison MR, Adzick NS, Flake AW, et al. Correction of congenital diaphragmatic hernia in utero. VI. Hard-earned lessons. J Pediatr Surg 1993;28:1411–8.
24. Harrison MR, Adzick NS, Bullard KM, et al. Correction of congenital diaphragmatic hernia in utero. VII. A prospective trial. J Pediatr Surg 1997;32:1637–42.
25. Wilson JM, DiFiore JW, Peters CA. Experimental fetal tracheal ligation prevents the pulmonary hypoplasia associated with fetal nephrectomy: possible application for congenital diaphragmatic hernia. J Pediatr Surg 1993;28:1433–40.
26. Adzick NS, Harrison MR, Glick PL, et al. Experimental pulmonary hypoplasia and oligohydramnios: relative contributions of lung fluid and fetal breathing movements. J Pediatr Surg 1984;19:658–65.
27. Bealer JF, Skarsgard ED, Hedrick MH, et al. The 'PLUG' odyssey: adventures in experimental fetal tracheal occlusion. J Pediatr Surg 1995;30:361–5.
28. DiFiore JW, Fauza DO, Slavin R, et al. Experimental fetal tracheal ligation reverses the structural and physiological effects of pulmonary hypoplasia in congenital diaphragmatic hernia. J Pediatr Surg 1994;29:248–56.
29. Hedrick MH, Estes JM, Sullivan KM, et al. Plug the lung until it grows (PLUG): a new method to treat congenital diaphragmatic hernia in utero. J Pediatr Surg 1994;29:612–7.
30. Beierle EA, Langham MR Jr, Cassin S. In utero lung growth of fetal sheep with diaphragmatic hernia and tracheal stenosis. J Pediatr Surg 1996;31:141–7.
31. Kitano Y, Davies P, von Allmen D, et al. Fetal tracheal occlusion in the rat model of nitrofen-induced congenital diaphragmatic hernia. J Appl Physiol 1999;87:769–75.
32. Lipsett J, Cool JC, Runciman SI, et al. Effect of antenatal tracheal occlusion on lung development in the sheep model of congenital diaphragmatic hernia: a morphometric analysis of pulmonary structure and maturity. Pediatr Pulmonol 1998;25:257–69.
33. Roubliova XI, Verbeken EK, Wu J, et al. Effect of tracheal occlusion on peripheric pulmonary vessel muscularization in a fetal rabbit model for congenital diaphragmatic hernia. Am J Obstet Gynecol 2004;191:830–6.
34. Kanai M, Kitano Y, von Allmen D, et al. Fetal tracheal occlusion in the rat model of nitrofen-induced congenital diaphragmatic hernia: tracheal occlusion reverses the arterial structural abnormality. J Pediatr Surg 2001;36:839–45.

35. Luks FI, Wild YK, Piasecki GJ, et al. Short-term tracheal occlusion corrects pulmonary vascular anomalies in the fetal lamb with diaphragmatic hernia. Surgery 2000;128:266–72.
36. Sylvester KG, Rasanen J, Kitano Y, et al. Tracheal occlusion reverses the high impedance to flow in the fetal pulmonary circulation and normalizes its physiological response to oxygen at full term. J Pediatr Surg 1998;33:1071–5.
37. DiFiore JW, Fauza DO, Slavin R, et al. Experimental fetal tracheal ligation and congenital diaphragmatic hernia: a pulmonary vascular morphometric analysis. J Pediatr Surg 1995;30:917–23.
38. Piedboeuf B, Laberge JM, Ghitulescu G, et al. Deleterious effect of tracheal obstruction on type II pneumocytes in fetal sheep. Pediatr Res 1997;41: 473–9.
39. O'Toole SJ, Karamanoukian HL, Irish MS, et al. Tracheal ligation: the dark side of in utero congenital diaphragmatic hernia treatment. J Pediatr Surg 1997;32: 407–10.
40. Bin Saddiq W, Piedboeuf B, Laberge JM, et al. The effects of tracheal occlusion and release on type II pneumocytes in fetal lambs. J Pediatr Surg 1997;32:834–8.
41. O'Toole SJ, Sharma A, Karamanoukian HL, et al. Tracheal ligation does not correct the surfactant deficiency associated with congenital diaphragmatic hernia. J Pediatr Surg 1996;31:546–50.
42. Kitano Y, Von Allmen D, Kanai M, et al. Fetal lung growth after short-term tracheal occlusion is linearly related to intratracheal pressure. J Appl Physiol 2001;90:493–500.
43. Nardo L, Maritz G, Harding R, et al. Changes in lung structure and cellular division induced by tracheal obstruction in fetal sheep. Exp Lung Res 2000;26: 105–19.
44. Banes AJ, Tsuzaki M, Yamamoto J, et al. Mechanoreception at the cellular level: the detection, interpretation, and diversity of responses to mechanical signals. Biochem Cell Biol 1995;73:349–65.
45. Harrison MR, Adzick NS, Flake AW, et al. Correction of congenital diaphragmatic hernia in utero. VIII. Response of the hypoplastic lung to tracheal occlusion. J Pediatr Surg 1996;31:1339–48.
46. Mychaliska GB, Bealer JF, Graf JL, et al. Operating on placental support: the ex utero intrapartum treatment procedure. J Pediatr Surg 1997;32:227–30.
47. Harrison MR, Mychaliska GB, Albanese CT, et al. Correction of congenital diaphragmatic hernia in utero. IX. Fetuses with poor prognosis (liver herniation and low lung-to-head ratio) can be saved by fetoscopic temporary tracheal occlusion. J Pediatr Surg 1998;33:1017–22.
48. Flake AW, Crombleholme TM, Johnson MP, et al. Treatment of severe congenital diaphragmatic hernia by fetal tracheal occlusion: clinical experience with fifteen cases. Am J Obstet Gynecol 2000;183:1059–66.
49. VanderWall KJ, Bruch SW, Meuli M, et al. Fetal endoscopic ('FETENDO') tracheal clip. J Pediatr Surg 1996;31:1101–4.
50. Golombeck K, Ball RH, Lee H, et al. Maternal morbidity after maternal-fetal surgery. Am J Obstet Gynecol 2006;194:834–9.
51. Deprest J, Gratacos E, Nicolaides KH. Fetoscopic tracheal occlusion (FETO) for severe congenital diaphragmatic hernia: evolution of a technique and preliminary results. Ultrasound Obstet Gynecol 2004;24:121–6.
52. Flageole H, Evrard VA, Vandenberghe K, et al. Tracheoscopic endotracheal occlusion in the ovine model: technique and pulmonary effects. J Pediatr Surg 1997;32:1328–31.

53. Chiba T, Albanese CT, Farmer DL, et al. Balloon tracheal occlusion for congenital diaphragmatic hernia: experimental studies. J Pediatr Surg 2000;35:1566–70.
54. Harrison MR, Albanese CT, Hawgood SB, et al. Fetoscopic temporary tracheal occlusion by means of detachable balloon for congenital diaphragmatic hernia. Am J Obstet Gynecol 2001;185:730–3.
55. Cortes RA, Keller RL, Townsend T, et al. Survival of severe congenital diaphragmatic hernia has morbid consequences. J Pediatr Surg 2005;40:36–45.
56. David AL, Weisz B, Gregory L, et al. Ultrasound-guided injection and occlusion of the trachea in fetal sheep. Ultrasound Obstet Gynecol 2006;28:82–8.
57. Chang R, Komura M, Andreoli S, et al. Rapidly polymerizing hydrogel prevents balloon dislodgement in a model of fetal tracheal occlusion. J Pediatr Surg 2004;39:557–60.
58. Davey MG, Danzer E, Schwarz U, et al. Prenatal glucocorticoids and exogenous surfactant therapy improve respiratory function in lambs with severe diaphragmatic hernia following fetal tracheal occlusion. Pediatr Res 2006;60:131–5.

Management of Fetal Lung Lesions

N. Scott Adzick, MD*

KEYWORDS

- Fetal surgery • Congenital cystic adenomatoid malformation
- Bronchopulmonary sequestration

Prenatal diagnosis provides insight into the in utero evolution of fetal thoracic lesions such as congenital cystic adenomatoid malformation (CCAM), bronchopulmonary sequestration (BPS), congenital lobar emphysema, and mediastinal teratoma. Serial sonographic study of fetuses with thoracic lesions has helped define the natural history of these lesions, determine the pathophysiologic features that affect clinical outcome, and formulate management based on prognosis.[1–6] A decade ago, the author and colleagues reported a series of more than 175 prenatally diagnosed cases from the Children's Hospital of Philadelphia and the University of California, San Francisco,[7] and the author's clinical experience over the past 14 years at the Center for Fetal Diagnosis and Treatment at the Children's Hospital of Philadelphia now extends to more than 600 cases. The author has found that the overall prognosis depends on the size of the thoracic mass and the secondary physiologic derangement. A large mass causes mediastinal shift, hypoplasia of normal lung tissue, polyhydramnios, and cardiovascular compromise leading to fetal hydrops and death. Hydrops is a harbinger of fetal or neonatal demise, and manifests itself as fetal ascites, pleural and pericardial effusions, and skin and scalp edema.

Smaller thoracic lesions can cause respiratory distress in the newborn period, and the smallest masses may be asymptomatic until later in childhood when infection, pneumothorax, or malignant degeneration may occur. Large fetal lung tumors may regress in size on serial prenatal sonography, illustrating that improvement occasionally can occur during fetal life.[8–10] In particular, many noncystic bronchopulmonary sequestration dramatically decrease in size before birth and may not need treatment after birth.[7]

The finding that fetuses with hydrops are at very high risk for fetal or neonatal demise led the author and colleagues to perform either fetal surgical resection of the massively enlarged pulmonary lobe (fetal lobectomy) for cystic/solid lesions, or

Center for Fetal Diagnosis and Treatment, Children's Hospital of Philadelphia, 34th and Civic Center Boulevard, Philadelphia, PA 19104, USA
* Center for Fetal Diagnosis and Treatment, Children's Hospital of Philadelphia, 34th and Civic Center Boulevard, Philadelphia, PA 19104.
E-mail address: adzick@email.chop.edu

Clin Perinatol 36 (2009) 363–376
doi:10.1016/j.clp.2009.03.001
0095-5108/09/$ – see front matter
© 2009 Elsevier Inc. All rights reserved.

thoracoamniotic shunting for lung lesions with a dominant cyst.[7,11–13] Lesions with associated hydrops diagnosed late in gestation may benefit from resection using an ex utero intrapartum therapy (EXIT) approach.[14] Recognition of cystic mediastinal masses also may occur first on fetal ultrasound. The fetus that develops progressive nonimmune hydrops, cardiac failure, or mediastinal shift with compression of developing lung tissue may benefit from in utero decompression or resection of a cystic mediastinal lesion.[15] The fetus with a lung mass but without hydrops has an excellent chance for survival with maternal transport, planned delivery, and neonatal evaluation and surgery.

PRENATAL DIAGNOSIS AND NATURAL HISTORY

CCAM is characterized by an adenomatoid increase of terminal respiratory bronchioles that form cysts of various sizes. Grossly, a CCAM is a discrete, intrapulmonary mass that contains cysts ranging in diameter from less than 1 mm to over 10 cm. Histologically, CCAM is distinguished from other lesions and normal lung by:

Polypoid projections of the mucosa
An increase in smooth muscle and elastic tissue within cyst walls
An absence of cartilage (except that found in entrapped normal bronchi)
The presence of mucous secreting cells
The absence of inflammation

Although the tissue within these malformations does not function in normal gas exchange, there are connections with the tracheobronchial tree as evidenced by air trapping that can develop during postnatal resuscitative efforts. Cha has identified two histologic patterns of fetal CCAM, pseudoglandular and canalicular.[16] Stocker originally defined three types of CCAM (types 1 to 3) based primarily on cyst size.[17] The author and colleagues have classified prenatally diagnosed CCAM into two categories based on gross anatomy and ultrasound findings.[1] Macrocystic lesions contain single or multiple cysts that are 5 mm in diameter or larger on prenatal ultrasound, whereas microcystic lesions appear as a solid echogenic mass on sonography. CCAM usually arises from one lobe of the lung, and bilateral lung involvement is rare. The author and colleagues have learned that the overall prognosis depends primarily on the size of the CCAM rather than on the lesion type, and the underlying growth characteristics are likely to be important.[18]

Resected large fetal CCAM specimens demonstrate increased cell proliferation and markedly decreased apoptosis compared with gestational age-matched normal fetal lung tissue.[19] Examination of factors that enhance cell proliferation or down-regulate apoptosis in CCAM may provide further insights into the pathogenesis of this tumor and may suggest new therapeutic approaches. With regard to cell proliferation, the author and colleagues examined the role of pneumocyte mitogens like keratinocyte growth factor (KGF) and platelet-derived growth factor (PDGF) in rapidly growing fetal CCAMs. CCAM-like lesions occur in transgenic mice that overexpress KGF,[20] but the author and colleagues found no differences in the expression of KGF protein or KGF mRNA in CCAM and normal lung. In contrast, fetal CCAMs that grew rapidly, progressed to hydrops, and required in utero resection showed increased PDGF-B gene expression and PDGF-BB protein production compared with either normal fetal lung or term CCAM specimens.[21] Flake's group showed that transuterine ultrasound-guided microinjections of adenoviral vector encoding the rfgf10 transgene leads to FGF10 overexpression and consequent CCAM lesions in fetal rat lung. Remarkably, FGF10 overexpression in the proximal tracheobronchial tree during the pseudoglandular stage of rat lung development resulted in large cysts, whereas FGF10 overexpression in the distal lung parenchyma during the canalicular stage resulted in small cysts, and the lesions showed the pathologic spectrum of human CCAM. These findings support a role for FGF10 in the induction of human-like CCAMs.[22]

Bronchopulmonary sequestrations are masses of nonfunctioning lung tissue that are supplied by an anomalous systemic artery and do not have a bronchial connection to the native tracheobronchial tree. On prenatal ultrasonography, a BPS appears as a well-defined echodense, homogeneous mass. Detection by color flow Doppler of a systemic artery from the aorta to the fetal lung lesion is a pathognomonic feature of fetal BPS.[23] If this Doppler finding is not detected, however, then an echodense microcystic CCAM and a BPS can have an identical prenatal sonographic appearance. Ultrafast fetal MRI may help differentiate CCAM from BPS.[24] Furthermore, the author and others also have described prenatally diagnosed lung masses that display clinicopathologic features of both CCAM and sequestration—hybrid lesions—suggesting a shared embryologic basis for some of these lung masses.[25,26] The ability to differentiate intralobar and extralobar sequestration before birth is limited unless an extralobar sequestration is highlighted by a pleural effusion or is located in the abdomen. There are no diagnostic hallmarks for the specific prenatal diagnosis of an intralobar sequestration.

Congenital lobar emphysema can be distinguished prenatally from other cystic lung lesions on ultrasonography by increased echogenicity and reflectivity compared with a microcystic CCAM and the absence of systemic arterial blood supply compared with a BPS.[27] Progressive enlargement of these lesions before 28 weeks gestation may be caused by fetal lung fluid trapping in the lobe analogous to the air trapping seen postnatally. Late in gestation, lobar emphysema may regress in the size and the character of the mass, rendering it indistinguishable from adjacent normal fetal lung.[28] Postnatal assessment is important because of the risk of postnatal air trapping in the emphysematous lobe. At the time of birth, the affected lobe may be radio-opaque on chest radiography because of delayed clearance of fetal lung fluid. Prenatally diagnosed mainstem bronchial atresia results in massive lung enlargement, hydrops, and fetal death; ultrafast fetal MRI demonstrates that the entire lung is involved and that there are dilated bronchi distal to the mainstem atresia.[29]

Huge fetal lung lesions have reproducible pathophysiologic effects on the developing fetus. Esophageal compression by the thoracic mass causes interference with fetal swallowing of amniotic fluid and results in polyhydramnios. Polyhydramnios is a common obstetric indication for ultrasonography, so a prenatal diagnostic marker exists for many large fetal lung tumors. Support for this concept comes from the absence of fluid in the fetal stomach in some of these cases, and the alleviation of polyhydramnios after effective fetal treatment.[2] The hydrops is secondary to vena caval obstruction and cardiac compression from large tumors causing an extreme mediastinal shift. Like CCAMs, a fetal BPS also can cause fetal hydrops, either from the mass effect or from a tension hydrothorax that is the result of fluid or lymph secretion from the BPS.[7] Although there is some association of both polyhydramnios and hydrops with fetal lung lesions, the author's experience indicates that either can occur independently of the other.

Although sonographic prenatal diagnosis is becoming increasingly sophisticated, diagnostic errors are possible. Diaphragmatic hernia can be distinguished by careful sonographic assessment or by ultrafast MRI.[24] The author and others have experience with other fetal thoracic masses including bronchogenic and enteric cysts, mediastinal cystic teratoma, congenital lobar emphysema, hemangioma, and bronchial atresia.[30]

The author and colleagues have described two cases of intrathoracic gastric duplication cyst associated with hydrops that were treated with placement of a thoracoamniotic shunt.[31] Several years ago, the author had an unusual case of unilateral pulmonary agenesis in which the prenatal sonographic findings included a densely echogenic left lung mass with flattening of the left hemidiaphragm and a marked mediastinal shift to the right. A chest radiograph after birth revealed right-sided pulmonary agenesis and hyperinflation of the remaining left lung. A bronchoscopic evaluation demonstrated a long area of tracheobronchial stenosis to the solitary left lung. Retention of fetal lung fluid with overdistention of the left lung secondary to the high-grade airway obstruction during fetal life resulted in sonographic findings similar to those of a large microcystic CCAM.

Associated anomalies in the author's experience are very uncommon compared with some other reports.[2] This difference may reflect a referral bias of cases to the author's center for possible fetal or postnatal treatment, such that fetuses with associated anatomic anomalies may not be referred.

Although a large pulmonary lesion diagnosed in utero is an ominous finding, the natural history of prenatally diagnosed pulmonary lesions is variable. Approximately 15% of the author's CCAM lesions decreased in size during gestation, and most (68%) of BPS lesions shrank dramatically before birth. Several other groups also reported the involution of some pulmonary lesions,[4,5,8–10] although the mass is invariably detectable by chest CT scan after birth.[32] Although regression of a lung lesion and associated hydrops has been reported, this is a rare circumstance.[6,33]

The exact mechanism by which these lesions shrink is unclear. The masses that shrank in the author's series and in other reported cases were usually echodense lesions. The echogenic appearance on ultrasonography is caused by the large number of tissue–fluid interfaces. As the lung lesions decreased in size, they also became less echogenic, implying that they were losing fluid/tissue interfaces. CCAMs and sequestrations usually do not communicate directly with the tracheobronchial tree, although abnormal channels to the airway and the gastrointestinal tract have been reported. Perhaps the lesions shrink because of decompression of fetal lung fluid through these abnormal channels. Another possible explanation is that the pulmonary lesions outgrow their vascular supply and involute. Initial impressions concerning the prognosis of large pulmonary lesions should be tempered with the understanding that they can shrink in size or even disappear.

Recently, the author and colleagues determined CCAM volume by sonographic measurement using the formula for a prolate ellipse (length × height × width × 0.52). A cystic adenomatoid malformation volume ratio (CVR) was obtained by dividing the CCAM volume by head circumference to correct for fetal size. The author and colleagues found that a CVR greater than 1.6 is predictive of increased risk of hydrops, with 80% of these CCAM fetuses developing hydrops. The CVR may be useful in selecting fetuses at risk for hydrops, thus needing close ultrasound observation and possible fetal intervention.[34] By performing serial CVR measurements, the author learned that CCAM growth usually reaches a plateau by 28 weeks gestation. For fetuses at less than 28 weeks, the author recommends twice weekly ultrasound surveillance if the CVR is greater than 1.6, and initial weekly surveillance for fetuses with smaller CVR values.

THE EXPERIMENTAL BACKGROUND FOR CLINICAL FETAL SURGERY

Experimental studies have elucidated the pathophysiologic consequences of fetal intrathoracic masses and have demonstrated that fetal pulmonary resection is straightforward. Simulation of the thoracic mass effect with an intrathoracic balloon in the third trimester fetal lamb resulted in pulmonary hypoplasia and death at term because of respiratory insufficiency, whereas lambs that underwent simulated resection of the mass by balloon deflation in the middle of the third trimester had sufficient lung growth to permit survival at birth.[35,36] In addition, the author and colleagues have shown that intrauterine pneumonectomy in fetal lambs is technically feasible at early and midgestation and can induce compensatory growth of the remaining lung by term.[37]

Hydrops caused by large CCAM lesions has been attributed to direct mediastinal compression, obstruction of venous return, protein loss from the tumor, or unspecified humoral factors that increase capillary permeability. To study the etiology of hydrops associated with huge fetal lung masses, the author and colleagues created a fetal sheep model in which a surgically implanted intrathoracic tissue expander was inflated over several days while monitoring fetal arterial, venous, intrathoracic, and intra-amniotic pressures and while monitoring for sonographic indications of hydrops.[38] The author and colleagues found that balloon inflation resulted in hydrops as a result of cardiac venous obstruction and increasing central venous pressure. Simulation of prenatal resection of the fetal thoracic mass by deflating the expander resulted in complete resolution of the hydrops and return of pressures to normal.

Experiments in nonhuman primates led to the development of the necessary surgical, anesthetic, and tocolytic techniques before clinical use and have shown that fetal intervention is safe for the mother and her future reproductive potential.[39–41] The salvage of human fetuses with various serious birth defects by in utero intervention established a sound basis for open fetal surgery based on extensive animal studies.[42]

THE FETAL SURGERY EXPERIENCE: TAPS, SHUNTS, RESECTIONS, AND EX UTERO INTRAPARTUM THERAPY

Fetuses with life-threatening lung lesions were selected for prenatal treatment according to predetermined guidelines, including the gestational age of the fetus, the size of the intrathoracic lesion, maternal health, and the development of fetal hydrops. The finding that fetuses with large tumors and hydrops are at high risk for fetal or neonatal demise led to several therapeutic maneuvers. Fetal thoracentesis alone was ineffective for treatment because of rapid reaccumulation of cyst fluid.[43] In rare cases, the aspirated cyst does not reaccumulate fluid. Thoracentesis, however, usually serves as a temporizing maneuver before shunt placement or resection. It is possible that administration of a short course of maternal betamethasone may impair CCAM growth in some cases and lead to amelioration of hydrops, so the author and colleagues recommend this therapy for fetal CCAM cases with a CVR greater than 1.4.[44]

Catheter Shunt Placement

Thoracoamniotic shunting was performed in cases that had a large predominant cyst as long as there was not a large solid component to the CCAM (**Figs. 1** and **2**). Twenty years ago, Clark documented resolution of hydrops after 3 weeks of catheter drainage,[45] and successful shunt placement has been reported in several other cases of unilocular CCAM lesions.[2,5,46] Eleven years ago, the author's group reported the management of nine hydropic CCAM pregnancies using thoracoamniotic shunting.[47] The mean pre- and postshunting mass volumes were 46.3 and 18.1 cc respectively, representing a 61% mean reduction in mass volume following shunt placement. Hydrops resolved following shunting in all cases. Average shunt-to-delivery time was

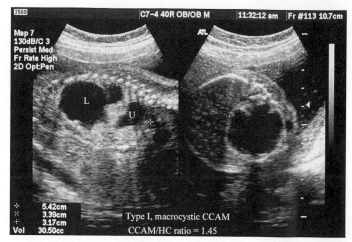

Fig. 1. Sonographic views of a 22-week gestation fetus with a congenital cystic adenomatoid malformation associated with ascites and polyhydramnios. Longitudinal view on the left shows two large cysts marked L (*lower*) and U (*upper*) that proved to communicate. Transverse view on the right shows the largest cyst. A thoracoamniotic shunt was placed.

13 weeks 2 days, and fetal or neonatal loss was 1 case out of 9. Five years ago, the author and colleagues reported 23 shunt cases with 17 survivors.[48] They also learned a gestational age of 20 weeks gestation or less at thoracoamniotic shunt placement may increase the risk of postnatal chest wall abnormalities.[49] Multicystic or predominantly solid CCAM lesions do not lend themselves to catheter decompression and require resection.

In 1998, the author and colleagues reported the treatment of three fetuses with a BPS and hydrops at 27, 29, and 30 weeks gestation.[7] The hydrops appeared to be a consequence of a tension hydrothorax from fluid or lymph secretion by the mass. The hydrops resolved after weekly fetal thoracenteses in one case and thoracoamniotic shunt placement in the two other cases. All three survived after delivery at 33 to 35 weeks gestation, required ventilatory support, and subsequently underwent BPS resection. Another fetus with sequestration, hydrops, and preterm labor

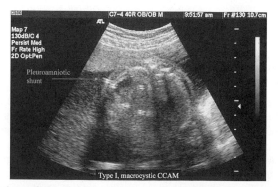

Fig. 2. Transverse view of the chest of the fetus shown in **Fig. 1.** A thoracoamniotic shunt (also known as a pleuroamniotic shunt) has been successfully placed percutaneously under sonographic guidance, resulting in complete decompression of the cysts in the fetal chest.

diagnosed at 34 weeks gestation was not treated prenatally, and this baby died from pulmonary hypoplasia despite postnatal resection and the use of extracorporeal membrane oxygenation (ECMO) for 3 weeks.

Open Fetal Surgery for Congenital Cystic Adenomatoid Malformation

For fetal surgery candidates, each family undergoes extensive discussion of the risks and benefits of fetal therapy for a lung tumor associated with hydrops. Fetal surgery candidates have a normal karyotype by amniocentesis or percutaneous umbilical blood sampling, and no other anatomic abnormalities are present on detailed sonographic and echocardiographic survey.[50] Fetal surgical techniques previously have been described in detail,[51] but in brief, indomethacin and antibiotics are given preoperatively. Isoflurane provides the necessary uterine relaxation and anesthesia for both mother and fetus, and a low transverse maternal laparotomy is performed. Sterile intraoperative sonography delineates both the fetal and placental position. The hysterotomy is facilitated by the placement of two large absorbable monofilament sutures parallel to the intended incision site and through the full-thickness of the uterine wall. A uterine stapler (US Surgical Corporation, Norwalk, Connecticut) with absorbable Lactomer staples[52] then is introduced directly through this point of fixation and into the amniotic cavity using a piercing attachment on the lower limb of the stapler. The stapler then is fired, thereby anchoring the amniotic membranes to the uterine wall and creating a hemostatic hysterotomy. The fetal chest is entered by a fifth intercostal space thoracotomy. Invariably, the lesion readily decompresses out through the thoracotomy wound consistent with increased intrathoracic pressure from the mass (**Fig. 3**). Using techniques developed in experimental animals, the appropriate pulmonary lobe(s) containing the lesion is resected.[7] The fetal thoracotomy is closed; the fetus is returned to the uterus. Warmed Ringer's lactate containing antibiotics is instilled into the amniotic cavity, and the uterine and abdominal incisions are closed in layers. Tocolysis with intravenous magnesium sulfate begins as the mother emerges from anesthesia. All fetal surgery mothers have a subsequent Cesarean delivery.

The knowledge that hydrops is highly predictive of fetal or neonatal demise led to fetal surgical resection of a massive multicystic or predominantly solid CCAM (fetal lobectomy) in 24 cases at 21 to 31 weeks gestation with 13 healthy survivors at 1 to

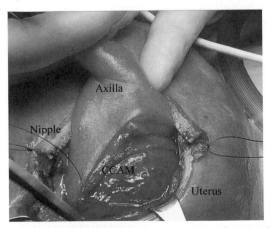

Fig. 3. Intraoperative photograph of a fetal surgical resection of congenital cystic adenomatoid malformation at 24 weeks gestation.

16 years follow-up. Resections involved a single lobectomy in 18 cases, right middle and lower lobectomies in four cases, extralobar BPS resection in one case, and one left pneumonectomy for CCAM. All cases had histologic confirmation of the diagnosis. In one multicystic case, a thoracoamniotic shunt failed to adequately decompress the mass effect before open fetal surgery. In the 13 fetuses that survived, fetal CCAM resection led to hydrops resolution in 1 to 2 weeks, return of the mediastinum to the midline within 3 weeks, and impressive in utero lung growth. Follow-up developmental testing has been normal in all survivors.

There were 11 fetal deaths in the fetal surgery resection cases. In the first case, the mother already had developed the maternal mirror syndrome.[53,54] The fetal operation was successful, and the hydrops improved. The placentomegaly and maternal hyperdynamic state remained, however, and the fetus was delivered 1 week later. In cases 6 and 16, 21-week gestation fetuses became bradycardic and died 8 and 12 hours postoperatively. Autopsy did not elucidate the cause of death in either case. In case 7, fetal death was caused by uncontrolled intraoperative uterine contractions, which hallmarks this limitation of fetal surgery. In case 18, postoperative chorioamnionitis 10 days postoperatively led to early delivery and neonatal demise. Finally, in six other cases, massive hydrops was present at 21 to 24 weeks gestation, and all fetuses died intraoperatively, usually after developing profound bradycardia after delivery of the mass from the fetal chest. The author and colleagues believe that mass delivery and abrupt removal of cardiac compression resulted in pathophysiology similar to relief of pericardial tamponade with fetal hemodynamic collapse and reactive bradycardia. As such, the author and colleagues have modified their approach before beginning the fetal operation. Prior to the fetal thoracotomy, the author and colleagues now obtain fetal intravenous access, check a fetal blood gas and hematocrit, and pretreat with intravenous atropine and fluid volume (usually warm, fresh blood). They also use fetal echocardiography on a routine basis for all fetal surgery cases regardless of lesion type to monitor fetal myocardial performance, particularly because maternal–fetal general anesthesia is a fetal myocardial depressant.[55]

With regard to maternal morbidity, there was one wound seroma and one wound infection that developed after cesarean delivery, and each required drainage. There were two maternal blood transfusions of packed red blood cells. Two cases of mild postoperative interstitial pulmonary edema responded to furosemide diuresis. There was one case of chorioamnionitis that led to neonatal death. In one case, a uterine wound dehiscence was evident at the time of cesarean delivery in each of her two subsequent pregnancies. Thirteen mothers have delivered normal babies by planned cesarean delivery subsequent to the fetal surgery pregnancy.

These results demonstrate that fetal CCAM resection is technically feasible, reasonably safe, reverses hydrops over 1 to 2 weeks, and allows sufficient lung growth to permit survival and normal postnatal development. The steep learning curve derived from the author's experience with more than 600 fetal surgery and fetoscopy cases for various fetal anomalies has provided invaluable lessons regarding optimal maternal anesthesia and uterine relaxation, hysterotomy and fetal exposure techniques, intraoperative fetal monitoring, and reliable methods for amniotic membrane and uterine closure.

In contrast, the unsuccessful fetal CCAM resection cases highlight remaining challenges. The author and colleagues learned in the first case that the maternal hyperdynamic state referred to as the mirror syndrome cannot be reversed solely by treatment of the underlying fetal condition. This preeclamptic state is associated with molar pregnancies and fetal conditions that cause placentomegaly, and may be caused by a factor released by poorly perfused placental tissue that leads to endothelial cell injury.[53,54] Until the pathophysiology of the maternal mirror syndrome is understood, earlier intervention before the onset of placentomegaly and the related maternal preeclamptic state may be the only approach to salvage these doomed fetuses. A subsequent case illustrated that placentomegaly can regress after fetal surgical CCAM resection if clinical signs of the maternal mirror syndrome are not present preoperatively.

The author's clinical focus has shifted from the technical details of the fetal surgical procedure to the crucial need for better postoperative maternal–fetal monitoring, reliable intraoperative fetal intravascular access for fetal blood sampling and infusions, and intraoperative fetal echocardiographic hemodynamic assessment. The detection and treatment of preterm labor remains the Achilles heel of fetal surgery. As a result of ongoing work in fetal animal models, the concept of a fetal intensive care unit with a specially trained cadre of physicians and nurses has become a clinical reality.

In the future, minimally invasive approaches to fetal lung lesions associated with hydrops may be possible. Laser therapy to fulgurate a fetal CCAM has been reported,[56,57] but the author believes that this approach is untenable given current technical limitations. For example, a mother carrying a 28-week gestation fetus with a large right-sided CCAM and hydrops was turned down for open fetal surgery by the author's group because of maternal psychosocial difficulties. She decided to seek YAG laser therapy at another medical center. Using a percutaneous technique under ultrasound guidance, a laser fiber was deployed in the fetal right chest, and the procedure was repeated twice during the next 4 weeks. After birth, the baby died from pulmonary hypoplasia and had a severely caved-in right chest with multiple rib fractures as a result of the prenatally applied laser energy. It is possible that laser therapy or techniques such as radiofrequency thermal ablation or sclerotherapy will be clinically useful for fetal lung lesions associated with fetal hydrops if the result is a decrease in mass effect, but experimental studies in animal models to rigorously test these techniques should be mandatory before clinical trials.[58]

The Ex Utero Intrapartum Therapy Procedure for High-Risk Fetal Lung Lesions

In clinical scenarios where the CVR continues to be large during the third trimester and it is anticipated that significant respiratory distress may be present at birth, the EXIT procedure is considered using placental bypass during the fetal thoracotomy and lobectomy. At the time of EXIT delivery, only the head, neck, and chest are delivered through the stapled hysterotomy (**Fig. 4**). The intrauterine volume is maintained with the lower fetal body and continuous amnioinfusion of warmed Ringer's lactate to prevent cord compression and hypothermia. Uterine relaxation is maintained by high concentration of inhalational anesthetics to preserve the utero–placental circulation and gas exchange between maternal, placental, and fetal compartments. The author and colleagues reported nine fetuses that underwent resection of fetal lung lesions during EXIT delivery.[14] The mean gestational age at EXIT delivery was 35.4 weeks. All lung masses remained large late in gestation, with a mean CVR of 2.5 at initial presentation and 2.2 at EXIT. Some of the nine fetuses demonstrated hydropic changes or polyhydramnios and had prenatal intervention including thoracentesis, thoracoamniotic shunt placement, amnioreduction, or maternal betamethasone administration. Eight of the nine neonates survived. The average time on placental bypass was 65 minutes. Postnatal complications included reoperation for air leak (n = 1) and death from bleeding and prematurity (n = 1). ECMO was used successfully in four neonates for persistent pulmonary hypertension. Maternal complications included polyhydramnios (n = 5), preterm labor (n = 4), and chorioamnionitis (n = 1). One mother required a perioperative blood transfusion. The author's total

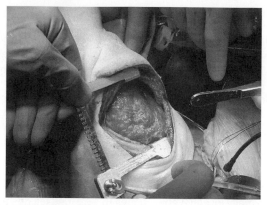

Fig. 4. Intraoperative photograph of a near-term resection of a large congenital cystic adenomatoid malformation during an ex utero intrapartum therapy (EXIT) procedure. The lower half of the fetus remains in the uterus, and the fetus remains connected to the maternal-placental-fetal circulation.

experience with 19 EXIT-to-lung lesion resections has confirmed that this approach allows for controlled resection of large fetal lung masses at delivery, avoiding acute respiratory decompensation related to mediastinal shift, air trapping, and compression of normal lung.

MANAGEMENT SUMMARY

The author and colleagues have learned from prenatal diagnosis that there is a wide spectrum of clinical severity for the fetus with a lung mass. Accurate prognostic information is necessary for providing appropriate management and parental counseling. If an associated life-threatening anomaly is present or if the mother is sick with the mirror syndrome, then the family may choose to terminate the pregnancy. If the fetus is not hydropic and an isolated fetal lung lesion is present, then the mother is followed by serial ultrasound, and arrangements are made for the best possible care after birth. Some CCAMs and many bronchopulmonary sequestrations will shrink in size, so it is important to try to differentiate these lesions using prenatal diagnostic criteria, although this is not always possible.[7]

All fetuses with fetal thoracic masses and without hydrops in the author's series survived in the setting of maternal transport, planned delivery, and postnatal evaluation at a facility with ECMO capability. Many of the babies with large lesions at the author's center required ventilatory support, and 10 babies needed treatment with extracorporeal membrane oxygenation. Interestingly, the author's impression is that these nonhydropic fetuses with lung masses have less lung hypoplasia and a much better prognosis than those with diaphragmatic hernia despite a similar degree of mediastinal shift as judged by prenatal sonography.

In asymptomatic neonates with a cystic lung lesion, the author and colleagues believe that elective resection is warranted because of the risks of infection and occult malignant transformation.[59–64] Malignancies consist mainly of pleuropulmonary blastoma in infants and young children, and bronchioloalveolar carcinoma in older children and adults. After confirmation of CCAM location by postnatal chest CT scan with intravenous contrast, the author and colleagues recommend elective resection at 1 month of age or older. This age has been chosen, because anesthetic risk in babies decreases after 4 weeks of age. An experienced pediatric surgeon can perform a lobectomy safely in infants with minimal morbidity by means of either a thoraco-scopic or muscle-sparing thoracotomy approach, with an average hospital stay of 3 days.[65] Early resection also maximizes compensatory lung growth. In contrast, the author and colleagues usually have followed patients with a tiny, asymptomatic, non-cystic EPS if they are confident of the diagnosis based on postnatal imaging studies. They do not favor the approach of catheterization and embolization for treating larger BPS lesions.

If the fetus is hydropic at presentation or if hydrops develops during serial follow-up, management depends upon the gestational age. For those hydropic fetuses greater than 32 weeks gestation, early delivery should be considered so that the lesion can be resected using an EXIT strategy with resection of the mass during the EXIT proce-dure. For those hydropic fetuses less than 32 weeks gestation, there is now an accepted therapeutic option—to treat the lesion before birth.

REFERENCES

1. Adzick NS, Harrison MR, Glick PL, et al. Fetal cystic adenomatoid malformation: prenatal diagnosis and natural history. J Pediatr Surg 1985;20:483–8.
2. Thorpe-Veeston JG, Nicolaides KH. Cystic adenomatoid malformation of the lung: prenatal diagnosis and outcome. Prenat Diagn 1994;14:677–88.
3. Sakala EP, Perrott WS, Grube GL. Sonographic characteristics of antenatally diagnosed extralobar pulmonary sequestration and congenital cystic adenoma-toid malformation. Obstet Gynecol Surv 1994;49:647–55.
4. Miller JA, Corteville JE, Langer JC. Congenital cystic adenomatoid malformation in the fetus: natural history and predictors of outcome. J Pediatr Surg 1996;31: 805–8.
5. Dommergues M, Louis-Sylvestre C, Mandelbrot L, et al. Congenital adenomatoid malformation of the lung: when is active fetal therapy indicated? Am J Obstet Gy-necol 1997;177:953–8.
6. Taguchi T, Suita S, Yamanouchi T. Antenatal diagnosis and surgical management of congenital cystic adenomatoid malformation of the lung. Fetal Diagn Ther 1995;10:400–7.
7. Adzick NS, Harrison MR, Crombleholme TM, et al. Fetal lung lesions: manage-ment and outcome. Am J Obstet Gynecol 1998;179:884–9.
8. Saltzman DH, Adzick NS, Benacerraf BR. Fetal cystic adenomatoid malformation of the lung: apparent improvement in utero. Obstet Gynecol 1988;71:1000–3.
9. MacGillivray TE, Harrison MR, Goldstein RB, et al. Disappearing fetal lung lesions. J Pediatr Surg 1993;28:1321–5.
10. Laberge JM, Flageole H, Pugash D. Outcome of the prenatally diagnosed congenital cystic adenomatoid lung malformation: a Canadian experience. Fetal Diagn Ther 2001;16:178–86.
11. Harrison MR, Adzick NS, Jennings RW, et al. Antenatal intervention for congenital cystic adenomatoid malformation. Lancet 1990;336:965–7.
12. Kuller JA, Yankowitz J, Goldberg JD, et al. Outcome of antenatally diagnosed cystic adenomatoid malformation. Am J Obstet Gynecol 1992;167:1038–41.
13. Adzick NS, Harrison MR, Flake AW, et al. Fetal surgery for cystic adenomatoid malformation of the lung. J Pediatr Surg 1993;28:806–12.
14. Hedrick HL, Flake AW, Crombleholme TM, et al. The ex utero intrapartum therapy (EXIT) procedure for high-risk fetal lung lesions. J Pediatr Surg 2005;40:1038–43.

15. Merchant AM, Hedrick HL, Crombleholme TM, et al. Management of fetal mediastinal teratoma: a report of two cases. J Pediatr Surg 2005;40:228–31.
16. Cha I, Adzick NS, Harrison MR, et al. Fetal congenital cystic adenomatoid malformations of the lung: a clinicopathologic study of eleven cases. Am J Surg Pathol 1997;21:537–44.
17. Stocker TJ, Manewell JE, Drake RM. Congenital cystic adenomatoid malformation of the lung: classification and morphologic spectrum. Hum Pathol 1977;8:155–71.
18. Krieger PA, Ruchelli ED, Mahboubi S, et al. Fetal pulmonary malformations: defining histopathology. Am J Surg Pathol 2005;30:643–9.
19. Cass DL, Yang EY, Liechty KW, et al. Increased cell proliferation and decreased apoptosis in congenital cystic adenomatoid malformation: insights into pathogenesis. Surg Forum 1997;47:659–61.
20. Simonet WS, DeRose ML, Bucay N. Pulmonary malformation in transgenic mice expressing keratinocyte growth factor in the lung. Proc Natl Acad Sci U S A 1995;92:12461–5.
21. Liechty KW, Quinn TM, Cass DL, et al. Elevated PDGF-B in congenital cystic adenomatoid malformations requiring fetal resection. J Pediatr Surg 1999;34: 805–10.
22. Gonzaga S, Henrique-Coelho T, Davey M, et al. Cystic adenomatoid malformations are induced by localized FGF10 overexpression in fetal rat lung. Am J Respir Cell Mol Biol 2008;39:346–55.
23. Hernanz-Schulman M, Stein SM, Neblett WW. Pulmonary sequestration: diagnosis with color Doppler sonography and a new theory of associated hydrothorax. Radiology 1991;180:817–21.
24. Quinn TM, Hubbard AM, Adzick NS. Prenatal magnetic resonance imaging enhances prenatal diagnosis. J Pediatr Surg 1998;33:312–6.
25. Cass DL, Crombleholme TM, Howell LJ, et al. Cystic lung lesions with systemic arterial blood supply: a hybrid of congenital cystic adenomatoid malformation and bronchopulmonary sequestration. J Pediatr Surg 1997;32:986–90.
26. Mackenzie TC, Guttenberg ME, Nissenbaum HL, et al. A fetal lung lesion consisting of bronchogenic cyst, bronchopulmonary sequestration, and congenital cystic adenomatoid malformation: the missing link? Fetal Diagn Ther 2001;16:193–5.
27. Ankermann T, Oppermann HC, Engler S, et al. Congenital masses of the lung, cystic adenomatoid malformation versus congenital lobar emphysema. J Ultrasound Med 2004;23:1379–84.
28. Olutoye O, Coleman B, Hubbard AM, et al. Prenatal diagnosis and management of congenital lobar emphysema. J Pediatr Surg 2000;35:792–5.
29. Keswani SG, Crombleholme TM, Johnson MP, et al. The prenatal diagnosis and management of mainstem bronchial atresia. Fetal Diagn Ther 2005;20:74–8.
30. Albright EB, Crane JP, Shackelford GD. Prenatal diagnosis of a bronchogenic cyst. J Ultrasound Med 1988;7:91–5.
31. Ferro MM, Milner R, Cannizzaro C, et al. Intrathoracic alimentary tract duplication cysts treated in utero by thoracoamniotic shunting. Fetal Diagn Ther 1998;13: 343–7.
32. Winters WD, Effmann EL, Nghiem HV. Disappearing fetal lung masses: importance of postnatal imaging studies. Pediatr Radiol 1997;27:535–9.
33. daSilva OP, Ramanan R, Romano W. Nonimmune hydrops fetalis, pulmonary sequestration, and favorable neonatal outcome. Obstet Gynecol 1996;88:681–3.
34. Crombleholme TM, Coleman BG, Howell LJ, et al. Elevated cystic adenomatoid malformation volume ratio (CVR) predicts outcome in prenatal diagnosis of cystic adenomatoid malformation of the lung. J Pediatr Surg 2002;37:331–8.

35. Harrison MR, Jester JA, Ross NA. Correction of congenital diaphragmatic hernia in utero I. The model: intrathoracic balloon produces fatal pulmonary hypoplasia. Surgery 1980;88:174–80.

36. Harrison MR, Bressack MA, Churg AM. Correction of congenital diaphragmatic hernia in utero II. Simulated correction permits fetal lung growth with survival at birth. Surgery 1980;88:260–8.

37. Adzick NS, Harrison MR, Hu LM, et al. Compensatory growth after pneumonectomy in fetal lambs: a morphologic study. Surg Forum 1986;37:309–11.

38. Rice HE, Estes JM, Hedrick MH, et al. Congenital cystic adenomatoid malformation: a sheep model. J Pediatr Surg 1994;29:692–6.

39. Harrison MR, Anderson J, Rosen MA. Fetal surgery in the primate I. Anesthetic, surgical, and tocolytic management to maximize fetal–neonatal survival. J Pediatr Surg 1982;17:115–22.

40. Nakayama DK, Harrison MR, Seron-Ferre M. Fetal surgery in the primate II. Uterine electromyographic response to operative procedure and pharmacologic agents. J Pediatr Surg 1984;19:333–9.

41. Adzick NS, Harrison MR, Anderson JV, et al. Fetal surgery in the primate III. Maternal outcome after fetal surgery. J Pediatr Surg 1986;21:477–80.

42. Adzick NS, Nance ML. Medical progress: pediatric surgery. N Engl J Med 2000; 342:1651–7, 1726–32.

43. Chao A, Monoson RF. Neonatal death despite fetal therapy for cystic adenomatoid malformation. J Reprod Med 1990;35:655–7.

44. Peranteau WH, Wilson W, Liechty KW, et al. The effect of maternal betamethasone on prenatal congenital cystic adenomatoid malformation growth and fetal survival. Fetal Diagn Ther 2005;20:74–8.

45. Clark SL, Vitale DJ, Minton SD, et al. Successful fetal therapy for cystic adenomatoid malformation associated with second trimester hydrops. Am J Obstet Gynecol 1987;157:294–7.

46. Bernaschek G, Deutinger J, Hansmann M, et al. Feto–amniotic shunting: report of the experience of four European centres. Prenat Diagn 1994;14:821–33.

47. Baxter JK, Johnson MP, Wilson RD, et al. Thoracoamniotic shunts: pregnancy outcome for congenital cystic adenomatoid malformation and pleural effusion. Am J Obstet Gynecol 1998;185:S245.

48. Wilson RD, Baxter JK, Johnson MP, et al. Thoracoamniotic shunts: fetal treatment of pleural effusions and congenital cystic adenomatoid malformations. Fetal Diagn Ther 2004;19:413–20.

49. Merchant AM, Peranteau WH, Wilson RD, et al. Postnatal chest wall deformities after fetal thoracoamniotic shunting for congenital cystic adenomatoid malformation. Fetal Diagn Ther 2007;22:365–71.

50. Mahle WT, Rychik J, Tian ZY, et al. Echocardiographic evaluation of the fetus with congenital cystic adenomatoid malformation. Ultrasound Obstet Gynecol 2000; 16:620–4.

51. Adzick NS, Harrison MR. Fetal surgical techniques. Semin Pediatr Surg 1993;2: 136–42.

52. Adzick NS, Harrison MR, Flake AW. Automatic uterine stapling devices in fetal operation: experience in a primate model. Surg Forum 1985;36:479–80.

53. Creasy R. Mirror syndromes. In: Goodlin RC, editor. Care of the fetus. New York: Masson; 1979. p. 48–50.

54. Langer JC, Harrison MR, Schmidt KG. Fetal hydrops and death from sacrococcygeal teratoma: rationale for fetal surgery. Am J Obstet Gynecol 1989;160: 1145–50.

55. Rychik J, Tian Z, Ewing S, et al. Acute cardiovascular effects of fetal surgery in the human. Circulation 2004;110:1549–56.
56. Fortunato S, Lombardo S, Dantrell J, et al. Intrauterine laser ablation of a fetal cystic adenomatoid malformation with hydrops: the application of minimally invasive surgical techniques to fetal surgery. Am J Obstet Gynecol 1997;177:S84.
57. Bruner JP, Jarnagin BK, Reinisch L. Percutaneous laser ablation of fetal congenital cystic adenomatoid malformation: too little, too late? Fetal Diagn Ther 2000; 15:359–63.
58. Milner R, Kitano Y, Olutoye O, et al. Radiofrequency thermal ablation (RTA): a potential treatment for hydropic fetuses with a large chest mass. J Pediatr Surg 2000;35:386–9.
59. Miniati DN, Chintaqumpala M, Langston C, et al. Prenatal presentation and outcome of children with pleuropulmonary blastoma. J Pediatr Surg 2006;41: 66–71.
60. Benjamin DR, Cahill JL. Bronchoalveolar carcinoma of the lung and congenital cystic adenomatoid malformation. Am J Clin Pathol 1991;95:889–92.
61. Murphy JJ, Blair GK, Fraser GC. Rhabdomyosarcoma arising within congenital pulmonary cysts: report of three cases. J Pediatr Surg 1992;27:1364–7.
62. d'Agnostino S, Bonoldi E, Dante S, et al. Embryonal rhabdomyosarcoma of the lung arising in cystic adenomatoid malformation. J Pediatr Surg 1997;32:1381–3.
63. Ribet ME, Copin MC, Soots JG, et al. Bronchioloalveolar carcinoma and congenital cystic adenomatoid malformation. Ann Thorac Surg 1995;60:1126–8.
64. Granata C, Gambini C, Balducci T, et al. Bronchioloalveolar carcinoma arising in a congenital cystic adenomatoid malformation in a child: case report and review of the literature. Pediatr Pulmonol 1996;25:62–6.
65. Tsai AY, Liechty KW, Hedrick HL, et al. Outcomes following postnatal resection of prenatally diagnosed asymptomatic cystic lung lesions. J Pediatr Surg 2008;43: 513–7.

Fetal Lower Urinary Tract Obstruction

Serena Wu, MD[a], Mark Paul Johnson, MD[b,c,d],*

KEYWORDS

- Obstructive uropathy • Lower urinary tract obstruction
- Antenatal diagnosis and management
- Fetal surgery/intervention • Bladder shunt

Prenatal ultrasonography often identifies fetal urinary tract anomalies, with detection possible as early as 12 to 14 weeks of gestation. Obstructive abnormalities of the urinary tract are common and observed in approximately 1% of pregnancies. Fortunately, most of these have little clinical significance, and only approximately 1 in 500 pregnancies is complicated by significant fetal urologic malformations. The challenge, however, is prenatal identification and development of a coordinated prenatal and postnatal management plan directed at optimizing clinical outcomes in cases with potential postnatal morbidity and mortality. This article focuses on the causes and consequences of lower urinary tract (urethral) obstructions (LUTOs).

EARLY EXPERIMENTAL MODELS
Natural History of Obstructive Uropathy

The natural history of obstructive uropathy is highly variable and depends on gender, severity, duration, and age of onset of the obstruction. Complete obstruction of the urethra early in gestation can lead to massive distention of the bladder, hydroureteronephrosis, and renal fibrocystic dysplasia. Inability of the urine to enter

---

[a] General Surgery, The Center for Fetal Diagnosis and Treatment, The Children's Hospital of Philadelphia, Philadelphia, 34th and Civic Center Boulevard, Philadelphia, PA 19104, USA
[b] Department of Obstetrics and Gynecology, University of Pennsylvania School of Medicine, The Center for Fetal Diagnosis and Treatment, The Children's Hospital of Philadelphia, 34th and Civic Center Boulevard, Philadelphia, PA 19104, USA
[c] Department of Surgery, University of Pennsylvania School of Medicine, The Center for Fetal Diagnosis and Treatment, The Children's Hospital of Philadelphia, 34th and Civic Center Boulevard, Philadelphia, PA 19104, USA
[d] Department of Pediatrics, University of Pennsylvania School of Medicine, The Center for Fetal Diagnosis and Treatment, The Children's Hospital of Philadelphia, 34th and Civic Center Boulevard, Philadelphia, PA 19104, USA
* Corresponding author. Department of Obstetrics and Gynecology, University of Pennsylvania School of Medicine, The Center for Fetal Diagnosis and Treatment, The Children's Hospital of Philadelphia, 34th and Civic Center Boulevard, Philadelphia, PA 19104.
E-mail address: johnsonm@email.chop.edu (M.P. Johnson).

Clin Perinatol 36 (2009) 377–390
doi:10.1016/j.clp.2009.03.010
0095-5108/09/$ – see front matter © 2009 Elsevier Inc. All rights reserved.

perinatology.theclinics.com

the amniotic space results in oligohydramnios, leading to pulmonary hypoplasia and secondary deformations of the face and extremities. Outcome is measured in terms of postnatal survival and depends on two factors: pulmonary development and renal function. Of these, pulmonary development may be the more critical for neonatal survival.

Pulmonary hypoplasia and prematurity are the leading causes of mortality in obstructive uropathy. In cases of posterior urethral valves (PUVs), there is a 45% mortality rate that can be directly attributed to pulmonary insufficiency.[1] This high mortality is generally not reflected in postnatal urologic series of lower urinary tract obstruction (LUTO); it represents the "hidden mortality" of this disorder, because these infants do not survive for transfer to a pediatric specialty center for treatment. Early midgestation oligohydramnios carries a poor prognosis for the fetus, and when associated with urethral obstruction, the mortality rate has been estimated to be as high as 95%.[2,3] Therefore, fetuses with oligohydramnios and LUTO represent the most severe end of the obstructive uropathy spectrum and are at highest risk for pulmonary hypoplasia and renal dysplasia.

A sheep model of surgically created urinary tract obstruction reflecting the pathophysiology observed in human fetuses was developed in the early 1980s.[4,5] The effects of ureteral ligation at 62 to 84 days of gestation (total gestation period in sheep is 144 days) on renal histologic findings were found to depend on when in gestation the ureteral obstruction occurred. Using a combination of urachal ligation and gradual occlusion of the urethra, pulmonary hypoplasia, bladder dilatation, hydroureters, and hydronephrosis resulted. This model produced histologic changes in the kidneys similar to those seen in humans, with increased fibrosis throughout the kidney, although no parenchymal disorganization or cysts were observed, which are frequent findings in humans. A sheep model was then developed to determine if in utero decompression was beneficial.[6] Urethral obstruction was established at 95 days, after which half of the animals underwent suprapubic cystostomy after 15 to 27 days of obstruction, allowing urine to flow freely from the obstructed fetal bladder. Cystostomy resulted in universal survival with minimal need for respiratory support, in contrast to high mortality and need for maximal respiratory support in the first 24 hours of life in those without decompression. These studies demonstrated that restoration of amniotic fluid volume (AFV) resulted in improved lung growth and pulmonary survival. All lambs that had undergone cystostomy had mildly dilated urinary tracts and minimal histologic renal parenchymal damage. Although no evidence of cystic dysplasia was observed, fibrosis was prominent throughout the kidneys of lambs that had not been decompressed.

Renal cystic dysplasia and disorganized architecture similar to those occurring in humans was produced in the sheep model when ureteral ligation was performed earlier in gestation (58–66 days of gestation). Fibrosis and parenchymal disorganization were present, and the medullary region contained abnormal-appearing ducts.[6] To determine whether in utero relief of obstruction would prevent renal dysplasia, unilateral ureteral obstruction at 58 to 66 days of gestation was performed, followed by end-ureterostomy to relieve obstruction at 20, 40, and 60 days after obstruction. Duration of obstruction was directly related to the likelihood of deterioration in renal function and occurrence of histologic change. Decompression, regardless of timing, improved histologic findings and function compared with controls that had not been decompressed, however, and provided evidence that in utero decompression of early obstruction could arrest histologic changes, prevent severe dysplastic damage, and potentially preserve renal function.

Experimental Studies for Evaluating Fetal Renal Function

Prenatal clinical determination of renal injury in obstructive uropathy has been problematic.[7–10] Several studies have assessed the predictive value of the sonographic appearance of the fetal kidneys as an indicator of damage. Such observational impressions lack the sensitivity and specificity for accurate correlation with renal function, however.[11–13] As renal function deteriorates, urine production diminishes and is reflected by a decline in AFV. Quantitative assessment of AFV alone is a poor measure of renal function, however, because renal dysplasia may already be irreversibly established by the time oligohydramnios is sonographically detected.[8,14]

Appropriate prenatal management in human fetuses would depend on the ability to determine the presence and extent of functional damage in the kidneys reliably so as to select those that might benefit from intervention to prevent further progressive damage. Severe oligohydramnios early in gestation, in addition to increased echogenicity and the presence of discrete parenchymal cysts, correlates with advanced renal damage.[12,15] Mild to moderate decreases in AFV and subtle renal parenchymal change on ultrasound are less reliable in predicting renal function and extent of damage, however. Therefore, a simple and safe method of reliably determining the degree of renal damage was required. The first useful approach was based on the review of electrolyte patterns from fetal urine obtained during clinical evaluation of obstructive uropathies. The University of California, San Francisco group reviewed data from 20 human fetuses and categorized outcomes as "poor function" (n = 10) or "good function" (n = 10) based on renal histologic findings at autopsy or biopsy or on renal and pulmonary function at birth.[16] Groups were compared for (1) amniotic fluid status at initial presentation, (2) ultrasound appearance of the kidney, (3) electrolyte composition of fetal urine obtained by vesicocentesis, and (4) fetal urine output. Fetuses categorized with poor function were found to have moderate to severely decreased AFV, echogenic or cystic kidneys on ultrasound, urine outputs less than 2 mL/h, sodium concentrations greater than 100 mEq/L, chloride concentrations greater than 90 mEq/L, and osmolality levels greater than 210 mOsm/L. Those fetuses grouped as having good function had normal to moderately decreased AFV, normal to mildly echogenic renal parenchyma, urine output greater than 2 mL/h, sodium concentrations less than 100 mEq/L, chloride concentrations less than 90 mEq/L, and osmolality values less than 210 mOsm/L. Numerous subsequent clinical series have supported and refined these predictive criteria, and evaluation of urinary components has continued to evolve, with the addition of other markers, such as urinary calcium, β_2-microglobulin, and total protein. Recently, there has been investigational interest in fetal cystatin-C in amniotic fluid as another biochemical marker for early identification of obstructive uropathies and postnatal renal function prediction.[17] Cystatin-C is a protein synthesized steadily and continuously by all nucleated cells that does not vary with gestational age and does not cross the placenta.[18] Although promising, its use as a prognostic tool is undetermined. Currently, there is a randomized trial underway that is evaluating these biochemical markers for correlation with postnatal renal function (percutaneous lower urinary tract obstruction [PLUTO]).[19] Finally, use of serial urine aspirations to document change in tonicity after repeated bladder drainage has significantly improved the predictive value and helped to select fetuses that would benefit from in utero treatment.[20]

LOWER URINARY TRACT ANOMALIES

LUTO generally involves developmental abnormalities of the penile urethra in male fetuses, with PUVs and urethral atresia being the most common causes for early-onset

LUTO. Other urethral anomalies, such as anterior urethral valves, meatal stenosis, and a narrow hypoplastic midurethra, have also been associated with LUTO. The typical prenatal sonographic features of LUTO include an enlarged fetal bladder, bilateral hydronephrosis, and decreased AFV. Normal AFV would indicate the absence of complete urethral obstruction and is more consistent with the diagnosis of urethral stricture, midurethral hypoplasia, or "incomplete" PUV. LUTO in female fetuses is generally associated with cloacal developmental abnormalities and is normally a component of syndromic conditions for which prenatal therapy has not been shown to be beneficial.[21] Finally, there are several genetic causes, such as megacystis-microcolon syndrome, megacystis-megaureter syndrome, and chromosomal aneuploidy (trisomy 21 and 18), that are associated with LUTOs. It is the heterogeneity of underlying causes that has made the prenatal evaluation and treatment of LUTO a challenge and has resulted in the highly variable renal outcomes reported for prenatal treatment of these disorders. It was not until recently that a stepwise algorithm for the prenatal evaluation and selection of fetuses for treatment was established. By following these guidelines, however, patient selection and predictive precision have improved in the evaluation of existing fetal renal function.[22]

Histologic Changes Associated with Lower Urinary Tract Obstruction

Complete urethral obstruction or significant restriction of urethral flow results in accumulation of urine within the fetal bladder, leading to marked distention. Prolonged obstruction results in smooth muscle hypertrophy and hyperplasia within the bladder wall and to eventual impairment of contractile capacity in addition to compliance and elasticity.[23] Bladder wall distortion-associated hypertrophy may contribute to loss of the physiologic ureterovesical valve mechanism, resulting in reflux and the development of hydroureters and progressive hydronephrosis.

Hydronephrosis develops from continued urine production with urethral obstruction. The renal pelvises and calyces of the upper collecting system become progressively distended and compress the renal parenchyma against the distended renal capsule. Histologic studies indicate progressive dilatation of the distal-to-proximal renal tubules, which is associated with the development of peritubular and interstitial fibrosis. Sonographically, the degree of compression, and associated fibrosis, is reflected by the development of an echogenic appearance of the parenchyma. Eventually, these processes may trigger cystic degeneration of the kidneys, with the appearance of discrete cysts in the renal cortex on ultrasound, and renal insufficiency at birth.

CONTEMPORARY APPROACH TO PRENATAL THERAPY

The use of a double-pigtail catheter, placed into the fetal bladder to allow obstructed urine to flow into the amniotic space, has met with inconsistent success. The criteria for in utero therapy used in early efforts were variable, and evaluation of the fetus before treatment was limited in many cases. Therefore, fetuses with underlying chromosomal abnormalities, other significant structural anomalies, and advanced renal dysplasia with a predictably poor outcome were treated unnecessarily. In 1994, an algorithm was proposed for the prenatal evaluation and selection of fetal candidates for prenatal therapy and exclusion of those in whom therapy would not improve the clinical outcome.[24] The three major components of this evaluation algorithm include obtaining (1) a fetal karyotype, (2) a detailed sonographic evaluation to rule out other structural anomalies that might have an impact on the prognosis for the fetus, and (3) a serial fetal urine evaluation to determine the extent of the underlying renal damage.

To be considered a candidate for prenatal treatment, the fetus must have a confirmed normal male karyotype and ultrasound must demonstrate oligohydramnios or anhydramnios or document decreasing AFV, in addition to absence of other fetal anomalies that would adversely affect the prognosis and clinical outcome for the infant. For fetuses that meet all other criteria but have urine values demonstrating minimal improvement and cluster around the threshold cutoffs, it can be counseled that placement of a vesicoamniotic shunt may help to ensure a live birth and reduce the risk for lethal pulmonary hypoplasia but that the infant would be expected to have renal insufficiency, likely require early dialysis, and may need early renal transplantation.

Amniocentesis to obtain a fetal karyotype is often not possible because of the associated oligohydramnios or anhydramnios. Therefore, transabdominal chorionic villus sampling (TA-CVS) or cordocentesis can be performed to obtain a fetal karyotype. Fetal blood sampling provides a rapid banded fetal karyotype in approximately 72 hours but carries a slightly higher complication risk than TA-CVS, which can provide a preliminary aneuploid screen using fluorescent in situ hybridization technology within 48 hours and a full-banded karyotype within 3 to 5 days. Documentation of a normal male karyotype is important, because female fetuses are usually not found to have simple urethral obstruction and typically have more complex developmental abnormalities of the cloaca and urogenital sinus resulting in urinary obstruction. Past attempts at in utero shunt therapy have proved unsuccessful in improving the outcomes for female fetuses; therefore, therapy is not indicated. Fetuses that have trisomy 21, trisomy 18, and Klinefelter syndrome with apparent isolated bladder distention, hydronephrosis, and decreased AFV in the absence of other major sonographic markers have been reported. The overall aneuploidy rate in the authors' LUTO patient database is 5%.

Role of Ultrasound in Evaluation

Detailed sonographic anatomic survey is necessary to rule out the presence of other anomalies, such as neural tube or cardiac defects, which occur at a higher frequency with LUTO and would have a dramatic impact on the prognosis for that infant. Certainly, in utero therapy would not be warranted when the fetus is affected with another life-threatening anomaly. Careful evaluation for other more subtle phenotypic signs, such as limb shortening or facial abnormalities, is required, because these findings may indicate the presence of an underlying genetic syndrome, altering the underlying long-term prognosis.

Detailed evaluation of the fetus in the presence of severe oligohydramnios or anhydramnios can be extremely difficult. The use of amnioinfusion to re-establish the fluid-tissue interface is recommended, allowing better sonographic evaluation of the fetus. Plain lactated Ringer's solution, warmed to 37°C, is infused through a closed sterile intravenous tubing system to restore AFVs to a low-normal level. In addition, the patient is given a 10- to 14-day course of oral antibiotics.[25]

The urinary tract must be carefully evaluated from the kidneys to the distal urethra for clues as to the underlying cause of obstruction and renal status. Long-axis measurement of the kidney is useful in evaluating underlying hydronephrosis, and, in general, kidneys that measure large for gestational age and are less echogenic are associated with a better prognosis. Kidneys that are hyperechogenic and measure small for gestational age are generally found to have poor underlying function because of renal fibrosis.

The renal parenchyma is examined for the degree of echogenicity, parenchymal compression, and presence or absence of discrete cortical cysts (**Fig. 1**). Care must be taken when possible cystic changes are found to ensure differentiation between

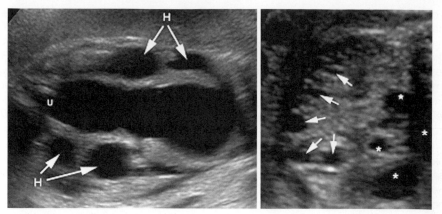

Fig. 1. (*Left*) Enlarged bladder with dilated proximal urethra (u) and bilateral hydroureters (H). (*Right*) Multiple cysts within the cortical region of the echogenic kidney (*arrows*, *dilated calyces), which was found to have characteristic fibrocystic dysplasia on autopsy.

cystic change and dilated calyces; the former is associated with advanced irreversible parenchymal damage, which renders the fetus not amenable to shunt therapy.

Next, the ureters should be evaluated for abnormalities. The presence of significant pyelectasis in the absence of hydroureters may indicate the presence of ureteropelvic junction (UPJ) obstruction. Megaureters and obvious distortion of the vesicoureteral junctions indicate severe reflux, which may be associated with more advanced renal damage and a poorer prognosis.

The bladder is carefully evaluated before and after complete drainage by fine-needle vesicocentesis. Before drainage, overall size is assessed in addition to degree of apparent proximal urethral dilation (ie, "keyhole sign"; **Fig. 2**) as an indicator of level

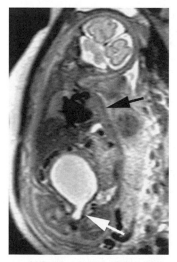

Fig. 2. Ultrafast fetal MRI image of bladder outlet obstruction and typical "keyhole" appearance of the dilated proximal urethra (*white arrow*). Also note the small chest, hypoplastic lungs (*black arrow*), and anhydramnios.

and cause of apparent obstruction. An abnormal bladder shape or urachal abnormalities may indicate the presence of an underlying developmental abnormality of cloacal differentiation, which represents more complex anomalies that have not benefited from simple shunt-diverting procedures. The shape of the bladder, before and after urine drainage, may provide a clue to the underlying source of obstruction (**Fig. 3**). Previous observations suggest that after drainage of the bladder by vesicocentesis, fetuses that have urethral atresia or complete obstructing PUVs demonstrate bladders that are symmetrically round and thick-walled. Bladders that are symmetrically thick-walled but elongated and somewhat tubular in appearance after drainage occur in fetuses with incomplete urethral obstruction, such as incomplete PUVs, urethral strictures, or urethral meatus abnormalities. Fetuses with patent but hypoplastic urethras demonstrate a more unusual appearance to the bladder, with it being somewhat elongated and segmented in appearance, giving rise to what the authors refer to as a "snowman" bladder. These particular bladders seem to demonstrate the typical thickening caused by hypertrophy and hyperplastic changes in the lower bladder neck region but have minimal thickening in the bladder dome, making them more susceptible to bladder rupture. This group of fetuses has been shown to have an underlying smooth muscle and connective tissue abnormality of the bladder.[24]

Finally, the penile urethra should be evaluated for clues to the cause of obstruction. Occasionally, the degree of proximal urethral dilation (keyhole sign) is mild to moderate, and a dilated membranous penile urethra can be traced to its distal end. Such a finding has been shown to be associated with anterior urethral valves or abnormalities of the tip of the penis, such as meatal stenosis or phimosis.

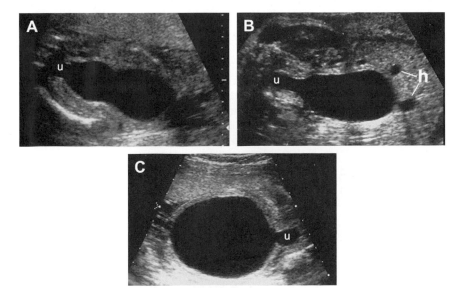

Fig. 3. Sonographic appearance of fetal bladders with urethral obstructions (u, proximal urethra; h, hydroureter). (*A*) Segmented ("snowman") shape of bladders seen in fetuses with urethral hypoplasia (TRIAD syndrome). (*B*) Elongated bladder with hydroureters seen in cases of incomplete PUVs. (*C*) Symmetric thick-walled bladder found in urethral atresia or completely obstructing PUVs.

Evaluation of Fetal Renal Function

The last, and perhaps most important, component of the prenatal evaluation is the serial analysis of fetal urine, obtained by ultrasound-guided fine-needle bladder drainage (vesicocentesis). The importance of serial sampling has been well described,[20] and it must be performed at set time intervals for the information to retain its predictive value. Complete bladder drainage at 24- to 48-hour intervals is recommended, as is the analysis of fetal urine for sodium, chloride, osmolality, calcium, β_2-microglobulin, and total protein (**Table 1**). A minimum of three bladder drainage procedures completed over 5 to 7 days is usually necessary to provide optimal predictive value. Additional vesicocenteses may be necessary to establish a clear pattern of decreasing or increasing hypertonicity, however. Reflux and urinary stasis cause increased intrarenal pressure, progressive dilatation of the renal tubules and collecting systems, and probable altered blood flow to the delicate proximal renal tubules, resulting in altered physiologic function. Decreased solute reabsorption, protein catabolism and subsequent increased loss of substances in the fetal urine results, and the degree of urine hypertonicity present have been positively correlated with the extent of underlying histologic renal damage.[26]

The initial bladder drainage procedure evaluates urine that has been present in the fetal bladder for an undetermined time and does not reflect present renal function. The second bladder drainage procedure represents urine from the upper tracts that has drained into the bladder and does not represent recent renal urine production. The third bladder drainage procedure, however, represents urine that has recently been formed by the kidneys, and is most reflective of the degree of underlying renal function and damage. In cases of severe renal damage, a decrease in hypertonicity is not observed and increasing values are reflective of progressive and more advanced renal disease. In select cases, however, a pattern of progressively decreasing hypertonicity and improving values that are lower than established thresholds can be observed, which indicates potential renal salvage and identifies fetuses that may benefit from in utero intervention (**Fig. 4**).

Technical Considerations and Surgical Approach in Vesicoamniotic Shunting

Vesicoamniotic shunting represents a temporary therapeutic intervention allowing simple diversion of fetal urine from the obstructed bladder into the amniotic space. It is essential that patients understand that such therapy is not curative but may be preventative and that the baby requires further evaluation and surgical treatment for the obstruction after birth. Pregnancies complicated by anhydramnios present

Table 1
Prognostic urine values for selection of fetuses for prenatal intervention[a]

	Good Prognosis	Poor Prognosis
Sodium	<90 mmol/L	>100 mmol/L
Chloride	<80 mmol/L	>90 mmol/L
Osmolality	<180 mOsm/L	>200 mOsm/L
Calcium	<7 mg/dL	>8 mg/dL
Total protein	<20 mg/dL	>40 mg/dL
β_2-microglobulin	<6 mg/L	>10 mg/L

[a] Based on the last urine specimen obtained by serial bladder drainage (three to four times) at 24- to 48-hour intervals between 18 and 22 weeks of gestational age.

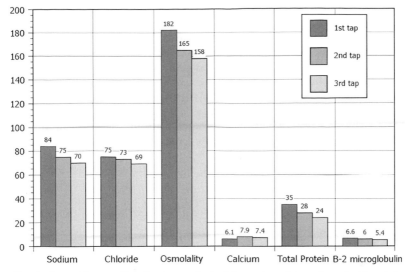

Fig. 4. Graph shows the results of urinary electrolyte and protein values from serial vesico-centesis. As shown in this case, the potential for renal salvage is good after successful in ute-ro shunt placement, because values decrease to lower than the established thresholds on sequential samplings.

a technical challenge when placing a vesicoamniotic shunt from a visualization perspective and because the distal end of the shunt catheter needs to be placed into a pocket of amniotic fluid. As noted previously, amnioinfusion at time of initial evaluation is used to assist sonographic evaluation; however, in most cases, the amniotic space must be re-expanded with fluid for successful shunt placement.

Paralysis of the fetus before vesicocentesis or the vesicoamniotic shunt placement procedure is not required. For shunt placement procedures, local anesthesia with 1% lidocaine is used, and intravenous maternal sedation using a combination of morphine (5–15 mg) and diazepam (5–15 mg), with the total dose depending on the initial maternal response and level of fetal and maternal sedation and pain relief required. This decreases fetal movement and provides pain relief for the mother and fetus.

Once the appropriate approach for optimal placement of the shunt into the lower bladder is chosen, maternal intravenous sedation is given and the maternal skin is anesthetized with 1% lidocaine. A small 3- to 4-mm stab wound is made through the maternal skin to allow easy passage of the shunt trocar, which is then introduced under continuous ultrasound guidance into the amniotic space near the lower fetal abdomen. An adequate pocket of amniotic fluid needs to be present in which to drop the distal end of the shunt catheter on exiting the fetal abdomen. If insufficient fluid space is present, additional amnioinfusion can be performed through the shunt trocar before entering the fetal abdomen and bladder. The tip of the trocar is positioned in the same manner as the vesicocentesis needle, and color Doppler is used to confirm that the trocar does not injure the umbilical arteries on passage through the bladder wall. The trocar is quickly inserted into the bladder and positioned into a central location. The catheter is then completely threaded into the trocar sheath. If the "rocket of London" two-push rod shunt procedure is utilized, a short push rod is introduced and used to push the proximal coiled segment of the catheter into the bladder. This is then removed, and a long push rod is gently introduced until it comes in contact with the distal tip of the shunt catheter within the trocar sheath. The push rod is then held in place while the shaft of the trocar sheath is slowly pulled back approximately 2 cm. At this point, the trocar sheath should lie just outside the fetal abdomen, with the straight segment of the shunt catheter traversing the region of abdomen between the bladder and amniotic space. Failure to perform this part of the maneuver properly may result in partial displacement of the proximal end of the catheter and increased risk for shunt displacement.

The trocar sheath is now directed away from the insertion site, and the long push rod is advanced to displace the distal end of the catheter into the amniotic space. The position of the proximal and distal coiled segments of the catheter and initiation of bladder drainage are confirmed sonographically. The patient is then placed on external fetal or uterine monitoring for 1 to 2 hours, and any evidence of uterine contractions is managed with tocolytic therapy, initially with subcutaneous terbutaline (0.25 mg) or oral nifedipine (20 mg administered every 4–6 hours).

Complications

Counseling of the patient before initiation of a course of prenatal evaluation includes discussion of potential complications of any invasive procedure, such as chorioamnionitis; premature rupture of fetal membranes; direct trauma to the fetus, including iatrogenic gastroschisis; and intraplacental bleeding and possible associated onset of preterm labor, particularly if a transplacental approach is necessary.[27]

After vesicocentesis, transient vesicoperitoneal fistulas can occur that result in urinary ascites. Such fistulas usually spontaneously close in 7 to 10 days, followed by re-enlargement of the bladder.

Vesicoamniotic shunt displacement is a common complication, occurring in approximately 40% of cases in clinical series. Despite the fact that the rocket of London catheter is designed so that the distal end curls to lie flat against the fetal abdomen, it may become entangled in fetal extremities or more directly dislodged by the movement of the fetus, necessitating replacement on recurrence of bladder distention. If the shunt catheter is placed too high within the distended bladder, it may be placed under stretch as the bladder shrinks with drainage and eventually displaced and possibly drawn within the fetal abdomen, resulting in massive urinary ascites.

The authors have had several cases of successful shunt placements at 19 to 21 weeks of gestation in which catheter placement and function were considered optimal, with decreasing hydronephrosis and maintenance of reasonable AFVs. At 27 to 29 weeks of gestation, however, AFVs decreased, renal parenchyma became increasingly echodense, and renal growth stopped and actually regressed over time. All these fetuses died near or shortly after birth. On autopsy, all demonstrated severe fibrocystic renal dysplasia and were found to have appropriately placed patent shunt catheters. The cause of this late-onset renal dysplasia, despite resolution of obstructive hydronephrosis, remains unclear.

Follow-up

After a fetal vesicoamniotic shunt procedure, a follow-up sonographic evaluation should be performed 24 to 48 hours later to confirm catheter placement and function. Weekly examinations are suggested for at least 4 weeks to confirm catheter placement and function, progressive resolution of the hydronephrosis, and maintenance of AFV. At that point, evaluation can be spaced to every 2 weeks depending on maintenance of AFV.

Prenatal consultation with the pediatric urologist and neonatologist who are going to care for the baby after birth is recommended so that issues of postnatal evaluation, management, and treatment options can be discussed with the patient.

Route of delivery should be dictated by routine obstetric indications and not influenced by the presence of the indwelling bladder catheter. Pregnancies that have undergone shunting typically experience spontaneous rupture of fetal membranes or onset of labor with vaginal delivery at 34 to 35 weeks of gestation. This gestational age for delivery has been found to be no different than that occurring in an age-matched cohort of unshunted fetuses with LUTO, but the family should be counseled about this tendency for early delivery in pregnancies complicated by LUTO.

Outcomes After Prenatal Intervention

Perhaps the most difficult question still confronting us is whether the contemporary approach to fetal evaluation and intervention actually improves postnatal renal outcomes.[28–31] Unfortunately, until recently, there have been no randomized trials or large multicenter studies to address this issue. Currently, a multicenter randomized controlled trial (PLUTO) is ongoing to answer some of these questions. This trial, a shunting for PLUTO randomized control trial, looks to evaluate the efficacy of vesicoamniotic shunting as compared with conservative treatment in perinatal and postnatal mortality and renal outcomes.[19] Nevertheless, two recent retrospective case series have reported on long-term outcomes after vesicoamniotic shunting in LUTO. The initial study in 1999 reported on a heterogeneous population of children in which the cause of LUTO varied.[32] The more recent study was designed to focus on the long-term outcomes of children with specific documented urethral obstructions (PUVs, urethral atresia, and prune-belly syndrome).[33] In this somewhat more homogeneous group of children selected for in utero intervention by established criteria, survival at 1 year was 91%, with two neonatal deaths occurring as a result of pulmonary hypoplasia. PUVs and prune-belly (TRIAD) syndrome were the most common final postnatal diagnosis (39% each). At a median follow-up age of 5.8 years, 44% of the entire group demonstrated acceptable renal function (creatinine clearance >70 mL/min), 22% demonstrated mild renal insufficiency (creatinine clearance <70 mL/min not requiring renal replacement), and 34% went on to require renal replacement. Persistent respiratory problems were present in 44% of children (most commonly, asthma and recurrent pulmonary infections), musculoskeletal problems were present in 50%, poor growth (height and weight <25th percentile) was present in 66.5%, and frequent urinary tract infections were present in 50%. Spontaneous voiding was experienced by 61% of the group. Interestingly, health-related quality of life assessed by the children and their parents did not differ from a healthy child population.

Little is known about the natural history of renal and bladder injury in cases of LUTO with normal AFV; as such, these pregnancies are generally excluded from fetal therapy, because pulmonary hypoplasia would not be expected and the risk for renal insufficiency is unproved. To determine whether such fetuses might be at risk for poor renal outcomes, and therefore warrant consideration for prenatal therapy, the North American Fetal Therapy Network (NAFTNet) is conducting an outcomes study ("natural history of lower urinary tract obstruction with normal amniotic fluid volume"[34]) that is gathering sonographic information on urinary tract status and markers of injury before birth and on renal, bladder, and pulmonary outcomes through 2 years of age.

FUTURE DIRECTIONS
In Utero Cystoscopic Treatment

Among the challenges for the future are efforts to refine the approach to intervention in LUTO further and to develop techniques to decrease the most frequent technical complications of shunt displacement and migration. One new technique being developed is the cystoscopic disruption of PUVs.[35–37] In this approach, microcystoscopy is performed and the proximal urethra is directly visualized. If the source of obstruction can be identified, features can be evaluated to determine whether they represent PUVs or urethral atresia. If valves can be confirmed, laser ablation or mechanical disruption may be technically possible. This approach has been used investigatively with mixed results, but the potential for the future is to relieve the obstruction without the need for a diverting catheter. Perhaps more importantly, it may allow for a more normal physiologic state of bladder cycling with storage and voiding, which has been suggested to play an important role in long-term bladder function.[38] After vesicoamniotic shunt placement, the bladder passively empties through the shunt, and therefore never cycles (fills and empties); as such, shunt placement may interfere with normal bladder development and maturation, contributing to the voiding dysfunction found in children surviving in utero therapy. As experience, instrumentation, and visualization improve, this may become the treatment of choice for fetuses with PUVs. For cases of LUTO attributable to other causes, diverting shunt therapy is likely to remain the intervention of choice.

SUMMARY

Although tremendous improvements in patient selection have resulted in more consistent selection in fetal therapy for LUTO, short-term outcomes remain highly variable among centers and long-term outcomes into the adolescent and young adult years remain to be confirmed. With careful prenatal evaluation and case selection, vesicoamniotic shunt placement has been shown to be successful in preventing the mortality associated with pulmonary hypoplasia and seems to result in improved postnatal renal and bladder function. Whereas shunt displacement remains an ongoing problem, fetal cystoscopy and endoscopic surgery may improve renal outcomes in the future. The results from the PLUTO trial may provide additional clinical data to determine the future role of in utero surgery for the treatment of LUTO.

REFERENCES

1. Nakayama DK, Harrison MR, deLorimier AA. Prognosis of posterior urethral valves presenting at birth. J Pediatr Surg 1986;21:43–5.
2. Mahony BS, Callen PW, Filly RA. Fetal urethral obstruction: ultrasound evaluation. Radiology 1985;157:221–4.
3. Housley HT, Harrison MR. Fetal urinary tract abnormalities. Natural history, pathophysiology, and treatment. Urol Clin North Am 1998;25:63–73.
4. Harrison MR, Filly RA. The fetus with obstructive uropathy: pathophysiology, natural history, selection, and treatment. In: Harrison MR, Golbus MS, Filly RA, editors. The unborn patient: prenatal diagnosis and treatment. 2nd edition. Philadelphia: WB Saunders Company; 1991. p. 328–93.
5. Harrison MR, Ross NA, Noall R, et al. Correction of urogenital hydronephrosis in utero. The model: fetal urethral obstruction produces hydronephrosis and pulmonary hypoplasia in fetal lambs. J Pediatr Surg 1983;18:247–56.

6. Glick PL, Harrison MR, Noall RA, et al. Correction of congenital hydronephrosis in utero III: early mid-trimester ureteral obstruction produces renal dysplasia. J Pediatr Surg 1983;18:681–7.

7. Kramer SA. Current status of fetal intervention for congenital hydronephrosis. J Urol 1983;130:641–6.

8. Bellinger MF, Comstock CH, Grosso D, et al. Fetal posterior urethral valves and renal dysplasia at 15 weeks gestational age. J Urol 1983;129:1238–9.

9. Wladimiroff JW. Effect of furosemide on fetal urine production. Br J Obstet Gynecol 1975;82:221–4.

10. Chinn DH, Filly RA. Ultrasound diagnosis of fetal genitourinary tract anomalies. Urol Radiol 1982;4:115–23.

11. Mahony BS, Fill RA, Callen PW, et al. Fetal renal dysplasia: sonographic evaluation. Radiology 1984;152:143–6.

12. Glazer GM, Filly RA, Callen PW. The varied sonographic appearance of urinary tract in the fetus and newborn with urethral obstruction. Radiology 1982;144:563–8.

13. Crombleholme TM, Harrison MR, Longaker MT, et al. Prenatal diagnosis and management of bilateral hydronephrosis. Pediatr Nephrol 1988;2:334–42.

14. Lumbers ER, Hill KJ, Bennett VJ. Proximal and distal tubular activity in chronically catheterized fetal sheep compared with the adult. Can J Physiol Pharmacol 1988; 66:697–702.

15. Adzick NS, Harrison MR, Flake AW, et al. Development of a fetal renal function test using endogenous creatinine clearance. J Pediatr Surg 1985;20:602–7.

16. Glick PL, Harrison MR, Golbus MS, et al. Management of the fetus with congenital hydronephrosis II. Prognostic criteria and selection for treatment. J Pediatr Surg 1985;20:376–87.

17. Mussap M, Fanos V, Pizzini C, et al. Predictive value of amniotic fluid cystatin C levels for the early identification of fetuses with obstructive uropathies. Br J Obstet Gynecol 2002;109:778–83.

18. Reed C. Diagnostic applications of cystatin C. Br J Biomed Sci 2000;57:323–9.

19. PLUTO Collaborative Study Group, Kilby M, Khan K, et al. PLUTO trial protocol: percutaneous shunting for lower urinary tract obstruction randomised controlled trial. Br J Obstet Gynecol 2007;114:904–5, e1–4.

20. Johnson MP, Corsi P, Badfield W, et al. Sequential urinalysis improves evaluation of fetal renal function in obstructive uropathy. Am J Obstet Gynecol 1995;173:59–65.

21. Tomlinson M, Johnson MP, Goncalves L, et al. Correction of hemodynamic abnormalities by vesicoamniotic shunting in familial congenital megacystis. Fetal Diagn Ther 1996;11:46–9.

22. Freedman AL, Bukowski TP, Smith CA, et al. Fetal therapy for obstructive uropathy: diagnosis-specific outcomes. J Urol 1996;156(Pt 2):720–3.

23. Freedman AL, Qureshi F, Shapiro E, et al. Smooth muscle development in the obstructed fetal bladder. Urology 1997;49:104–7.

24. Johnson MP, Bukowski TP, Reitleman C, et al. In utero surgical treatment of fetal obstructive uropathy: a new comprehensive approach to identify appropriate candidates for vesicoamniotic shunt therapy. Am J Obstet Gynecol 1994;170:1770–6.

25. Feldman B, Hassan S, Kramer RL, et al. Amnioinfusion in the evaluation of fetal obstructive uropathy: the effect of antibiotic prophylaxis on complication rates. Fetal Diagn Ther 1999;14:172–5.

26. Qureshi F, Jacques SM, Seifman B, et al. In utero fetal urine analysis and renal histology do correlate with the outcome in fetal obstructive uropathies. Fetal Diagn Ther 1996;11:306–12.

27. Hassan S, Mariona L, Kasperski S, et al. Complications of vesicoamniotic shunting. Am J Obstet Gynecol 1997;176:583 [abstract].
28. Manning FA, Harrison MR, Rodeck D. Catheter shunts for fetal hydronephrosis and hydrocephalus: report of the international fetal surgery registry. N Engl J Med 1986;315:336–40.
29. Crombleholme TM, Harrison MR, Golbus MS, et al. Fetal intervention in obstructive uropathy: prognostic indicators and efficacy of intervention. Am J Obstet Gynecol 1990;162:1239–44.
30. Sholder AJ, Maizels M, Depp B, et al. Caution in antenatal intervention. J Urol 1988;139:1026–9.
31. Coplen DE, Hare JY, Zderic SA, et al. 10-year experience with prenatal intervention for hydronephrosis. J Urol 1996;156:1142–5.
32. Freedman AL, Johnson MP, Smith CA, et al. Long-term outcome in children after antenatal intervention for obstructive uropathies. Lancet 1999;345:374–7.
33. Biard J, Johnson MP, Carr MC, et al. Long-term outcomes in children treated by prenatal shunting for lower urinary tract obstruction. Obstet Gynecol 2005;106: 503–8.
34. NAFTNet. Available at: www.naftnet.org. Accessed June 3, 2009.
35. Quintero RA, Johnson MP, Romero R, et al. In utero percutaneous cystoscopy in the management of fetal lower obstructive uropathy. Lancet 1995;346:537–40.
36. Quintero RA, Hume R, Smith C, et al. Percutaneous fetal cystoscopy and endoscopic fulguration of posterior urethral valves. Am J Obstet Gynecol 1995; 172(Pt 1):206–9.
37. Clifton MS, Harrison MR, Ball R, et al. Fetoscopic transuterine release of posterior urethral valves: a new technique. Fetal Diagn Ther 2008;23:89–94.
38. Close CE, Carr MC, Burns MW, et al. Lower urinary tract changes after early valve ablation in neonates and infants: is early diversion warranted? J Urol 1997;157: 984–8.

Twin-to-Twin Transfusion Syndrome: A Comprehensive Update

Mounira Habli, MD[a,b,c,d], Foong Yen Lim, MD[a,b,d],
Timothy Crombleholme, MD[a,b,d],*

KEYWORDS

- TTTS • Recipient • Cardiomyopathy • Laser • Amnioreduction

In 2005, the total twin birth rate in the United States was 32.2 twins per 1000 births.[1] The twin birth rate has risen steadily since the 1980s with a 70% increase since 1980.[1] Human twins are generally either monozygotic or dizygotic. The occurrence of dizygotic twinning varies widely between populations, ranging from about 6 per 1000 in Asia to 10 to 20 per 1000 in the United States and Europe and as high as 40 per 1000 in Africa.[2] Twin pregnancies are characterized by an increased incidence of both fetal and maternal complications especially in monozygotic twins. In monozygotic twins, the majority of monochorionic twins have vascular anastomoses, and this shared blood supply can result in twin-to-twin transfusion syndrome (TTTS), a condition characterized by unequal sharing of the maternal blood supply, which results in asymmetrical fetal growth and fetal mortality in 80% or more of untreated cases, particularly if problems develop before 28 weeks' gestation.[3–5]

TTTS is a serious complication in about 10% to 20% of monozygous twin gestations[6] with an incidence of 4% to 35% in the United States.[7] Severe TTTS is reported to occur in 5.5% to 17.5% of cases.[8] The relatively broad incidence range of TTTS likely reflects differences in clinical criteria used to make the diagnosis. TTTS is a progressive disease in which sudden deteriorations in clinical status can occur, leading to death of a co-twin. Up to 30% of survivors may have abnormal neurodevelopment as a result of the combination of profound antenatal insult and the complications of severe prematurity.[9]

[a] The Fetal Care Center of Cincinnati, Cincinnati Children's Hospital, University of Cincinnati, MLC 2023, 3333 Burnet Ave, Cincinnati, OH 45229 3039, USA
[b] Division of Pediatric General, Thoracic and Fetal Surgery, Cincinnati Children's Hospital, Cincinnati, OH 45229, USA
[c] Maternal Fetal Medicine, University of Cincinnati, College of Medicine, ML0528, Cincinnati, OH 45219, USA
[d] University of Cincinnati, College of Medicine, OH, USA
* Corresponding author. The Fetal Care Center of Cincinnati, MLC 2023, 3333 Burnet Ave, Cincinnati, OH 45229 3039.
E-mail address: timothy.crombleholme@cchmc.org (T. Crombleholme).

Clin Perinatol 36 (2009) 391–416
doi:10.1016/j.clp.2009.03.003
0095-5108/09/$ – see front matter © 2009 Elsevier Inc. All rights reserved.
perinatology.theclinics.com

Historically, the diagnosis of TTTS was made based on neonatal criteria of greater than 20% discordance in birth weight, and greater than 5 g/dL discordance in cord hemoglobin levels.[8] These criteria have now been recognized to be insufficient for midgestation diagnosis of TTTS.[8] They have been replaced with more stringent ultrasound-based criteria, with particular attention to amniotic fluid discordance, bladder volumes, and fetal echocardiography and Doppler studies.

In this article, we present an overview of what is known about the pathophysiology and the diagnosis of TTTS, the role of echocardiography in TTTS, treatment options available for TTTS, complications of treatment for TTTS, and short- and long-term outcomes of TTTS.

PATHOPHYSIOLOGY

TTTS is a complex and dynamic pathologic condition that involves placental intertwin vascular anastomoses; fetal humoral, biochemical, and functional changes; and fetal hemodynamic changes. These changes appear to be responsible for the progression and outcome of TTTS.

Placental Architectural Changes

Placental vascular anastomoses, unequal placental sharing, and abnormalities in umbilical cord insertions are all associated with TTTS. It is believed that almost all monochorionic twins have intertwin vascular anastomoses.[10] These vascular anastomoses can be either direct, superficial anastomoses between the twins' umbilical cord branch vessels on the chorionic plate surface; or "deep" anastomoses, wherein the arterial vessels from one twin's cord pierce the chorionic plate to supply a placental cotyledon drained by the venous system of its co-twin; or both. In regard to type of anastomoses, vascular communications between the recipient and donor twin may be artery to artery, vein to vein, or artery to vein within a placental cotyledon. Depending on the number and type of anastomoses present, the exchange of blood may be balanced or unbalanced. Shifts in blood flow between the twins may be acute, as in the case of co-twin demise, or chronic. Both ex vivo injection studies and in vivo studies have demonstrated such anastomosis.[11,12] Artery-to-artery and vein-to-vein anastomoses are superficial anastomoses with bidirectional flow, but artery-to-vein anastomoses are deep anastomoses with unidirectional flow from one twin to the other. It is thought that TTTS is more likely to develop when there is a paucity of bidirectional artery-to-artery and vein-to-vein anastomoses that can assist with regulation of intertwin circulatory imbalances. It has been suggested that artery-to-artery and vein-to-vein anastomoses when present are protective.[13–16] The antenatal detection of artery-to-artery anastomoses with color Doppler ultrasound is associated with a nine-fold reduction in the likelihood of developing chronic TTTS.[17]

The percent of each type of anastomoses ranges from 20% to 90% based on whether the vascular connection was determined by pathologic examination or from fetoscopic studies.[15,17] Recent evidence suggests that vascular diameter, vascular resistance, and chorionic plate pattern may be as important as the number and type of anastomoses in development, timing, and severity of TTTS.[14,18] In a mathematical model of monochorionic placental circulation, Umur and colleagues[15] reported that vascular diameter and resistance are important determinants of hemodynamic imbalance in diamniotic-monochorionic placentas, especially in blood vessels with a high pressure differential, such as artery-to-vein anastomoses. De Paepe and colleagues,[14] in a retrospective study of placental pathology and placental vascular injection of TTTS patients, reported a higher incidence of what is termed the *magistral* vascular pattern (≥75% of the vascular territory showing relatively large vessels extending from the insertion of the cord to the periphery without a significant reduction of diameter) as compared to *dispersed* vascular pattern (≥75% made up of a superficial vascular arrangement characterized by regular, near-symmetric dichotomous branching, resulting in a progressive diminution of vascular caliber).

Several studies have reported the relationship of vascular anastomoses and perinatal outcome in monochorionic twins and TTTS. In a retrospective study of placental angioarchitecture in relation to survival in monochorionic twins, fetal survival in monochorionic twins was higher in pregnancies with artery-to-artery anastomoses but lower with a vein-to-vein anastomoses.[11,19–22] Bajoria and colleagues[19] reported that TTTS with unidirectional artery-to-vein anastomoses had a worse perinatal outcome. However, placental vascular anastomoses by themselves do not explain the pathophysiology of TTTS. Other factors, such as cord insertion and placental sharing, may also play an important role.

Fetal Adaptive Responses

The unbalanced blood shunting from donor to recipient has been reported to cause hormonal, hemodynamic, and biochemical fetal changes. This shunting creates a hydrostatic difference between the recipient and donor twins. The recipient becomes hyperdynamic and hypervolumic. The donor becomes hypovolumic and hypodynamic. This donor hypovolumia causes a decrease in renal perfusion, thus activating the renin-angiotensin-aldosterone system, which is a hormone system that regulates blood pressure and water (fluid) balance by increasing renin enzyme and angiotensin II (a vasoconstrictor), which in turn stimulates the secretion of the hormone aldosterone (increases fluid volume) from the adrenal cortex.[23–26] This donor hypovolumia is also associated with a number of renal structural and functional aberrations, especially in severe TTTS, including renal tubular degeneration and cellular apoptosis, loss of glomeruli or reduction in tubular number, and maldevelopmental progression to renal dysgenesis.[23,24] Thus, in TTTS, donors have an increase in renin-secreting cells with up-regulation of renin synthesis system and an increase in angiotensin II, aldosterone, and antidiuretic hormones as an adaptive mechanism to restore euvolemia.[23–26] With progression of TTTS or in severe TTTS cases, further fetal vasoconstriction mediated by angiotensin II compromises renal and placental blood flow, leading to worsening oliguria, oligohydramnios, and growth restriction in the donor. In contrast, recipient fetuses demonstrate down-regulation of renin expression with elevation in renin levels and glomerular and arterial lesions in the kidneys, suggestive of hypertension-induced microangiopathy. These findings suggest that hypertensive changes in the recipient twin may be due to vascular shunting of renin from the donor, leading to these hormonal changes.[23–26] These studies, however, do not take into account the possibility that the placenta could be a source for these vasoactive substances.

These vasoactive hormonal changes are likely a contributing factor in worsening hypervolemia and polyuria/polyhydramnios in recipients. In addition to these vasoactive substances, the recipient has increased cardiac synthesis and secretion of natriuretic peptides. Natriuretic peptides are endogenous hormones released by the heart in response to myocardial stretch, volume overload, hyperosmolality, hypoxia, and vasoconstrictors, such as angiotensin II, vasopressin, and endothelin-1.[27] These natriuretic peptides, mainly atrial natriuretic peptide (ANP) and brain natriuretic peptide (BNP), regulate blood pressure and body fluid homeostasis through their diuretic, natriuretic, vasorelaxant, and anti-hypertensive effects. These natriuretic peptides also exert antiproliferative effects on cardiovascular/mesenchymal tissue.[27] In the fetus, ANP and BNP expression has been detected as early as postconception week 8 to 9. Normal concentrations of ANP and BNP were found to be higher than those in adult humans, and concentrations in the fetus declined with advancing gestational age.[27] Data also show that fetal ANP and BNP behave similar to adult natriuretic system.[27] Little information is known about the role of the natriuretic system in TTTS. Bajoria and colleagues[28–30] demonstrated that recipient twins in TTTS have higher concentrations of ANP, BNP, and endothelin-1 than their co-twin donors or diamniotic monochorionic twins without TTTS, and that high concentrations of BNP and endothelin-1 are particularly correlated with cardiac dysfunction in the recipient. The investigators suggested that these compounds might be used as early markers of cardiac compromise.

Consistent with the hypothesis that vasoactive mediators play an important role in TTTS, Bajoria and colleagues[31] reported that endothelin-1, a potent vasoconstrictor, is 2.5-fold higher in the serum of recipient twins than in donor twins. Moreover, plasma endothelin-1 levels were significantly higher in the recipient twins with hydrops than those with mild or no hydrops.[31] Endothelin-1 may also be important for the regulation of amniotic fluid volume.[28] Both endothelin-1 and BNP amniotic fluid levels correlate with amniotic fluid index in TTTS. Recipient twin amniotic fluid levels of endothelin-1 and human BNP are the highest, followed by amniotic fluid levels from non-TTTS monochorionic twins, followed by amniotic fluid levels from donor twins.[30]

In addition to the renin-angiotensin-aldosterone system, natriuretic peptides, and other vasoactive mediators, several other angiogenic and antiangiogenic mediators and hormonal systems have been studied in relation to TTTS. Recently, Kusanovic and colleagues[32] conducted a case-control study that included monochorionic-diamniotic pregnancies between 16 and 26 weeks with and without TTTS. The investigators reported that maternal plasma concentrations of soluble vascular endothelial growth factor receptor–1 and soluble endoglin were higher, and that placental growth factors had a lower median than those without TTTS. The investigators suggested that TTTS could be an antiangiogenic state.[32] Moreover, insulinlike growth factors and receptors leptin and erythropoietin have all been suggested to play a role in TTTS.[33–37]

DIAGNOSIS AND STAGING OF TWIN-TO-TWIN TRANSFUSION SYNDROME

Diagnosis of TTTS is one of exclusion based upon ultrasound findings. Although not all of the following sonographic criteria are necessary for a diagnosis of TTTS, the following findings are suggestive of the diagnosis: (1) monochorionicity, (2) discrepancy in amniotic fluid between the amniotic sacs with polyhydraminos of one twin (deepest vertical pocket >8 cm) and oligohydraminos of the other (deepest vertical pocket <2 cm), (3) discrepancy in size of the umbilical cords, (4) presence of cardiac dysfunction in the polyhydramniotic twin, (5) characteristically abnormal umbilical artery or ductus venosus Doppler velocimetry, and (6), less specifically, significant growth discordance (often ≥20%). The differential diagnosis of TTTS includes uteroplacental insufficiency, growth disturbances due to abnormal cord insertions, discordant manifestation of intrauterine infection, preterm premature rupture of membranes of one twin, and discordant chromosomal or structural anomalies of one twin.[38,39]

TTTS has at least four staging systems available: the Quintero staging system (**Table 1**), the Cincinnati staging system (**Table 2**), the cardiovascular profile scoring (CVPS) system (**Table 3**), and the Children's Hospital of Philadelphia (CHOP) system (**Table 4**). The Quintero staging system is based solely on ultrasound findings, including mainly Doppler waveform changes with disease progression. The Cincinnati

Table 1
Quintero staging system

Stages	Donor Bladder	Amniotic Fluid: Donor/Recipient	Doppler Wave Forms	Other
		Observations		
I	Visible	Oligohydramnios/ polyhydramnios	Normal	
II	Not visible	Oligohydramnios/ polyhydramnios	Normal	
III	Visible or not visible	Oligohydramnios/ polyhydramnios	Abnormal	
IV				Fetal hydrops or abdominal ascites
V				Demise of either fetus

Abnormal Doppler waveform defined as absent or reverse end-diastolic flow in the umbilical artery, reverse flow in the ductus venosus, or pulsatile umbilical venous flow.
From Quintero RA. Twin-twin transfusion syndrome. Clin Perinatol 2003;30:591–600; with permission.

staging system, a modification of the Quintero staging system, incorporates fetal echocardiographic findings. The CVPS and the CHOP systems are based on echocardiographic findings of both twins. The importance of each component of these systems is discussed below.

Table 2
Cincinnati staging system

Stage	Donor	Recipient	Recipient Cardiomyopathy
I	Oligohydramnios (deepest vertical pocket <2 cm)	Polyhydramnios (deepest vertical pocket >8 cm)	No
II	Bladder not visible	Bladder visible	No
III	Abnormal Doppler	Abnormal Doppler	None
IIIA			Mild
IIIB			Moderate
IIIC			Severe
IV	Hydrops	Hydrops	
V	Death	Death	
Variables			
Cardiomyopathy	Mild	Moderate	Severe
AV regurgitation	Mild	Moderate	Severe
RV/LV thickness[a]	>2 + Z-score	>3 + Z-score	>4 + Z-score
MPI[a,b]	>2 + Z-score	>3 + Z-score	Severe biventricular dysfunction

Abbreviations: AV, atrial-ventricular valve; MPI: myocardial performance index; RV/LV, right ventricular/left ventricular.
[a] Reference for normal values:[116–118]
[b] Normal RV MPI is 0.32 ± 0.08. Normal LV MPI is 0.33 ± 0.05.
From Harkness UF, Crombleholme TM. Twin–twin transfusion syndrome: Where do we go from here? Seminars in Perinatology 2005;29:296–304; with permission.

Table 3 CVPS system			
Findings	Normal (2 Points Each)	1-Point Deduction	2-Point Deduction
Hydrops fetalis	None	Ascites; pleural and pericardial effusion	Skin edema
Venous Doppler	Normal	Ductus venosus atrial systolic reversal	Umbilical venous pulsation
Cardiothoracic ratio	<0.35	>0.35 and <0.5	>0.5
Cardiac function	Ventricular SF >0.28 and valve regurgitation	SF <0.28 or TR or semilunar valve regurgitation	TR plus dysfunction or any mitral regurgitation
Arterial Doppler	Normal	Absent end-diastolic flow in the umbilical artery	Reverse end-diastolic flow in the umbilical artery

Abbreviations: SF, shortening fraction; TR, tricuspid regurgitation.

Data from Hofstaetter C, Hansmann M, Eik-Nes SH, et al. A cardiovascular profile score in the surveillance of fetal hydrops. J Matern Fetal Neonatal Med 2006;19(7):407–13; and Shah AD, Border WL, Crombleholme TM, et al. Initial fetal cardiovascular profile score predicts recipient twin outcome in twin-twin transfusion syndrome. J Am Soc Echocardiogr 2008;21(10):1105–8.

Characteristic Doppler Changes in Twin-to-Twin Transfusion Syndrome

Since the 1980s, Doppler waveforms had been used to quantitatively assess placental anastomoses in twins and TTTS pregnancies in relation to fetal growth.[40,41] Several case series earlier reported that TTTS pregnancies have an abnormal pulsatility index of umbilical artery Doppler waveforms; abnormal middle cerebral artery systolic velocities; and pulsatile waveforms in the ductus venosus, hepatic vein, and umbilical veins. Early investigators concluded that Doppler waveforms of the umbilical artery, umbilical vein, ductus venosus, and middle cerebral artery may play a role in diagnosis, prognosis, survival, treatment selection, and follow up after treatment.[42–47] In 1999, Doppler waveforms of the ductus venosus, umbilical artery, and umbilical vein were an integral part of the Quintero TTTS staging system.[8] The investigator incorporated Doppler changes in severe stages of TTTS based on the natural history of the disease.

These Doppler changes in TTTS pregnancies are clinically a reflection of the histopathologic placental vascular communication among the donor, the recipient, and the shared cardiac circulatory system. Thus, umbilical vein, umbilical artery, ductus venosus, and middle cerebral artery Doppler waveforms are reflective of the fetal circulatory and cardiac status.[48–53]

Since the advent of laser therapy as an acceptable primary treatment of TTTS, several investigators have reported changes in the Doppler waveforms after laser therapy as a clinical reflection of interruption of intervascular anastomoses between both twin placentas.

A decrease in the ductus venosus pulsatility index was consistently reported in the recipient after laser therapy. Meanwhile, measurements taken both before and after laser therapy found no significant change or a decrease in umbilical vein flow volume and an inconsistent change in the pulsatility index of the umbilical artery with either worsening or no change or improvement.[54,55] These changes in the recipient twin are reflective of a progressive improvement of previous signs of right-sided cardiac

Table 4 CHOP system			
Recipient	**0 Point**	**1 Point**	**2 Points**
Ventricular findings			
Cardiac enlargement	None	Mild	> Mild
Systolic dysfunction	None	Mild	> Mild
Ventricular hyperterophy	None	Present	
Valve function			
Tricuspid regurgitation	None	Mild	> Mild
Mitral regurgitation	None	Mild	> Mild
Venous Doppler findings			
Tricuspid valve inflow	2 Peaks	1 Peak	
Mitral valve inflow	2 Peaks	1 Peak	
Ductus venosus	All forward	Decreased atrial contraction	Reversal
Umbilical vein	No pulsation	Pulsations	
Great vessel findings			
Outflow tracts	PA > AO	PA = AO	PA < AO, RVOTO
Pulmonary insufficiency	Absent	Present	
Donor twin			
Umbilical artery	Normal	Decreased diastole	Absent or reverse end-diastolic flow

Abbreviations: AO, aorta; PA, pulmonary artery; RVOTO, right ventricular outflow obstruction.
From Rychik J, Tian Z, Bebbington M, et al. The twin-twin transfusion syndrome: spectrum of cardiovascular abnormality and development of a cardiovascular score to assess severity of disease. Am J Obstet Gynecol 2007;197(4):392.e1–8; with permission.

dysfunction as a result of interruption of vascular anastomoses with laser. As for donors, measurements after laser therapy showed a decrease in the umbilical artery pulsatility index, a transient increase in ductus venosus pulsatility index, and an increase in umbilical vein flow volume as compared to preoperative changes. These changes imply the presence of an adequate placental territory and removal of donor hypotension post–laser therapy.[54,55] Thus, laser therapy consistently affects the donor and recipient in opposite ways, inducing hemodynamic variations in TTTS that eliminate the initial hemodynamic imbalance. These changes are mainly in severe TTTS stages in both staging systems.

Quintero Staging System

In 1999, Quintero[8] proposed a staging system for TTTS that considered a sequence of progressive ultrasonographic features (see **Table 1**). Like staging systems for many other medical disorders, this staging system for TTTS was developed to assist in assessing prognosis, survival, treatment selection, and communication among centers. For a staging system to be useful, it not only needs to distinguish good prognoses from bad prognoses at the time the disease is diagnosed, but must also accurately document disease progression or regression. Taylor and colleagues,[56] in a prospective observational study of 52 consecutive TTTS cases, reported that the Quintero staging system did not predict survival at time of presentation nor at treatment of TTTS. However, survival was found to be significantly poorer when stage increased rather than decreased. These investigators concluded that the Quintero staging system should be used cautiously for determining prognosis at the time of diagnosis, suggesting that it may be better suited for monitoring disease progression.[56] Duncombe and colleagues[57] also showed a correlation of Quintero stage at initial presentation and perinatal survival. In another study, Luks and colleagues[58] showed that this staging system is not reflective of progression of disease. To address the controversy in validation of this staging system in regard to disease prognosis and treatment selection, Crombleholme and colleagues[6] suggested a modified staging system that integrates fetal echocardiography. This system is based on the echocardiographic findings and the significance of these findings at each TTTS stage.

Recipient Echocardiographic Findings

TTTS is a progressive disease secondary to interplacental vascular anastomoses leading to functional and structural cardiac changes in the recipient, but seldom in the donor. For donor twins, Doppler echocardiographic changes are rare, and ventricular function and atrioventricular valve competence are usually preserved.[28]

Cardiovascular compromise occurs in most recipient twins, is a major cause of death for these fetuses, and contributes to morbidity and mortality in the donor co-twin.[59] As early as 1992, specific recipient echocardiographic abnormalities were reported. These abnormalities are tricuspid regurgitation, ventricular hypertrophy, increased cardiothoracic ratio, and pulmonary stenosis.[60,61] An echocardiographic examination of the twins is thus an essential component of the initial workup of TTTS. Then, during the antenatal and postnatal periods, follow-up evaluation for progression of the disease is also necessary. The recipient twin manifests a cardiomyopathy that is progressive in nature. At first, right ventricular dilatation and hypertrophy can be identified to a greater degree than ventricular dilatation and hypertrophy in the left ventricle. However, as the process progresses, right and left ventricular hypertrophy become more pronounced. This hypertrophy is associated with atrioventricular valve regurgitation involving first tricuspid regurgitation and then mitral valve regurgitation. Estimates of right ventricular pressures based on flow velocity of tricuspid regurgitation jet suggest that recipient cardiomyopathy is a hypertensive cardiomyopathy. Right ventricular pressures in excess of 70 mm Hg are common. The cause of this hypertensive cardiomyopathy is postulated to be due to vasoactive substances from the placenta or donor twin. The recipient twin experiences an increase in blood volume, vasoconstriction, and ventricular hypertrophy, possibly mediated by angiotensin II and endothelin-1.[27,62]

The most common recipient cardiovascular abnormalities in TTTS are unilateral or bilateral ventricular hypertrophy (ranges 18%–49%), increased cardiothoracic ratio as high as 47%, ventricular dilation (ranges 17%–31%), tricuspid regurgitation (ranges 35%–52%), and mitral regurgitation (ranges 13%–15%).[59,63,64] These abnormalities are more common with advanced stages of disease. Finally, several cases of acquired pulmonary atresia/stenosis with intact ventricular septum have been described in the recipient twin.[59,65]

The reported prevalence of pulmonary stenosis in TTTS is fourfold greater than in non-TTTS.[66] The proposed pathophysiology is that worsening right ventricular hypertrophy, reduced right ventricular systolic function, and severe tricuspid regurgitation result in progressively diminished flow across the pulmonic valve, resulting in stenosis or atresia and, with increase severity, resulting in right ventricular outflow tract obstruction. The incidence of right ventricular outflow tract obstruction in TTTS is as high as 9.6%.[65] These observations are not consistent with primary structural heart disease but rather acquired valvular atresia/stenosis related to TTTS, a unique form of "acquired congenital" heart disease. As for congenital heart diseases, there is a 15- to 23-fold higher risk of congenital heart disease with TTTS over that of singletons, and a 2.78 times more frequent occurrence of congenital heart disease in the setting of TTTS as compared to monochorionic twins without TTTS.[66] The most common structural heart defects in TTTS twins are ventricular septal defects and atrial septal defects.[67]

Echocardiographic Significance in Twin-to-Twin Transfusion Syndrome Staging

The Quintero staging system is a useful basic framework but it ignores the fundamental cardiovascular elements of the disease, which are present in 50% to 60% of Quintero stages I and II.[68] Progression of TTTS-recipient cardiomyopathy is associated with disease stage.[59,64,68] Michelfelder and colleagues,[68] in a recent retrospective study of 42 TTTS patients, looked at the cardiac spectrum changes in relation to the Quintero staging system. The investigators reported that 50% to 61% of recipients as early as stage I and II had functional and quantitative cardiac dysfunction. They concluded that the Quintero system does not reflect the functional and cardiac changes in TTTS. Thus, incorporation of these finding are important in risk stratification and treatment selection.

Hofstaetter and colleagues[69] suggested the CVPS system for fetal heart failure (see **Table 3**). This system has been modified and assessed in TTTS.[70] This CVPS system is a simple system that reflects the functional as well as the structural status of the fetus. This CVPS system is a 10-point scale that incorporates the presence or absence of hydrops, abnormal venous and arterial Doppler findings, cardiomegaly, atrioventricular valve regurgitation, and cardiac dysfunction. There are 1-point to 2-point deductions from the total score, depending on the extent of cardiovascular abnormalities noted.[69] Shah and colleagues,[70] in a retrospective study, assessed the severity of recipient cardiomyopathy at presentation characterized by the CVPS system, and evaluated the relationship of the CVPS system score with recipient-twin survival. The investigators reported that a normal 10-point CVPS system score in the recipient TTTS predicts a recipient survival rate of 75%. By comparison, a recipient with a 1-point deduction had a 55% chance of survival, and a recipient with a 2-point deduction had a 35% chance of survival. Thus, incorporating fetal echocardiographic parameters in TTTS staging can help in predicting prognosis and survival and may also help guide treatment selection.

Rychik and colleagues,[67] (see **Table 4**) of Children's Hospital of Philadelphia, suggested a cardiovascular scoring system to assess the severity of recipient cardiomyopathy. The CHOP scoring system is composed of nine recipient echocardiographic parameters (ventricular hypertrophy, cardiac dilation, ventricular dysfunction, tricuspid valve regurgitation, mitral valve regurgitation, tricuspid valve inflow, mitral valve inflow, right-sided outflow tract, and pulmonary regurgitation) and four ultrasonographic parameters (recipient ductus venoses; recipient umbilical vein; donor umbilical artery). Each parameter was given a numeric value based on its presence, absence, or degree of severity of the finding with a total of 20 points. The investigators reported, as had previous investigators, that the Quintero system does not fully reflect the severity of TTTS. The CHOP scoring system is a comprehensive system but it has several limitations. These limitations include the echocardiographic training required to properly apply the system and the time needed per patient to complete the survey. In addition, before the CHOP scoring system is incorporated in TTTS staging, it needs to be validated in regard to disease prognosis, progression, and relation to survival and treatment.

The Quintero staging system is heavily weighted towards findings in the donor and ignores the cardiovascular impact of TTTS, particularly in the recipient. In stage I, there is only fluid discordance but no assessment of fetal echocardiography findings. Similarly, stage II is reached only when the bladder of the donor cannot be visualized, and stage III mainly reflects changes in Doppler waveforms. While Doppler changes can be in either donor or recipient, the most commonly observed Doppler finding is absent end-diastolic flow in the umbilical artery in the donor. Doppler waveform findings in the recipient twin, such as pulsatile umbilical vein, absent or reversal of a wave in the ductus venosus, or absent or reversal of end-diastolic flow in the umbilical artery, are late findings in the recipient and usually are indicators of severe TTTS cardiomyopathy. Even in stage I with only fluid discordance, 55% of patients have characteristic echocardiographic findings of TTTS cardiomyopathy.[70]

The standard Quintero staging is limited in its ability to predict outcome or progression of disease, is heavily weighted toward findings in the donor twin, and ignores cardiovascular changes in the recipient twin. Cardiac assessment by the CVPS system may improve clinical decision-making and the timing of fetal interventions because most of the parameters used in the CVPS system reflect more advanced disease and do not fully capture the subtle cardiovascular changes in TTTS cardiomyopathy.

Cincinnati Staging System

The Fetal Care Center of Cincinnati[6] incorporated fetal echocardiography in staging TTTS using three parameters to define mild, moderate, and severe cardiomyopathy (see **Table 2**). Echocardiographic features include the presence and severity of atrioventricular valvar incompetence, ventricular wall thickening, and ventricular function, as assessed by the myocardial performance index (also known as the Tei index). The echocardiographic findings in this staging system have been validated in relation to survival,[64] treatment,[64] prognosis, and progression of disease.[59,64,68-70] Also, other groups have demonstrated the impact of these echocardiographic findings in TTTS. Furthermore, the National Institutes of Health (NIH)–sponsored TTTS trial found that the recipient echocardiographic abnormalities were the best predictor of recipient survival.[17]

TREATMENT OPTIONS

Numerous treatments for TTTS have been proposed, including selective feticide, cord coagulation, sectioparva (removing one fetus), placental blood letting, maternal digitalis, maternal indomethacin, serial amnioreduction, microseptostomy of the intertwin membrane, and nonselective or selective fetoscopic laser photocoagulation. For decades in the United States, serial amnioreduction has been the most prevalent therapy for TTTS, but in recent years, selective fetoscopic laser photocoagulation has become more widely accepted and in many centers is the primary treatment offered.

Amnioreduction

Amnioreduction was employed initially for maternal comfort and as a means to control polyhydramnios in the hope of prolonging the pregnancy until the risks of extreme prematurity were lessened. In addition, amnioreduction improves uteroplacental blood flow, likely by reducing intra-amniotic pressure from polyhydramnios. In uncontrolled series, amnioreduction improved survival compared with the natural history of untreated TTTS. Moise,[71] in a review of 26 reports dating from the 1930s of 252 fetuses, found an overall survival of 49%. The survival in more recent series, with more consistently aggressive serial amnioreduction to reduce amniotic fluid volume to normal, have ranged from as low as 37% to as high as 83%.[5,72–76] However, these retrospective series are made up of few patients and those patients represent a range of gestational ages and cover the spectrum of TTTS severity. Severity of TTTS and gestational age at diagnosis may have a profound impact on the observed mortality with any treatment strategy. The earlier in gestation that TTTS presents, the worse is the prognosis. Mari and associates[77] found that patients presenting with advanced TTTS prior to 22 weeks' gestation and absent end-diastolic flow in the recipient umbilical artery had a survival of both twins with aggressive amnioreduction of only 13%; with absent end-diastolic flow in the donor umbilical artery, survival was 33%.

Microseptostomy

The paradoxic resolution of oligohydramnios after a single amnioreduction was suggested initially by Saade and associates[4] to be due to inadvertent puncture of the intertwin membrane. Intertwin septostomy was proposed specifically as a treatment for TTTS to restore amniotic fluid dynamics without the need for repeated amnioreduction. One objection to this approach is that it possibly results in a large septostomy, creating an essentially monoamniotic sac with the attendant risk of cord entanglement. In their small multicenter series of 12 patients, Saade and associates[4] reported an 81% survival with microseptostomy. However, not only was this series small and uncontrolled, but there was no report of neurologic or cardiac morbidity. In a direct comparison in a small retrospective single-institution series of serial amnioreduction and microseptostomy, Johnson and colleagues[78] observed no survival advantage with either therapy. This was confirmed in a subsequent study by Moise and colleagues,[79] who reported the results of a multicenter prospective randomized clinical trial comparing amnioreduction to septostomy. The survival in each arm of the study was 65%, consistent with the concept that the effect of amnioreduction may be inadvertent septostomy. These studies, however, cannot prove that intertwin microseptostomy is the mechanism by which amnioreduction works. The use of ultrasonographically guided microseptostomy has fallen out of favor largely because of the risk of creating a monoamniotic gestation and the attendant risk of cord entanglement and cord accident.[80]

Fetoscopic Laser Photocoagulation

The first treatment for TTTS that attempted to treat the anatomic basis for the syndrome was reported by De Lia and colleagues,[81] who described fetoscopic laser photocoagulation of vessels crossing the intertwin membrane. This treatment option should be superior, at least in theory, because it not only arrests shunting of blood between twins, but it also halts transfer of potentially vasoactive mediators. In their small series, these investigators reported a survival of 53% in 26 patients. Although survival was not significantly better than those in previous reports with serial amnioreduction, the "neurologic outcome" in 96% of survivors was "normal," as assessed by head ultrasonography. Other groups from Europe have reported similar survival with nonselective laser photocoagulation. Ville and colleagues[82] reported 53% survival with a fetoscopic laser technique, which was better than the survival observed with historical controls at the same center with serial amnioreduction (37%). They also observed a lower incidence of abnormalities detected by neonatal head ultrasonography compared with historical controls.

The nonselective fetoscopic laser technique photocoagulates all vessels crossing the intertwin membrane.[83] This approach may be problematic because the intertwin membrane often bears no relationship to the vascular equator of the placenta. Thus, nonselective laser photocoagulation of all vessels crossing the intertwin membrane may sacrifice vessels not responsible for the TTTS, resulting in a higher death rate of the donor twin from acute placental insufficiency.[84] More recently, Quintero and colleagues[84] described a selective approach to fetoscopic laser photocoagulation in TTTS that does not photocoagulate every vessel crossing the intertwin membrane. Only direct, artery-to-artery and vein-to-vein connections are photocoagulated, along with, more commonly, any unpaired artery going to a cotyledon drained by a corresponding unpaired vein (and vice versa) going to the opposite (co-twin's) umbilical cord. Vessels on the chorionic plate can be differentiated endoscopically because arteries usually cross over veins and are darker because of lower oxygen saturation. In a prospective, but nonrandomized, comparison of patients treated by serial amnioreduction at one center and selective laser photocoagulation at another, the overall survival was not statistically significantly different (61% for laser versus 51% for serial amnioreduction). However, the survival of at least one twin with laser photocoagulation was 79% compared with 60% for serial amnioreduction ($P<.05$).

Quintero and colleagues[84] retrospectively examined data from 78 patients treated by serial amnioreduction and 95 patients treated with selective laser photocoagulation. They found no significant difference in patient distribution by stage. Perinatal survival was not significantly different in the laser versus the amnioreduction group (64.2% versus 57.7%), although there was an inverse relationship between fetal survival and stage in the amniocentesis group but not in the laser group. For stage IV disease, fetal survival in the amnioreduction group was significantly lower than in the laser group (20.6% versus 63.6%, $P<.001$). This information has important implications for evaluation of treatment options and the development of stage-based treatment protocols. One potential limitation to the success of laser treatment is the presence of deep vascular arteriovenous anastomoses that cannot be identified endoscopically. In one study, vascular casts of 8 of 15 placentas (53%) demonstrated potentially significant atypical arteriovenous anastomoses such that two apparently normal cotyledons actually communicated below the chorionic surface.[85] A second type of atypical arteriovenous anastomoses was noted in 11 of the 15 placentas (73%) in which shared cotyledons arose within larger apparently normal cotyledons. Such anastomoses would appear as shared cotyledons on endoscopy, and ablating these has the potential to destroy some surrounding normal cotyledon that, in the donor's territory, could contribute to placental insufficiency.[85] In up to 20% of cases, communicating vessels on the chorionic plate are missed at the time of fetoscopic laser treatment,[85] but only 5% of these cases were associated with persistence of TTTS. These observations point to the necessity of a careful fetoscopic inspection of the chorionic plate to be certain that no vessel is missed.

Fetoscopic Cord Coagulation

Some centers have taken the view that the most definitive approach to treating TTTS is selective reduction using fetoscopic cord ligation or coagulation. The rationale is that cord occlusion and sacrifice of one twin arrests the syndrome, prolongs the gestation, and maximizes the outcome for the surviving twin. Crombleholme and colleagues[6] have reserved this approach for instances in which advanced TTTS cardiomyopathy has irretrievably compromised the recipient twin and there is no hope for salvage. In cases where there is also evidence of placental insufficiency due to unequal sharing between the donor and recipient, the selective fetoscopic laser procedure may result in death of the donor twin from acute placental insufficiency within hours of the procedure and death of the recipient twin from progressive TTTS cardiomyopathy. In this situation, fetoscopic cord coagulation may be the best option available. Cord coagulation preserves the vascular communications between the donor twin and the placenta in the recipient twin's domain. In their series of 19 of 20 such cases, these investigators observed rebound fetal growth and restoration of amniotic fluid volume, and delivery of a neurologically intact donor twin at a mean gestational age of 34 weeks was achieved.[17] One survivor had grade I intraventricular hemorrhage but is otherwise doing well.

Sequential Treatment

The approach at the Fetal Care Center of Cincinnati has been to offer sequential therapy tailored to the needs of a given set of twins based on gestational age at presentation and evidence of progression of hemodynamic compromise according to Doppler velocimetry and echocardiographic changes.[64] In this approach, only those cases in which less invasive approaches have failed are offered the more invasive fetoscopic treatments. For patients who present later than 24 weeks of gestation, we have favored amnioreduction because of the usually more favorable prognosis in these patients except in cases of severe TTTS cardiomyopathy. For patients presenting prior to 24 weeks' gestation in which advanced cardiac changes are not seen in the recipient (stages I, II, III, IIIA), we have tended toward amnioreduction as an initial therapy with serial echocardiographic surveillance. For patients who have echocardiographic evidence of moderate or severe TTTS cardiomyopathy (stages IIIB, IIIC, IV), we favor selective fetoscopic laser treatment because there is insufficient time to see if the pregnancy will respond to amnioreduction before TTTS cardiomyopathy worsens. Patients presenting earlier in gestation tend to develop signs of more rapid hemodynamic progression of TTTS despite less abnormal amniotic fluid dynamics. For this reason, all pregnancies treated by amnioreduction undergo close serial ultrasonographic and echocardiographic surveillance for progressive cardiac and hemodynamic changes, which are indications to go on to selective fetoscopic laser surgery. We reserve fetoscopic cord coagulation in TTTS for instances in which cotwin demise is imminent and fetoscopic laser surgery might adversely affect the available placental mass in the donor fetus, predisposing to acute placental insufficiency and risking demise of the donor as well. The one downside to an initial trial of amnioreduction is chorioamnionic separation, which occurred in one patient in this series (3%); chorioamnionic separation precludes a fetoscopic procedure. Fortunately, this patient had responded to amnioreduction.

Complications Following Laser Treatment

Few studies have addressed laser complications in TTTS pregnancies and identified predisposing factors. Yamamoto and colleagues,[86] in a retrospective study of 175 TTTS pregnancies treated with laser, reported that the most frequent complication was premature rupture of membranes, which occurred in 28% of the cases. However, premature rupture of membranes occurred within 3 weeks after laser therapy in only 12% of the cases. The entry of the trocar was transplacental in 48 cases (27%), but it was not associated with adverse outcome.

A few case series reported late complications of laser photocoagulation, such as monoamniotic gestation, amniotic band syndrome, and ischemic limb or bowel atresia from vascular accidents, which can also occur in monochorionic twins without TTTS. All laser-treated cases should be followed closely with weekly surveillance of ultrasound to detect any late complications. In a large cohort of 151 cases, Robyr and colleagues[87] demonstrated that progression of the disease occurred in 14% of cases and 13% developed reversal of TTTS (ie, the recipient twin behaves like the donor and the donor develops TTTS like the recipient twin). In addition, twin anemia polycythemia sequence has been reported in up to 13% of cases following TTTS. Habli and colleagues[88] recently reported the early and late complication rates with selective fetoscopic laser photocoagulation (SFLP) from the Fetal Care Center of Cincinnati in a cohort of 139 consecutively treated cases. In this series, progression or persistence of TTTS occurred in only 2 cases (1.4%). Twin anemia polycythemia sequence occurred in only 3 cases (2.2%). The low rate of complications related to missed vascular connections was attributed to a stringent mapping protocol used by this group during SFLP.

NEONATAL MORTALITY AND MORBIDITY IN TWIN-TO-TWIN TRANSFUSION SYNDROME

Compared to mothers of dichorionic twins, mothers of monochorionic twins are six times more likely to miscarry before 24 weeks, have a higher prevalence of preterm delivery before 32 weeks (9% versus 6%), and are more likely to have both twins small for gestational weight (8% versus 2%).[89] Monochorionic pregnancies have a perinatal mortality rate three times higher[90] and are eight times more likely to have cerebral palsy[91] than dichorionic pregnancies. The higher rates of perinatal mortality and morbidity are due to almost ubiquitous vascular anastomoses.[11,92–94] The complications in monochorionic twins with TTTS should be interpreted in the light of a baseline greater risk of complications in monochorionic twins without TTTS.

Short-Term Outcome

Despite improved survival after fetoscopic laser treatment, the optimal treatment for TTTS, neonates of TTTS pregnancies still suffer severe neonatal morbidities secondary to prematurity in addition to TTTS-related conditions (**Table 5**). TTTS pregnancies have a high prevalence of adverse neonatal outcome as compared to non-TTTS monochorionic pregnancies. The reported miscarriage rate in TTTS ranges between 3.5% and 17%. Preterm premature rupture of fetal membranes in TTTS occurs earlier than 24 weeks in 1% to 13% and later than 24 weeks in 5% to 9.8%. In addition, preterm labor, defined as labor occuring prior to 33 weeks, occurs in TTTS in 27% to 44%.[57,94–98] Furthermore, TTTS neonates in neonatal intensive care units have a 4.8% to 7% rate of acute renal failure, a 3% to 4% rate of necrotizing enterocolitis, a 27% to 62% rate of respiratory distress syndrome with a 4% to 34% prevalence of intraventricular hemorrhage grade 3 to 4. There are also some reported cases of persistent pulmonary hypertension (3%) in pregnancies complicated with TTTS. This wide range in frequency of neonatal morbidity is mainly due inadequate sample size; different outcome measure definitions; and varying experience, treatment modalities, and management among centers.[57,94–99]

Fetal/neonatal survival

The Eurofoetus trial[100] was the first prospective randomized trial to compare the efficacy and safety of treatment of TTTS with laser therapy to serial amnioreduction. Women presenting between 15 and 26 weeks' gestation with polyhydramnios in the recipient twin and oligohydramnios in the donor twin participated in the trial. The patients were staged according to Quintero criteria: 52% were stage I or II, 47% were stage III, and 1% were stage IV. Enrollment was halted after a planned interim analysis revealed a significantly higher likelihood of survival of at least one twin to 28 days of age (76% versus 56%, P<.009) and to 6 months of age (76% versus 51%, P<.002) in the laser group compared with the amnioreduction group. In addition, more infants were alive without neurologic abnormalities detected on neuroimaging studies in the laser group (52% versus 31%, P<.003). The overall survival in the laser

Table 5
Short-term neonatal outcome in TTTS

| Author/Year | TTTS Pregnancy (n) | Gestational Age at Delivery (wk) | Delivery Mode | | Preterm Labor <33 wk (%) | Acute Renal Failure (%) | Necrotizing Enterocolitis (%) | Respiratory Distress Syndrome (%) | Intraventricular Hemorrhage Grade 3–4 (%) |
			Spontaneous Vaginal Delivery (%)	Cesarean Section (%)					
Dickson/2000[103]	112	29	NA	NA	NA	7	3	27	16
Duncomb/2003[113]	69	29.4	NA	NA	NA	4.8	2.9	62	5.8
Lepoir/2005[104]	85	32.6	34	66	NA	NA	3	34	14
Lufti/2005[106]	48	NA	27	73	27	5.2	NA	27	13
Acosta/2007[107]	101	33	NA	NA	44	NA	4.3	43	4
Lenclen/2007[108]	79	29	NA	NA	NA	NA	NA	NA	NA

Abbreviation: NA, data not available.

arm was 57%, which was consistent with survival rates in previous reports of nonselective fetoscopic laser treatment (53%).[82,101] This rate is significantly lower, however, than the survival reported with SFLP (64%–68%).[95,102] Of particular concern is the poor survival observed in the amnioreduction arm of 39%, which is significantly lower than previously reported (60%–65%).[74,75,77,102] Antenatal, peripartum, and neonatal care was provided by the referring hospital, and lack of standardization may explain some of these differences.[103] The decreased survival in the amnioreduction group may reflect the higher pregnancy termination rate in the amnioreduction group (16 versus 0 in the laser group). The terminations were requested after the diagnosis of severe fetal complications. It would be instructive to know whether these women were offered cord coagulation as a means of rescuing one baby.[102] Reliable assessment of neurologic outcome is critical when assessing efficacy of treatment for TTTS. Although the rate of abnormality on neurologic imaging was lower in the laser group (7% versus 17%), long-term neurodevelopmental assessment has revealed no difference in outcome between survivors treated by fetoscopic laser and those treated by amnioreduction.[104]

The NIH-sponsored TTTS trial is the only other prospective randomized trial after the Eurofetus trial comparing survival among those receiving amnioreduction versus SFLP.[17] This trial differed from the Eurofoetus trial in several important aspects. First, to qualify for the NIH trial, the TTTS patient had to fail to respond to a qualifying amniocentesis. The rationale for this requirement was to eliminate those who were more likely to respond to amnioreduction, the so-called "single amnio paradox." Second, patients were candidates only if the TTTS presented earlier than 22 weeks of gestation, and no stage I patients were candidates for the trial. These two requirements were substantially different from those of the Eurofoetus trial, in which women were randomized into the trial up to 26 weeks of gestation, and 52% of those entered were stage I or II.[100] The NIH study was stopped early, after 42 women were randomized, when the trial oversight committee detected a trend in adverse fetal outcome affecting the recipient twin in one treatment arm and recommended to the data safety monitoring board that the trial be stopped to allow biostatistical analysis of the adverse trend. Results of the NIH TTTS trial showed no statistically significant difference in overall neonatal survival to 30 postnatal days (60% versus 43%, P not significant) or neonatal survival of one or both twins in the same pregnancy (75% versus 65%, P not significant) in cases of severe TTTS treated by either amnioreduction or SFLP. Despite these overall results, a statistically significant worse fetal survival was observed among recipient twins in pregnancies treated by SFLP compared with those treated by amnioreduction. This apparent conundrum can be accounted for by recipient fetal losses in the SFLP arm being balanced by increased treatment failures among recipients in the amnioreduction arm. These results suggest that, in these highly selected cases of severe TTTS, neither treatment is superior to the other. Once TTTS reaches this degree of severity, the mortality among recipients is considerable, but the losses may occur at different times, depending on treatment. The impact of TTTS severity on fetal survival is supported further by the significantly worse fetal survival among recipient twins in stages III and IV compared with those in stage II. The strongest predictor of recipient demise in this trial is echocardiographic evidence of TTTS cardiomyopathy.

The losses of fetal recipients treated by SFLP usually occur within 24 hours of the procedure. In contrast, the recipients treated by amnioreduction are not lost following the procedure, but there is progressive TTTS cardiomyopathy, as reflected by more recipients in the amnioreduction arm meeting criteria to be declared treatment failures. In every case, findings in the recipient twin met criteria for treatment failure. Taken together, these data suggest a disproportionate impact of TTTS cardiomyopathy on recipient survival in advanced stages of TTTS no matter what treatment they receive.

Recently, Rossi and D'Addario[105] reported the results of a Cochrane review of TTTS with a meta-analysis that included data from both the Eurofoetus and NIH trials. The conclusion drawn from this analysis was that SFLP of TTTS is preferred over amnioreduction when it is available and amnioreduction is preferred when SFLP is not available. The results of this analysis are likely to be skewed toward fetoscopic laser based on the small numbers of individuals included from the NIH trial (n = 40) compared with the number included from the Eurofoetus trial (n = 142). Amnioreduction is readily available, less costly, and less invasive; laser therapy is only available at select institutions and requires specialized training. Although it makes sense to use amnioreduction where treatment options give similar results, it would be prudent to move promptly to laser therapy in the setting of advanced disease.

In our experience, for patients who respond to amnioreduction, the overall survival rate has been 88%.[104] In those cases in which echocardiographic progression is detected despite amnioreduction, the overall survival rate when SFLP is performed is 80%. The difference in survival between responders to amnioreduction and those who progress to SFLP are not statistically significantly different, suggesting that survival was not compromised by an initial trial of amnioreduction before progressing to SFLP.

Long-Term Outcome

Renal outcomes in twin-to-twin transfusion syndrome
The donor twin in TTTS pregnancies secondary to vascular anastomoses suffers from hypovolemia, hypotension, and oliguria, which predispose the donor to acute and possible chronic renal insufficiency. There is little information about the impact of such hemodynamic derangement in TTTS on the donor kidney in the short and long term. Beck and colleagues[106] conducted a retrospective chart review of 18 surviving twin pairs of TTTS treated with laser photocoagulation followed up over a range of 1 to 9 years. The investigators reported no significant renal impairment between donors and recipients.

Although, this series reported complete recovery of donor kidney status, other investigators have reported the development of renal failure requiring dialysis in TTTS survivors. Thus, renal function should be monitored carefully at birth in TTTS twins.

Cardiovascular outcomes in twin-to-twin transfusion syndrome
Information concerning the long-term cardiovascular implications of TTTS is scarce, as are data on the effect of various treatment modalities for TTTS on cardiovascular compromise and progression. Two main theories have been suggested to explain the etiology of cardiovascular morbidities in the recipient twin. One theory suggests that increased preload due to hypervolemia in the recipient is a major cause of cardiac hypertrophy. The second theory is that increases in afterload due to increases to vasoactive substances either endogenously secreted in recipient or due to cross-passage from the donor could cause a hypertensive state in the recipient.

Few studies have looked at the impact of the above changes on the cardiac function of the recipient postnatally and during infancy. Fesslova and colleagues,[107] in a retrospective chart review of 17 TTTS pregnancies with 6 severe cases treated with amnioreduction, found no specific cardiac involvement in donor twins in utero or after birth. All recipient twin fetuses showed variable degrees of biventricular hypertrophy and dilation with tricuspid regurgitation. These cardiac features of the 11 surviving recipient infants gradually regressed and returned completely to normal within 40 days to 6 months after birth.

Herberg and colleagues[108] reported long-term cardiac function in a prospective study of 89 survivors (38 donors, 51 recipients) of 73 severe TTTS pregnancies at 21 month of age. All TTTS pregnancies were treated with fetoscopic laser photocoagulation. The investigators reported 11.2% incidence of structural heart disease and specifically a 7.8% pulmonary stenosis rate, which are higher than in the general population. Eighty-seven percent of the survivors had a normal cardiac examination. Despite the high rate and severity of prenatal cardiac impairment in recipients, systolic or diastolic ventricular function completely normalizes over the long term. While these reports are useful, sufficient information is still lacking in regard to response to treatment modality and impact of stage on both donor and recipient cardiac function.

Neurodevelopmental outcomes in twin-to-twin transfusion syndrome

Brain injury in TTTS fetuses can occur if both twins survive or a co-twin dies. If both twins survive, brain damage in the recipient twin could be related to polycythemia and venous stasis. In the donor, neurologic injury may be due to anemia or hypotension. If one co-twin dies, an acute fall in blood pressure may causes a decrease in placental resistance resulting in decrease in cerebral perfusion pressure of the surviving twin, leading to neurologic ischemic insult. The neurologic morbidity among survivors, regardless of treatment modality, is an underappreciated sequela of TTTS.

Neurodevelopmental outcomes in twin-to-twin transfusion syndrome treated with amnioreduction

The International Amnioreduction Registry tracked 223 women who had TTTS diagnosed before 28 weeks' gestation and were treated with serial aggressive amnioreduction.[77] Of those infants who survived to 4 weeks, 26 recipients (26/109 = 24%) and 22 donors (22/88 = 25%) had abnormal findings after ultrasound scanning. Findings included severe intraventricular hemorrhage, ventricular dilation, cerebral echogenic foci, cerebral cysts, and periventricular leukomalacia, among other less common lesions. Eighty infants died before reaching 4 weeks of age, and how many of these would have had abnormal imaging if cranial ultrasonography had been performed is unknown.

Among patients in the TTTS Registry from Australia and New Zealand, most of whom had been treated with amnioreduction, the rate of abnormal cranial ultrasonography findings was similar at 27.3%.[102] The rate of periventricular leukomalacia in this group was 10.8%, which is particularly important because of the association of this lesion with cerebral palsy. In another small series of patients treated with amnioreduction, the rate of abnormal neonatal cranial ultrasonography findings was as high as 58%.[109] However, neuroimaging does not always correlate with neurodevelopmental outcome.

Only a few studies have reported longer-term neurodevelopmental outcome. The incidence of severe neurodevelopmental abnormalities in monochorionic twins without TTTS is 4% to 8%.[91] In one small study that followed TTTS survivors for a mean of 6.2 years (range 4–11 years), the incidence of cerebral palsy was 26% (5 of 19 infants) in the group treated by serial amnioreduction. Studying infants from pregnancies complicated by TTTS and treated with amnioreduction, Mari and colleagues[77] detected a rate of cerebral palsy of 4.7% (2 of 42 infants) in those children who survived to more than 24 months of age.

Wee and colleagues[90] studied the long-term neurologic outcome of 52 children from 31 TTTS pregnancies who survived to more than 18 months. Most of the mothers of these children had been treated with amnioreduction. The comparison was a regional cohort of term and preterm infants, with most born very preterm. In addition, the TTTS babies were compared with matched singleton and twin control groups. The mean IQ of TTTS survivors was significantly lower than that of the comparison cohort, due primarily to a 13-point IQ reduction in those children born before 33 weeks' gestation. There was no difference in the rate of cerebral palsy (5.8% for TTTS versus 4.9% for very preterm twins versus 3.3% for very preterm singletons) or behavioral test results in the TTTS survivors. This was a small study, however, and not sufficiently powered to demonstrate differences in cerebral palsy.

Neurodevelopmental outcomes in twin-to-twin transfusion syndrome treated with laser

Few studies have examined the long-term outcome of survivors of TTTS treated with intrauterine laser photocoagulation therapy. Banek and colleagues[110] reported that in 89 such children, 78% showed normal development at a median age of 22 months. Eleven percent had minor neurologic abnormalities, including strabismus, mildly delayed motor development, or mildly abnormal speech. The remaining 11% suffered significant neurologic deficiencies, including cerebral palsy, hemiparesis, and spastic quadriplegia.

The findings of this study are consistent with those of Sutcliffe and colleagues,[111] who reported a cerebral palsy rate of 9% in children after in utero treatment with laser therapy for TTTS. Graef and coworkers,[112] in a report of 167 TTTS survivors who had been treated by fetoscopic laser, found normal neurodevelopmental testing results in 86.8% of cases, with 7.2% of infants having minor neurologic deficiencies and 6% having major neurologic deficiencies, such as cerebral palsy, hemiparesis, and quadriplegia. These findings were not unlike those in follow-up of monochorionic twins without TTTS, and the most severely affected children were delivered prior to 28 weeks' gestation, suggesting an important influence of gestational age on neurodevelopmental outcome.

Similarly, Ortqvist and colleagues[113] reported the neurodevelopmental outcome of 114 survivors treated in the Eurofoetus trial, in which 13.2% had evidence of a major neurodevelopmental abnormality. However, there was no difference between those who had been treated by laser and those treated by amnioreduction. Lastly, Lopriore and colleagues[114] published a detailed neurological, mental, and psychomotor follow-up of 115 laser-treated TTTS survivors at 2 years of age corrected for prematurity. The incidence of neurodevelopmental impairment was 17% (19 of 115) and was due to cerebral palsy (n = 8), mental developmental delay (n = 9), psychomotor developmental delay (n = 12), and deafness (n = 1). Perinatal factors, including gestational age at delivery and Apgar score, correlated with adverse outcome. Earlier and more sensitive antenatal detection of central nervous system injury[7,115] has been reported recently with the adjunct use of MRI techniques. MRI has enabled the detection of dilated cerebral venous sinus and more clearly delineated central nervous system lesions in up to 8% of TTTS fetuses prior to treatment. The improvements in antenatal detection may result in further improvements in clinical management[7] and reduced morbidity and its severity in survivors.

REFERENCES

1. Martin JA, Hamilton BE, Sutton D, Centers for Disease Control and Prevention National Center for Health Statistics National Vital Statistics System, et al. Births: final data for 2005. Natl Vital Stat Rep 2007;56(6):1–103.
2. Hall JG. Twinning. Lancet 2003;362:735–43.

3. Fieni S, Gramellini D, Piantelli G, et al. Twin-twin transfusion syndrome: a review of treatment option. Acta Biomed 2004;75:34–9.
4. Saade GR, Belfort MA, Berry DL, et al. Amniotic septostomy for the treatment of twin oligohydramnios-polyhydramnios sequence. Fetal Diagn Ther 1998;13: 86–93.
5. Urig MA, Clewell WH, Elliot JP. Twin-twin transfusion syndrome. Am J Obstet Gynecol 1990;163:1522–6.
6. Harkness UF, Crombleholme TM. Twin–twin transfusion syndrome: Where do we go from here? Semin Perinatol 2005;29:296–304.
7. Crombleholme TM. The treatment of twin-twin transfusion syndrome. Semin Pediatr Surg 2003;12:175–81.
8. Quintero RA. Twin-twin transfusion syndrome. Clin Perinatol 2003;30:591–600.
9. Haverkamp F, Lex C, Hanisch C, et al. Neurodevelopmental risks in twin-to-twin transfusion syndrome: preliminary findings. Europ J Paediatr Neurol 2001;5: 21–7.
10. Denbow ML, Cox P, Taylor M, et al. Placental angioarchitecture in monochorionic twin pregnancies: relationship to fetal growth, fetofetal transfusion syndrome, and pregnancy outcome. Am J Obstet Gynecol 2000;182:417–26.
11. De Paepe ME, Burke S, Luks FI, et al. Demonstration of placental vascular anatomy in monochorionic twin gestations. Pediatr Dev Pathol 2002;5:37–44.
12. Jain V, Fisk NM. The twin-twin transfusion syndrome. Clin Obstet Gynecol 2004; 47:181–202.
13. De Lia J, Fisk N, Hecher K, et al. Twin-to-twin transfusion syndrome—debates on the etiology, natural history and management. Ultrasound Obstet Gynecol 2000; 16:210–3.
14. De Paepe ME, DeKoninck P, Friedman RM. Vascular distribution patterns in monochorionic twin placentas. Placenta 2005;26:471–5.
15. Umur A, van Gemert MJ, Nikkels PG, et al. Monochorionic twins and twin-twin transfusion syndrome: the protective role of arterio-arterial anastomoses. Placenta 2002;23:201–9.
16. Taylor MJ, Denbow ML, Duncan KR, et al. Antenatal factors at diagnosis that predict outcome in twin-twin transfusion syndrome. Am J Obstet Gynecol 2000;183(4):1023–8.
17. Crombleholme TM, Shera D, Lee H, et al. A prospective, randomized, multi-center trial of amnioreduction vs selective fetoscopic laser photocoagulation for the treatment of severe twin-twin transfusion syndrome. Am J Obstet Gynecol 2007;197:396e1–9.
18. Luks FI, Carr SR, De Paepe ME, et al. What—and why—the pediatric surgeon should know about twin-to-twin transfusion syndrome. J Pediatr Surg 2005;40: 1063–9.
19. Bajoria R, Wee LY, Anwar S, et al. Outcome of twin pregnancies complicated by single intrauterine death in relation to vascular anatomy of the monochorionic placenta. Hum Reprod 1999;14(8):2124–30.
20. Lopriore E, Sueters M, Middeldorp JM, et al. Velamentous cord insertion and unequal placental territories in monochorionic twins with and without twin-to-twin-transfusion syndrome. Am J Obstet Gynecol 2007;196(2):159e1–5.
21. Bajoria R. Vascular anatomy of monochorionic placenta in relation to discordant growth and amniotic fluid volume. Hum Reprod 1998;13:2933–40.
22. Bruner JP, Anderson TL, Rosemond RL. Placental pathophysiology of the twin oligohydramnios-polyhydramnios sequence and the twin-twin transfusion syndrome. Placenta 1998;19:81–6.

23. Kilby MD, Platt C, Whittle MJ, et al. Renin gene expression in fetal kidneys of pregnancies complicated by twin-twin transfusion syndrome. Pediatr Dev Pathol 2001;4:175–9.
24. De Paepe ME, Stopa E, Huang C, et al. Renal tubular apoptosis in twin-to-twin transfusion syndrome. Pediatr Dev Pathol 2003;6:215–25.
25. Mahieu-Caputo D, Dommergues M, Delezoide AL, et al. Twin-to-twin transfusion syndrome. Role of the fetal renin angiotensin system. Am J Pathol 2000;156: 629–63.
26. Mahieu-Caputo D, Muller F, Joly D, et al. Pathogenesis of twin-twin transfusion syndrome: the renin-angiotensin system hypothesis. Fetal Diagn Ther 2001;16: 241–4.
27. Cameron VA, Ellmers LJ. Minireview: natriuretic peptides during development of the fetal heart and circulation. Endocrinology 2003;144(6):2191–4, Review.
28. Bajoria R, Ward S, Chatterjee R. Brain natriuretic peptide and endothelin-1 in the pathogenesis of polyhydramnios-oligohydramnios in monochorionic twins. Am J Obstet Gynecol 2003;189:189–94.
29. Bajoria R, Ward S, Chatterjee R. Natriuretic peptides in the pathogenesis of cardiac dysfunction in the recipient fetus of twin-twin transfusion syndrome. Am J Obstet Gynecol 2002;186:121–7.
30. Bajoria R, Ward S, Sooranna SR. Atrial natriuretic peptide mediated polyuria: pathogenesis of polyhydramnios in the recipient twin of twin-twin transfusion syndrome. Placenta 2001;22:716–24.
31. Bajoria R, Sullivan M, Fisk NM. Endothelin concentrations in monochorionic twins with severe twin-twin transfusion syndrome. Hum Reprod 1999;14(6):1614–8.
32. Kusanovic JP, Romero R, Espinoza J, et al. Twin-to-twin transfusion syndrome: an antiangiogenic state? Am J Obstet Gynecol 2008;198:382e1–8.
33. Gohlke BC, Huber A, Hecher K, et al. Fetal insulin-like growth factor (IGF)-I, IGF-II, and ghrelin in association with birth weight and postnatal growth in monozygotic twins with discordant growth. J Clin Endocrinol Metab 2005;90:2270–4.
34. Street ME, Seghini P, Fieni S, et al. Changes in interleukin-6 and IGF system and their relationships in placenta and cord blood in newborns with fetal growth restriction compared with controls. Eur J Endocrinol 2006;155:567–74.
35. Davidson S, Hod M, Merlob P, et al. Leptin, insulin, insulinlike growth factors and their binding proteins in cord serum: insight into fetal growth and discordancy. Clin Endocrinol (Oxf) 2006;65:586–92.
36. Hoggard N, Haggarty P, Thomas L, et al. Leptin expression in placental and fetal tissues: Does leptin have a functional role? Biochem Soc Trans 2001;29:57–63.
37. Sooranna SR, Ward S, Bajoria R. Discordant fetal leptin levels in monochorionic twins with chronic midtrimester twin-twin transfusion syndrome. Placenta 2001; 22:392–8.
38. Brennan JN, Diwan RV, Rosen MG, et al. Fetofetal transfusion syndrome: prenatal ultrasonographic diagnosis. Radiology 1982;143(2):535–6.
39. Uotila J, Tammela O. Acute intrapartum fetoplacental transfusion in monochorionic twin pregnancy. Obstet Gynecol 1999;5:819–21.
40. Gerson AG, Wallace DM, Bridgens NK, et al. Duplex Doppler ultrasound in the evaluation of growth in twin pregnancies. Obstet Gynecol 1987;70(3 Pt 1): 419–23.
41. Pretorius DH, Manchester D, Barkin S, et al. Doppler ultrasound of twin transfusion syndrome. J Ultrasound Med 1988;7(3):117–24, Review.
42. Yamada A, Kasugai M, Ohno Y, et al. Antenatal diagnosis of twin-twin transfusion syndrome by Doppler ultrasound. Obstet Gynecol 1991;78(6):1058–61.

43. Hecher K, Ville Y, Nicolaides KH. Color Doppler ultrasonography in the identification of communicating vessels in twin-twin transfusion syndrome and acardiac twins. J Ultrasound Med 1995;14(1):37–40.
44. Hecher K, Ville Y, Nicolaides KH. Fetal arterial Doppler studies in twin-twin transfusion syndrome. J Ultrasound Med 1995;14(2):101–8.
45. Hecher K, Ville Y, Snijders R, et al. Doppler studies of the fetal circulation in twin-twin transfusion syndrome. Ultrasound Obstet Gynecol 1995;5(5):318–24.
46. Bower SJ, Flack NJ, Sepulveda W, et al. Uterine artery blood flow response to correction of amniotic fluid volume. Am J Obstet Gynecol 1995;173(2):502–7.
47. Zikulnig L, Hecher K, Bregenzer T, et al. Prognostic factors in severe twin-twin transfusion syndrome treated by endoscopic laser surgery. Ultrasound Obstet Gynecol 1999;14(6):380–7.
48. Badeer HS. Hemodynamics for medical students. Adv Physiol Educ 2001;25: 44–52.
49. Gosling RG, King DH. Ultrasound angiology. In: Marcus AW, Adamson L, editors. Arteries and veins. Edinburgh (UK): Churchill Livingstone; 1975. p. 61–98.
50. van Gemert MJC, Sterenborg HJCM. Hemodynamic model of twin–twin transfusion syndrome in monochorionic twin pregnancies. Placenta 1998;19:195–208.
51. Wee LY, Taylor MJ, Vanderheyden T, et al. Transmitted arterio-arterial anastomosis waveforms causing cyclically intermittent absent/reversed end-diastolic umbilical artery flow in monochorionic twins. Placenta 2003;24:772–8.
52. Kiserud T, Eik-Nes SH, Blaas HG, et al. Ultrasonographic velocimetry of the fetal ductus venosus. Lancet 1991;338:1412–4.
53. Baschat AA. Relationship between placental blood flow resistance and precordial venous Doppler indices. Ultrasound Obstet Gynecol 2003;22:561–6.
54. Kontopoulos EV, Quintero RA, Chmait RH, et al. Percent absent end-diastolic velocity in the umbilical artery waveform as a predictor of intrauterine fetal demise of the donor twin after selective laser photocoagulation of communicating vessels in twin-twin transfusion syndrome. Ultrasound Obstet Gynecol 2007;30(1):35–9.
55. Gratacós E, Van Schoubroeck D, Carreras E, et al. Impact of laser coagulation in severe twin-twin transfusion syndrome on fetal Doppler indices and venous blood flow volume. Ultrasound Obstet Gynecol 2002;20(2):125–30.
56. Taylor MJ, Govender L, Jolly M, et al. Validation of the Quintero staging system for twin-twin transfusion syndrome. Obstet Gynecol 2002;100(6):1257–65.
57. Duncombe GJ, Dickinson JE, Evans SF. Perinatal characteristics and outcomes of pregnancies complicated by twin-twin transfusion syndrome. Obstet Gynecol 2003;101:1190–6.
58. Luks FI, Carr SR, Plevyak M, et al. Limited prognostic value of a staging system for twin-to-twin transfusion syndrome. Fetal Diagn Ther 2004;19(3):301–4.
59. Barrea C, Alkazaleh F, Ryan, et al. Prenatal cardiovascular manifestations in the twin-to-twin transfusion syndrome recipients and the impact of therapeutic amnioreduction. Am J Obstet Gynecol 2005;192:892–902.
60. Zosmer N, Bajoria R, Weiner E, et al. Clinical and echographic features of in utero cardiac dysfunction in the recipient twin in twin-twin transfusion syndrome. Br Heart J 1994;72(1):74–9.
61. Achiron R, Rabinovitz R, Aboulafia Y, et al. Intrauterine assessment of high-output cardiac failure with spontaneous remission of hydrops fetalis in twin-twin transfusion syndrome: use of two-dimensional echocardiography, Doppler ultrasound, and color flow mapping. J Clin Ultrasound 1992;20(4):271–7.

62. Iwai N, Shimoike H, Kinoshita M. Cardiac renin–angiotensin system in the hypertrophied heart. Circulation 1995;92:2690–6.

63. Sueters M, Middeldorp JM, Vandenbussche FP, et al. The effect of fetoscopic laser therapy on fetal cardiac size in twin-twin transfusion syndrome. Ultrasound Obstet Gynecol 2008;31(2):158–63.

64. Habli M, Michelfelder E, Livingston J, et al. Acute effects of selective fetoscopic laser photocoagulation on recipient cardiac function in twin-twin transfusion syndrome. Am J Obstet Gynecol 2008;199(4):412e1–6.

65. Lougheed J, Sinclair BG, Fung KFK, et al. Acquired right ventricular outflow tract obstruction in the recipient twin in twin-twin transfusion syndrome. J Am Coll Cardiol 2001;38:1533–8.

66. Bahtiyar MO, Dulay AT, Weeks BP, et al. Prevalence of congenital heart defects in monochorionic/diamniotic twin gestations: a systematic literature review. J Ultrasound Med 2007;26:1491–8.

67. Rychik J, Tian Z, Bebbington M, et al. The twin-twin transfusion syndrome: spectrum of cardiovascular abnormality and development of a cardiovascular score to assess severity of disease. Am J Obstet Gynecol 2007;197(4): 392e1–8.

68. Michelfelder E, Gottliebson W, Border W, et al. Early manifestations and spectrum of recipient twin cardiomyopathy in twin-twin transfusion syndrome: relation to Quintero stage. Ultrasound Obstet Gynecol 2007;30(7):965–71.

69. Hofstaetter C, Hansmann M, Eik-Nes SH, et al. A cardiovascular profile score in the surveillance of fetal hydrops. J Matern Fetal Neonatal Med 2006;19(7): 407–13.

70. Shah AD, Border WL, Crombleholme TM, et al. Initial fetal cardiovascular profile score predicts recipient twin outcome in twin-twin transfusion syndrome. J Am Soc Echocardiogr 2008;21(10):1105–8.

71. Moise KJ Jr. Polyhydramnios: problems and treatment. Semin Perinatol 1993;17: 197–209.

72. Rodestal A, Thomassen PA. Acute polyhydramnios in twin pregnancy. A retrospective study with special reference to therapeutic amniocentesis. Acta Obstet Gynecol Scand 1990;69:297–300.

73. Mahony BS, Petty CN, Nyberg DA, et al. The "stuck twin" phenomenon: ultrasonographic findings, pregnancy outcome, and management with serial amniocenteses. Am J Obstet Gynecol 1990;163:1513–22.

74. Elliott JP, Urig MA, Clewell WH. Aggressive therapeutic amniocentesis for treatment of twin-twin transfusion syndrome. Obstet Gynecol 1991;77:537–40.

75. Pinette MG, Pan Y, Pinette SG, et al. Treatment of twin-twin transfusion syndrome. Obstet Gynecol 1993;82:841–6.

76. Reisner DP, Mahony BS, Petty CN, et al. Stuck twin syndrome: outcome in thirty-seven consecutive cases. Am J Obstet Gynecol 1993;169:991–5.

77. Mari G, Roberts A, Detti L, et al. Perinatal morbidity and mortality rates in severe twin-twin transfusion syndrome: results of the International Amnioreduction Registry. Am J Obstet Gynecol 2001;185:708–15.

78. Johnson JR, Rossi KQ, O'Shaughnessy RW. Amnioreduction versus septostomy in twin-twin transfusion syndrome. Am J Obstet Gynecol 2001;185:1044–7.

79. Moise KJ Jr, Dorman K, Lamvu G, et al. A randomized trial of amnioreduction versus septostomy in the treatment of twin-twin transfusion syndome. Am J Obstet Gynecol 2005;193:701–7.

80. Ross M, van den Wijngaard JP, van Gemert MJ. TTTS amnioreduction versus setostomy. Am J Obstet Gynecol 2006;195:881–2.

81. De Lia JE, Cruikshank DP, Keye WR Jr. Fetoscopic neodymium: YAG laser occlusion of placental vessels in severe twin-twin transfusion syndrome. Obstet Gynecol 1990;75:1046–53.
82. Ville Y, Hyett J, Hecher K, et al. Preliminary experience with endoscopic laser surgery for severe twin-twin transfusion syndrome. N Engl J Med 1995;332:224–7.
83. Quintero RA, Morales WJ, Mendoza G, et al. Selective photocoagulation of placental vessels in twin-twin transfusion syndrome: evolution of a surgical technique. Obstet Gynecol Surv 1998;53:S97–103.
84. Quintero RA, Dickinson JE, Morales WJ, et al. Stage-based treatment of twin-twin transfusion syndrome. Am J Obstet Gynecol 2003;188:1333–40.
85. Wee LY, Taylor M, Watkins N, et al. Characterisation of deep arterio-venous anastomoses within monochorionic placentae by vascular casting. Placenta 2005;26:19–24.
86. Yamamoto M, El Murr L, Robyr R, et al. Incidence and impact of perioperative complications in 175 fetoscopy-guided laser coagulations of chorionic plate anastomoses in fetofetal transfusion syndrome before 26 weeks of gestation. Am J Obstet Gynecol 2005;193(3 Pt 2):1110–6.
87. Robyr R, Lewi L, Salomon LJ, et al. Prevalence and management of late fetal complications following successful selective laser coagulation of chorionic plate anastomoses in twin-to-twin transfusion syndrome. Am J Obstet Gynecol 2006;194(3):796–803.
88. Habli Mounira, Bombrys Annette, Lewis David, et al. Prevalence of complications in twin-twin transfusion syndrome following selective fetoscopic laser photocoagulation: a single center experience 2008;199(6 Suppl 1):S177.
89. Sebire NJ, Snijders RJ, Hughes K, et al. The hidden mortality of monochorionic twin pregnancies. Br J Obstet Gynaecol 1997;104:1203–7.
90. Dube J, Dodds L, Armson BA. Does chorionicity or zygosity predict adverse perinatal outcomes in twins? Am J Obstet Gynecol 2002;186:579–83.
91. Adegbite AL, Castille S, Ward S, et al. Neuromorbidity in preterm twins in relation to chorionicity and discordant birth weight. Am J Obstet Gynecol 2004;190:156–63.
92. Taylor M. Haemodynamic causes and consequences of twin–twin transfusion syndrome [thesis]. London: University of London; 2003.
93. Fick A, Norton ME, Feldstein V, et al. Twin–twin transfusion syndrome and placental anastomoses in a large unselected cohort of monochorionic twins. Am J Obstet Gynecol 2005;191(6 Suppl 1):S67.
94. Umur A, van Gemert MJ, Nikkels PG. Monoamniotic versus diamniotic-monochorionic twin placentas: anastomoses and twin–twin transfusion syndrome. Am J Obstet Gynecol 2003;189:1325–9.
95. Dickinson JE, Evans SF. Obstetric and perinatal outcomes from the Australian and New Zealand twin-twin transfusion syndrome registry. Am J Obstet Gynecol 2000;182(3):706–12.
96. Lopriore E, Sueters M, Middeldorp JM, et al. Neonatal outcome in twin-to-twin transfusion syndrome treated with fetoscopic laser occlusion of vascular anastomoses. J Pediatr 2005;147(5):597–602.
97. Lutfi S, Allen VM, Fahey J, et al. Twin-twin transfusion syndrome: a population-based study. Obstet Gynecol 2004;104(6):1289–97 [erratum in: Obstet Gynecol 2005 Feb;105(2):451].
98. Acosta-Rojas R, Becker J, Munoz-Abellana B, et al. Twin chorionicity and the risk of adverse perinatal outcome. Int J Gynaecol Obstet 2007;96(2):98–102 [Epub 2007 Jan 23].

99. Lenclen R, Paupe A, Ciarlo G, et al. Neonatal outcome in preterm monochorionic twins with twin-to-twin transfusion syndrome after intrauterine treatment with amnioreduction or fetoscopic laser surgery: comparison with dichorionic twins. Am J Obstet Gynecol 2007;196(5):450e1–7.

100. Senat MV, Deprest J, Boulvain M, et al. Endoscopic laser surgery versus serial amnioreduction for severe twin-to-twin transfusion syndrome. N Engl J Med 2004;351:136–44.

101. De Lia JE, Kuhlmann RS, Harstad TW, et al. Fetoscopic laser ablation of placental vessels in severe previable twin-twin transfusion syndrome. Am J Obstet Gynecol 1995;172:1202–8.

102. Hecher K, Plath H, Bregenzer T, et al. Endoscopic laser surgery versus serial amniocenteses in the treatment of severe twin-twin transfusion syndrome. Am J Obstet Gynecol 1999;180:717–24.

103. Fisk NM, Galea P. Twin-twin transfusion—as good as it gets? N Engl J Med 2004; 351:182–4.

104. Cromblehome TM, Livingston JC, Polzin W, et al. Multimodality and sequential therapy for twin-twin transfusion syndrome (TTTS): a stage and gestational age based approach to the use of amnioreduction (AR), selective fetoscopic laser photocoagulation (SFLP), and intrafetal radiofrequency ablation (RFA). Am J Obstet Gynecol 2007;197(Suppl):S202.

105. Rossi AC, D'Addario V. Umbilical cord occlusion for selective feticide in complicated monochorionic twins: a systematic review of literature. Am J Obstet Gynecol 2009;200(2):123–9.

106. Beck M, Gräf C, Ellenrieder B, et al. Long-term outcome of kidney function after twin-twin transfusion syndrome treated by intrauterine laser coagulation. Pediatr Nephrol 2005;20(11):1657–9.

107. Fesslova V, Villa L, Nava S, et al. Fetal and neonatal echocardiographic findings in twin-twin transfusion syndrome. Am J Obstet Gynecol 1998;179(4): 1056–62.

108. Herberg U, Gross W, Bartmann P, et al. Long term cardiac follow up of severe twin to twin transfusion syndrome after intrauterine laser coagulation. Heart 2006;92(1):95–100.

109. Denbow ML, Battin MR, Cowan F, et al. Neonatal cranial ultrasonographic findings in preterm twins complicated by severe fetofetal transfusion syndrome. Am J Obstet Gynecol 1998;178:479–83.

110. Banek CS, Hecher K, Hackeloer BJ, et al. Long-term neurodevelopmental outcome after intrauterine laser treatment for severe twin-twin transfusion syndrome. Am J Obstet Gynecol 2003;188:876–80.

111. Sutcliffe AG, Sebire NJ, Pigott AJ, et al. Outcome for children born after in utero laser ablation therapy for severe twin-to-twin transfusion syndrome. Br J Obstet Gynaecol 2001;108:1246–50.

112. Graef C, Ellenrieder B, Hecher K, et al. Long-term neurodevelopmental outcome of 167 children after intrauterine laser treatment for severe twin-twin transfusion syndrome. Am J Obstet Gynecol 2006;194:303–8.

113. Ortqvist LCS, Chevret S, Bussieres L, et al. Long-term neurodevelopmental outcome in twin-to-twin transfusion syndrome in the Eurofoetus trial. Am J Obstet Gynecol 2006;195(Suppl 1):S3.

114. Lopriore E, Nagel HT, Vandenbussche FP, et al. Longterm neurodevelopmental outcome in twin-to-twin transfusion syndrome. Am J Obstet Gynecol 2003;189: 1314–9.

115. Quarello E, Molho M, Ville Y. Incidence, mechanisms, and patterns of fetal cerebral lesions in twin-to-twin transfusion syndrome. J Matern Fetal Neonatal Med 2007;20:589–97.
116. Tsutsumi T, Ishii M, Eto G, et al. Serial evaluation for myocardial performance in fetuses and neonates using a new Doppler index. Pediatr Int 1999;41:722–7.
117. Tei C, Ling LH, Hodge DO, et al. New index of combined systolic and diastolic myocardial performance: a simple and reproducible measure of cardiac function—a study in normals and dilated ardiomyopathy. J Cardiol 1995;26:357–66.
118. Tan J, Silverman NH, Hoffman JI, et al. Cardiac dimensions determined by cross-sectional echocardiography in the normal human fetus from 18 weeks to term. Am J Cardiol 1992;70:1459–67.

Complicated Monochorionic Twin Pregnancies: Updates in Fetal Diagnosis and Treatment

Larry Rand, MD[a,b,]*, Hanmin Lee, MD[c]

KEYWORDS

- Monochorionic • Twins
- Relatively undergrown with normal twin
- Intrauterine growth retardation
- Twin reversed arterial perfusion • Demise

Complications of monochorionic twinning are the most common reason for referral to a Fetal Care Center.[1–4] The diagnosis of some monochorionic twin anomalies, such as Twin-Reversed Arterial Perfusion (TRAP) sequence, is relatively clearly defined. Other anomalies of monochorionic twinning, such as Twin-to-Twin Transfusion Syndrome (TTTS) or that of unequal placental sharing, may have subtleties that are harder to differentiate at first glance, but the understanding of which make all the difference in terms of selecting the appropriate treatment. To further complicate diagnosis and appropriate management, many patients will have overlapping elements of multiple complications of monochorionic twinning. In this article, the authors review the diagnosis and treatment of TRAP sequence, unequal placental sharing, and discordant monochorionic twins, as well as a limited review of TTTS (which is discussed in further detail in another article elsewhere in this issue). Correctly diagnosing the specific abnormality that may occur in MC twins leads to optimal management protocols, counseling, and treatment options.

It is estimated that up to 10% of MC twins develop TTTS.[2,5] More than half of all MC twins are complicated by some degree of pathologic condition resulting from their

[a] Division of Perinatology and Genetics, Fetal Treatment Center, University of California, San Francisco, 505 Parnassus Avenue, Box 0132, San Francisco, CA 94143, USA
[b] Department of Obstetrics, Gynecology, and Reproductive Sciences, University of California, San Francisco, San Francisco, CA, USA
[c] Fetal Treatment Center, Division of Pediatric Surgery, Department of Surgery, University of California, San Francisco, 513 Parnassus Avenue, Suite HSW 1601, San Francisco, CA 94143, USA
* Corresponding author. Division of Perinatology and Genetics, Fetal Treatment Center, University of California, San Francisco, 505 Parnassus Avenue, Box 0132, San Francisco, CA 94143.
E-mail address: randl@obgyn.ucsf.edu (L. Rand).

Clin Perinatol 36 (2009) 417–430
doi:10.1016/j.clp.2009.03.014   perinatology.theclinics.com
0095-5108/09/$ – see front matter © 2009 Elsevier Inc. All rights reserved.

monochorionicity, however.[6] MC twins may display a variety of discordances with signs that may have overlap with TTTS but are not necessarily associated with the diagnosis of TTTS. These include discordant growth disorders (eg, selective growth restriction, unequal placental sharing, relative undergrowth of one twin [with a normal cotwin]), reversed arterial perfusion of an acardiac twin, and discordant anomalies.[1–3] Discordant growth is commonly defined as a greater than 20% difference between the twins as calculated by means of the following formula: [(Larger EFW−Smaller EFW)/ Larger EFW] × 100, where EFW is estimated fetal weight.

Management protocols and treatment options vary depending on the diagnosis. Currently, the most effective treatment for stage II, III, and IV TTTS is generally considered to be fetoscopic placental laser ablation.[7,8] MC twins that are severely discordant for growth or demonstrate anomalies may undergo selective reduction by means of a variety of different techniques. At the authors' institution, radiofrequency ablation (RFA) of the abnormal twin is most frequently used. RFA of the acardiac twin has also proved to be an effective method of improving survival of the pump twin in the TRAP sequence. When unequal placental sharing is differentiated from TTTS, expectant management or avoidance of invasive therapy may offer excellent outcomes as long as the pregnancy is carefully monitored with ultrasound, echocardiography, and nonstress testing.

Adverse outcomes in expectantly and invasively managed MC twins include demise and morbidities incurred with dual or single survival, including neurologic and other end-organ damage. Assessment in such situations may involve additional imaging modalities, such as fetal MRI, and risk counseling can be quite difficult. As such, care for these complex pregnancies is ideally a coordinated multidisciplinary effort between perinatology, pediatric/fetal surgery, pediatric neurology, radiology/ultrasound, genetics, social services, neonatology, and labor and delivery.

TWIN-TO-TWIN TRANSFUSION SYNDROME

TTTS is reviewed in depth in another article in this issue. For clarity and comparison with other MC twin disorders, the key diagnostic criterion is the requisite sonographic finding of concomitant polyhydramnios (deepest vertical pocket >8 cm) and oligohydramnios (<2 cm).[1,6] A large number of fetuses that have TTTS may also have a size discrepancy, but this is not required for, or a part of, the diagnosis. True TTTS carries a dual mortality risk of up to 90% if untreated, and donors and recipients who survive face the risk for morbidity in various organ systems (ie, brain, cardiac, renal, bowel). Differentiating true TTTS from other MC twin disorders allows improved management and more specific tailoring of treatment.

PLACENTAL VASCULAR ANATOMY

The placenta is designed to support one fetus. When two fetuses develop circulations within one placenta, there is no established or predictable pattern for the vasculature to follow; each shared MC placenta is akin to a snowflake. Understanding the angioarchitecture of how the two circulations interact within one placenta is key to understanding the pathophysiology underlying the ensuing symptoms.

Counter to common perception, there is usually a significant amount of "crosstalk" or connectivity between the vasculature of each fetus even in uncomplicated MC pregnancies.[5] Unlike a dichorionic placentation, there is no embedded "barrier" to prevent the vessels from establishing anastomoses. Communication between the two circulations, however, does not equate with development of disease. Instead, development of disease depends, in large part, on the number and type (ie, arterial, venous) of intertwin vascular connections and the net direction of flow they create between the fetuses.

NORMAL ANGIOARCHITECTURE (PAIRED VESSELS)

Deoxygenated blood travels from the fetus to the umbilical cord by way of the two umbilical arteries, which wrap around the umbilical vein in a spiral. Once they reach the placenta's umbilical cord insertion site, they travel along the surface of the placenta as a pair and then dive down beneath the surface, where gas exchange occurs between them within a capillary network. After this capillary exchange, oxygenated blood enters the vein and then travels back up along the same route to the surface of the placenta so that it may make its way back to the umbilical cord (**Fig. 1**). The unit that describes this path—artery entering into the placenta, travel toward a microvascular network, gas exchange, and return of the vein back to the surface of the placenta—is called a cotyledon. Normal angioarchitecture for a given twin is identifiable by a set of paired vessels, an artery and a vein, situated next to one another as they come out of (and return to) the umbilical cord insertion site and travel to the cotyledon. Such paired vessels belong to one twin's circulation and do not represent communication between the twins but just a normal communication between a single fetus's artery and vein.[5]

ABNORMAL ANGIOARCHITECTURE (UNPAIRED VESSELS)

The hallmark of abnormal angioarchitecture in an MC placenta is identification of unpaired vessels. A single artery emerges from the cord of one fetus and travels to a cotyledon alone (unpaired); rather than connecting to a vein that travels back to the fetus along the same path, however, it connects with a single unpaired vein from the other fetus, creating an arteriovenous (AV) anastomosis between the twins (**Fig. 2**).[9]

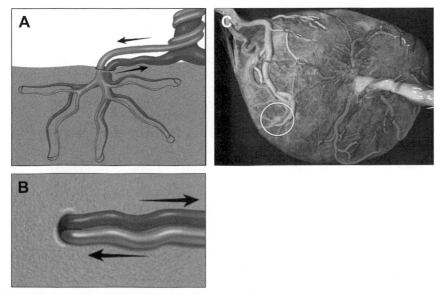

Fig. 1. (*A*) Normal angioarchitechture (cotyledon). (*Courtesy of* V. Feldstein, MD, San Francisco, CA.) (*B*) Superficial view of bidirectional flow into and out of a cotyledon. (*Courtesy of* V. Feldstein, MD, San Francisco, CA.) (*C*) Normal arteriovenous pair on placental pathology specimen. (*Courtesy of* G. Machin, MD, Toronto, Ontario, Canada.)

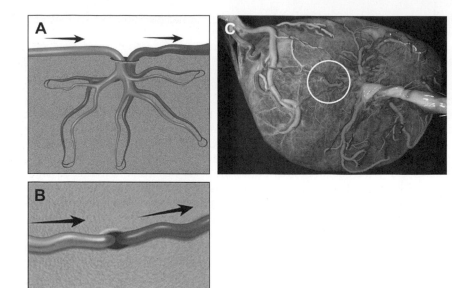

Fig. 2. (*A*) Abnormal intertwin connection: AV anastomosis. (*Courtesy of* V. Feldstein, MD, San Francisco, CA.) (*B*) Superficial view of unidirectional flow into and out of the cotyledon as a result of the intertwin AV anastomosis. (*Courtesy of* V. Feldstein, MD, San Francisco, CA.) (*C*) AV anastomosis seen superficially on placental pathology specimen. (*Courtesy of* G. Machin, MD, Toronto, Ontario, Canada.)

A variety of combinations exist in terms of vascular connections between the two fetal circulations. Most commonly, as described previously, an artery communicates with a vein (AV anastomosis), but it may also connect to another artery (arterioarterial [AA] anastomosis) or a vein may communicate with another vein (venovenous anastomosis). Because the artery determines direction of flow, an AV connection represents unidirectional flow from the artery of one fetus to the vein of the other (see **Fig. 2**A, B). The artery of an AV pair sends blood to the cotyledon, and the vein anastomosing with it accepts this blood and transfuses it to the other fetus rather than allowing it to return in its usual circuit back to the originating fetus. Unidirectional flow may occur from and to either fetus, as determined by which fetus the artery originates from.[5]

As noted previously, it is the norm to have many such vascular connections between fetuses in an MC placenta (crosstalk). There is no anatomic barrier between the circulations, and each MC placenta develops its vascular tree uniquely, easily impinging on the other. Yet, true TTTS only develops in an estimated 10% of MC twins—when the net flow of blood between fetuses is unbalanced.[10] Most commonly, vascular connections run in both directions (ie, an AV anastomosis from twin A to B is balanced out by flow from an AV anastomosis that runs from twin B to twin A). Therefore, despite the presence of many such unidirectional communications, in terms of total fluid dynamics, a net balance in blood flow results. In many instances, there may be several unidirectional AV anastomoses that are balanced by the presence of an AA connection. A significant net imbalance in flow is hypothesized to be one of the characteristic causes of TTTS.

In an AA anastomosis, an artery from each fetus meets, and because arteries are relatively high-pressure vessels, a turbulent bidirectional flow results. These connections are end to end and course along the surface of the placenta. They do not penetrate into the placental parenchyma (**Fig. 3**A, B). AAs are often larger than AVs, and

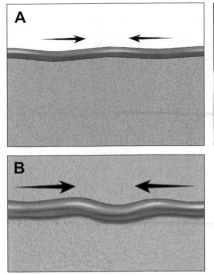
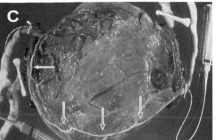

Fig. 3. (A) AA anastomosis. (*Courtesy of* V. Feldstein, MD, San Francisco, CA.) (B) Superficial view of bidirectional flow in AA anastomosis. (C) Superficial view of AA anastomosis (*arrows*) between cord insertions (both marginal) on placental pathology specimen. (*Courtesy of* G. Machin, MD, Toronto, Ontario, Canada.)

whereas several AVs may be present in a given MC placenta, pathologic correlation studies have shown that there is usually only one AA, which is present in 75% of MC placentas (see **Fig. 3**C). The presence of an AA anastomosis may provide enough balance of flow in an MC twin pregnancy to mitigate the development of true TTTS. This may account for the "near-TTTS" cases with discordant amniotic fluid that are so often referred and followed but never meet definitive criteria for true TTTS and do not seem to carry the same morbidity typically described for TTTS.[11]

If an AA anastomosis is present, it may often balance out the abnormal "transfusion" the AV anastomoses cause. An AA anastomosis may not be enough to protect the fetuses from displaying some degree of symptoms, and there may be signs of unequal placental sharing and discordant fluid volume, but emerging evidence suggests that the protective effect of the AA anastomosis may be enough to keep the fetuses from developing full-blown TTTS.[12] In a series of 639 placentas that underwent pathologic examination and were correlated with clinical outcomes, the presence of an AA anastomosis reduced the risk for TTTS. When an AA anastomosis was not found, the rate of TTTS was 47%, whereas it was only 5% if an AA anastomosis was present.[13]

This is helpful information if the presence of an AA anastomosis can be determined during antenatal evaluation; fortunately, with proper training, AA anastomoses may be detected by Doppler interrogation with ultrasound (**Fig. 4**). In a series of 40 MC twin pairs, 21 (53%) were found to have an AA anastomosis with ultrasound. Once again, 58% of those without an AA anastomosis developed TTTS, whereas only 5% of patients with an AA anastomosis went on to have TTTS.[14] As such, the presence, or absence, of an AA anastomosis may be helpful in prognosticating and managing these pregnancies. It should be noted that in addition to the anatomic circulatory connections, vasoactive mediators have been implicated in the fetal response seen in this condition.[15–17]

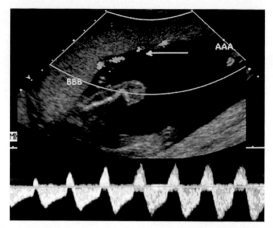

Fig. 4. Doppler ultrasound interrogation of AA anastomosis (*arrow*). (*Courtesy of* V. Feldstein, MD, San Francisco, CA.)

UNEQUAL PLACENTAL SHARING

A single placenta is meant to sustain a single fetus. When two fetuses share a single placenta, there is no set blueprint for how to achieve this successfully so that each fetus retains an equal share. The umbilical cords may insert anywhere on the placenta (eg, central, marginal, velamentous). A line perpendicular to the midpoint between the two cord insertions may be considered the vascular equator between the circulations. As such, if the cord of one twin inserts centrally and the others twin's cord inserts anywhere eccentrically (eg, peripheral, marginal, velamentous), the equator would, by definition, result in an unequal placental share for the fetus with the eccentric cord insertion. This may predispose to decreased growth potential and selective intrauterine growth retardation (S-IUGR) of the twin with a smaller share.[6,12] Most often, the smaller share is sufficient to support growth up to a certain point. It may well be that when the fetus reaches a certain size and its "demand" outstrips the fixed supply of that limited placental share, growth restriction ensues. This underlying mechanism may be largely responsible for discordant fetal size (and amniotic fluid volume) in MC twins. S-IUGR has been defined as growth estimated at less than 10% in one twin of an MC pair, and it is often accompanied by abnormal umbilical artery Doppler flow patterns. S-IUGR can be severe enough to be accompanied by oligohydramnios, giving the appearance of discordant fluid volumes and suspicion of TTTS. In this case, however, it is not attributable to TTTS; rather, the pathophysiology is one of a growth-restricted twin with oligohydramnios as compared with the unrestricted cotwin, who has normal amniotic fluid.[18]

Many MC twins with true TTTS also have underlying unequal placental sharing. When they are effectively dichorionized after fetoscopic laser ablation, the smaller of an extremely discordant pair (usually with a marginal or velamentous cord insertion) may be left with an extremely small placental share. Although the smaller donor twin would seem to benefit from dividing the circulations and halting the process of TTTS, this is not always so. In some cases, laser division of the placenta may put the smaller twin at added risk for further growth restriction and even demise. The mechanisms and circumstances for when laser placental division helps or hurts the growth restriction of the smaller twin remain incompletely understood. Some centers have proposed fetoscopic laser dichorionization in the setting of non-TTTS S-IUGR to prevent ensuing neurologic damage to a surviving cotwin in the event of demise of the growth-restricted fetus; in fact, there is currently an ongoing trial to evaluate the efficacy of fetoscopic laser for S-IUGR. As described previously, however, the small placental share associated with the S-IUGR fetus may predispose it to a significantly higher risk for demise.[19] Patients must be appropriately counseled to determine their objective in treatment (ie, avoiding risk for neurologic morbidity versus dual survival).

RELATIVELY UNDERGROWN FETUS WITH NORMAL TWIN

In the authors' experience, a significant proportion of patients are referred for suspected TTTS but are found to have discordant amniotic fluid volumes that do not meet requisite sonographic criteria for TTTS, discordant fetal weights alone, or both. The most frequent initial finding is that of one small fetus and one normal-sized fetus. Amniotic fluid may be normal or low in the smaller twin; however, in contradistinction to TTTS, it is normal in the larger twin (not polyhydramnios). Because these patients do not meet criteria for interventional therapy for TTTS, they are followed with close expectant management. The authors investigated the outcomes of this subset of patient referrals.[20]

Seven hundred seven such MC twins referred to one center for "suspected TTTS" were prospectively followed. The authors recorded their cord insertion sites; respective EFWs and trends in discordance; the presence of an AA anastomosis; trends in Doppler ultrasound; the gestational age at referral and delivery; and the indication for delivery. A significant number of such patients were identified; however, to minimize confounding factors, the cohort was limited to include only patients who were followed and delivered at the referral institution and did not undergo an invasive procedure. Fifteen such patients were preliminarily identified.

To distinguish them from TTTS, these MC twin pregnancies were referred to as relatively undergrown with normal twin (RUNT). Almost all had AA anastomoses on Doppler ultrasound interrogation. The smaller twin consistently had a peripheral cord insertion, whereas its cotwin's cord inserted centrally. The mean gestational age for delivery of these pregnancies was at 33.7 weeks, always prompting a rapidly increasing discordance trend and S-IUGR (<10%) in the smaller twin, with absent or reversed end-diastolic umbilical artery Doppler flow. Clinicians used these markers of fetal well-being to determine need for delivery.

These pregnancies are de facto likely at high risk for developing TTTS based on their vascular communications; however, the presence of an AA anastomosis may be what protects them from incurring a net transfusion. The unequal placental share seen in these twins likely contributes significantly to the resultant pathophysiology. More than two thirds of RUNTs progressed to development of S-IUGR (EFW <10%) in the smaller twin. Pregnancies were referred at a mean gestational age of 21 weeks; importantly, the mean gestational age for diagnosis of S-IUGR was not until nearly 30 weeks. Once S-IUGR was diagnosed, these fetuses underwent close antenatal surveillance. The latency period from diagnosis of S-IUGR to delivery was 3 weeks. Abnormal Doppler findings (specifically, absent or reversed end-diastolic flow) were noted even earlier than was the S-IUGR, at a mean gestational age of 24 weeks. Abnormal Doppler flow in the setting of an AA anastomosis was a more forgiving finding than we might usually expect, with a long latency period of 8 weeks between diagnosis and delivery. As such, clinicians did not act on abnormal Doppler findings in isolation; delivery was prompted only in the presence of S-IUGR and abnormal Doppler flow.

The results of this preliminary prospective cohort indicate that MC twin pregnancies referred for features inconsistent with TTTS often meet criteria for RUNT. With expectant management of such pregnancies (including antenatal surveillance in the setting of S-IUGR and abnormal Doppler flow patterns), there was 100% dual survival at a relatively reassuring mean delivery gestational age of 33.5 weeks. Again, almost all had AA anastomoses identified with antenatal obstetric ultrasound. Most importantly, all these patients avoided invasive intervention and its attendant risks to the pregnancy.

Thus, it is imperative to consider the causative pathophysiologic mechanisms in twins discordant for size or fluid volume, especially if they do not meet defining criteria for TTTS. The location of placental cord insertions, EFWs, and interrogation for AA anastomosis provide important clues as to the type of underlying angioarchitecture in a given shared MC placenta.

TWIN REVERSED ARTERIAL PERFUSION SEQUENCE/ACARDIAC TWIN

One percent of all MC twin pregnancies are complicated by a structurally normal twin perfusing an acardiac cotwin, often anencephalic, by means of a unique set of vascular connections.[21] Importantly, the acardiac twin has no placental share whatsoever. Umbilical artery flow, which normally runs from the fetus toward the placenta, is instead reversed in the acardiac twin, flowing toward it rather than away from it (**Fig. 5**). It receives all its blood volume from the so-called "pump" twin through this reversed arterial connection. Because of the enormous strain of this work, in addition to chronic hypoxia from the double-deoxygenated blood the acardiac twin sends back to the pump, the otherwise normal pump twin has greater than 50% mortality.[22] This is most often manifest as high-output cardiac failure, hydrops, and polyhydramnios in the pump twin (**Fig. 6**). The polyhydramnios serves to complicate matters further by increasing the risk for preterm labor and preterm rupture of the membranes. Overall prognosis depends on the size and vascularity of the acardiac mass.

Intervention in the setting of the TRAP sequence/acardiac twin first began with open hysterotomy and selective delivery of the acardiac mass so as to remove the burden on the otherwise normal pump twin (**Fig. 7**). This evolved to umbilical cord ligation by means of fetoscopy and, ultimately, to less invasive ultrasound-guided methods. Such therapies have included bipolar coagulation, fetoscopic laser, harmonic scalpel, and, most recently, devices causing thermal coagulation by means of RFA. A recent study of 26 MC TRAP pregnancies that underwent treatment with RFA of the acardiac twin's cord showed a survival rate of 92% of the pump twin with a mean gestational age at delivery of 35.5 weeks.[23]

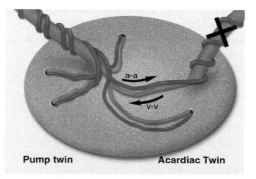

Fig. 5. Vasculature in TRAP/acardiac twin. a-a, arterioarterial; v-v, venovenous. (*Courtesy of* V. Feldstein, MD, San Francisco, CA.)

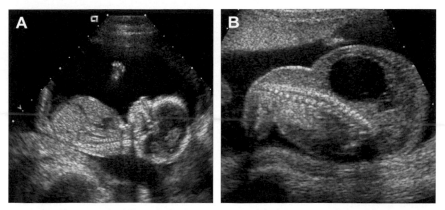

Fig. 6. TRAP donor twin (*A*) and TRAP pump twin (*B*). (*Courtesy of* V. Feldstein, MD, San Francisco, CA.)

RFA of the umbilical cord is now most commonly performed with a 17-gauge device (**Fig. 8**A). Under ultrasound guidance, the tip of the device is commonly inserted into the fetal abdominal wall at the level of the umbilical cord insertion. The device is then deployed, releasing an umbrella-shaped trio of three metallic tips, which, together, help to coagulate a 2-cm diameter of tissue thermally (see **Fig. 8**B). Because there is no beating heart in the acardiac twin, energy is applied until complete obliteration of flow through the umbilical cord is demonstrated by umbilical artery Doppler interrogation.

DISCORDANT TWINS

RFA devices may be used in other complicated MC twin settings in which one twin is severely affected, whereas the other twin is not affected at all, such as severely discordant growth and discordant structural anomalies (selective termination of anomalous twin; **Fig. 9**). RFA has also been described as a potential alternative therapy to laser photocoagulation in severely affected TTTS cases. The procedure-related loss risk for the 17-gauge RFA device independent of TRAP pregnancies has not yet been determined.

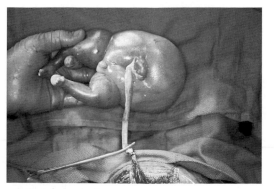

Fig. 7. Open selective delivery of acardiac twin. (*Courtesy of* M. Harrison, MD, San Francisco, CA.)

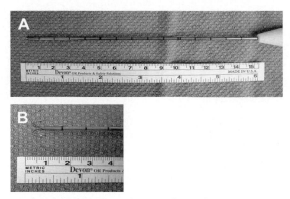

Fig. 8. (*A*) RFA device. (*B*) Umbrella-shaped tines of RFA device.

The long-term neurologic outcomes in the surviving twin after RFA cord coagulation have not yet been studied. Theoretically, there is some potential for such risk depending on the size of and amount of blood flow in the acardiac mass at the time of RFA. The major difference between RFA for TRAP pregnancies and RFA for other MC pregnancies is the consideration of placental share. In non-TRAP pregnancies, the fetus to be reduced has placental share, and there is a theoretic risk for blood loss from the viable twin and its placental share into the placental share of the reduced twin. Because the acardiac twin in a TRAP pair has no placental share, this potential risk for hypotension to the remaining twin is absent. Theoretically, to minimize potential neuromorbidity, the fetal circulations could be dichorionized by laser before performing RFA of one twin's cord. This would necessitate two invasive procedures rather than one, however, and laser scope equipment has a considerably larger diameter when compared with that of RFA (3 mm versus 17 gauge).

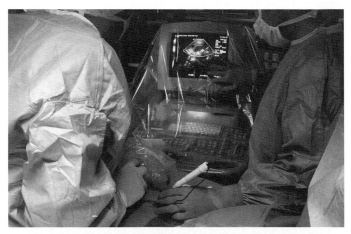

Fig. 9. Ultrasound-guided RFA selective termination of anomalous twin procedure. (*Courtesy of* V. Feldstein, MD, San Francisco, CA.)

COTWIN DEMISE

Any complicated MC twin pregnancy has an increased baseline risk for adverse events and may result in demise of one or both twins. When demise of one twin occurs, the well-being and long-term outcome of the surviving cotwin are of significant concern. Demise may occur spontaneously, during expectant management, or after an invasive procedure (ie, fetoscopic laser coagulation, ultrasound-guided RFA cord coagulation).

The literature on the morbidities of the surviving cotwin is incomplete, complex, and confounded, and it makes counseling challenging. There is up to an estimated 40% risk for adverse neurologic outcome in an MC survivor after cotwin demise.[24] What was once theorized as damage attributable to the passage of thrombotic emboli from one fetus to the other is now widely thought to be secondary to ischemic physiology. With demise of one twin in a vascularly interconnected pair, the often severe and sudden decrease in blood pressure causes a sieve-like massive transfusion to the demised twin. This equilibrates within a few minutes; however, depending on the severity and duration of the ischemic period, it may result in end-organ damage. As such, delivery of the surviving cotwin is not recommended as a way to reduce morbidity to the surviving cotwin. In the management of a complicated MC twin pair, the risk for a potential invasive intervention is constantly weighed against the potential risk incurred by a surviving cotwin if a spontaneous demise is allowed to occur.

Given the potential risk for organ damage, particularly neurologic damage, improving evaluation and assessment of a surviving cotwin are important adjuncts to treatment of MC twins after spontaneous or procedure-related demise. Antenatal ultrasound has been widely used, utilizing fetal neurosonography for signs of ischemic or other pathologic findings. Unfortunately, many such lesions are sonographically occult, because ultrasound is an excellent tool for the diagnosis of hemorrhage and ventriculomegaly but far less so for ischemic white matter injury. Added to the operator-dependent nature of ultrasound, these limitations can make prenatal diagnosis quite challenging.

Because MRI is the only sensitive imaging modality for the diagnosis of ischemic white matter injury, fetal MRI has recently been added in an attempt to improve antenatal neurologic risk assessment (**Fig. 10**). In a series of 47 cotwin demises at the authors' center, 21 occurred spontaneously (in pregnancies without intervention). Imaging findings after spontaneous demise and those after an invasive procedure were studied separately. In the spontaneous group, all twin pairs underwent fetal ultrasound and MRI. One third of the MRI scans were abnormal, most (66%) of which had normal ultrasound findings. Even in those fetuses with abnormal or suspicious ultrasound findings, MRI added additional information and detail, supporting MRI's greater sensitivity in detecting ischemic brain injury.[25]

All cotwin survivors of demise after an ablative procedure (laser photocoagulation or RFA) also underwent evaluation with ultrasound and MRI. None of the surviving cotwins had an abnormal ultrasound scan. One of these survivors had a small germinal matrix hemorrhage on MRI; otherwise, there were no abnormal MRI findings in any of these surviving cotwins.[26]

Further studies to elucidate the sensitivity, specificity, and predictive value of fetal MRI for neurologic outcome are certainly warranted, as is the long-term neurologic correlation of children with "normal" and "abnormal" MRI findings.

The ideal timing of when to perform this imaging after demise still remains unclear. Currently, the authors' typical protocol is assessment 2 weeks after injury/cotwin

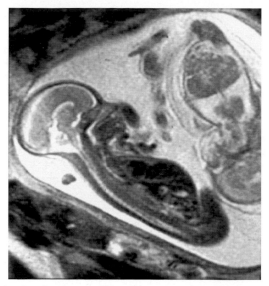

Fig. 10. Fetal MRI of twins. (*Courtesy of* O. Glenn, MD, San Francisco, CA.)

demise. This is modified depending on how close the pregnancy is to the legal limit of termination if that is a concern for the parents. MRI evidence of injury has been shown as early as 1 day after injury, and all insults were visible by 2 weeks.[25] Moreover, it should be noted that as gestational age increases, image quality on MRI improves vastly.

SUMMARY

MC twin pregnancies are at risk for developing significant complications, and although TTTS has become the most familiar to obstetricians and patients alike, a significant percentage of patients referred for suspected TTTS have a different underlying pathologic condition. Understanding and differentiating the subcategories of MC pathophysiologic conditions may significantly alter treatment course and outcome. When clinically appropriate, expectant noninvasive management or RFA of one twin's umbilical cord is an alternative to fetoscopic laser ablation. Data on RFA for TRAP have recently shown this to be an effective treatment strategy. The key to understanding complicated MC pregnancies lies in the placental angioarchitecture and the arrangement of intertwin vascular communications between the fetuses. Further research regarding long-term outcomes (especially neurologic) for complicated MC pregnancies undergoing treatment or managed expectantly is needed to improve counseling.

REFERENCES

1. Egan JFK, Borgida AF. Ultrasound evaluation of multiple pregnancies. In: Callen PW, editor. Ultrasonography in obstetrics ad gynecology. 5th edition. Philadelphia: Saunders Elsevier; 2008. p. 266–96.
2. Sebire NJ, Snijders RJ, Hughes K, et al. The hidden mortality of monochorionic twin pregnancies. Br J Obstet Gynaecol 1997;104:1203–7.
3. Taylor MJ. The management of multiple pregnancy. Early Hum Dev 2006;82:365–70.

4. Benirschke K, Kim CK. Multiple pregnancy. N Engl J Med 1973;288:1276–84.
5. Machin GA, Keith LG. An atlas of multiple pregnancy: biology and pathology. New York: Parthenon Publishing Group; 1999.
6. Blickstein I, Keith LG. Prenatal assessment of multiple pregnancy. London: Informa; 2007. p. 15–44.
7. Senat MV, Deprest J, Boulvain M, et al. Endoscopic laser surgery versus serial amnioreduction for severe twin-twin perfusion syndrome. N Engl J Med 2004; 351:136–44.
8. Yamamoto M, Ville Y. Recent findings on laser treatment of twin-to-twin transfusion syndrome. Curr Opin Obstet Gynecol 2006;18:87–92.
9. Bajoria R, Wuggkesworth J, Fisk N. Angioarchitecture of monochorionic placentas.
10. Denbow ML, Cox P, Taylor M, et al. Placental angioarchitecture in monochorionic twin pregnancies: relationship to fetal growth, fetofetal transfusion syndrome, and pregnancy outcomes. Am J Obstet Gynecol 2000;182:417–26.
11. Taylor MJ, Denbow ML, Duncan KR, et al. Antenatal factors at diagnosis that predict outcome in twin-twin transfusion syndrome. Am J Obstet Gynecol 2000; 183:1023–8.
12. Fick AL, Feldstein VA, Norton ME, et al. Unequal placental sharing and birth-weight discordance in monochorionic diamniotic twins. Am J Obstet Gynecol 2006;195:178–83.
13. Fick AL, Norton ME, Machin GA, et al. Twin-twin transfusion syndrome and placental anastomoses in a large unselected cohort of monochorionic twins. Journal of Ultrasound Medicine, submitted for publication.
14. Taylor MJ, Denbow ML, Tanawattanacharoen S, et al. Doppler detection of arterio-arterial anastomosis in monochorionic twins: feasibility and clinical application. Humanit Rep 2000;15:1632–6.
15. Soorana SR, Ward S, Bajora R. Discordant fetal leptin levels in monochorionic twins with chronic midtrimester twin-twin transfusion syndrome. Placenta 2001; 22:392–8.
16. Bajoria R, Gibrson MJ, Ward S, et al. Placental regulation of insulin-like growth factor axis in monochorionic twins with chronic twin-twin transfusion syndrome. J Clin Endocrinol Metab 2001;86:3150–6.
17. Bajoria R, Hancock M, Ward S, et al. Discordant amino acid profiles in monochorionic twins with twin-twin transfusion syndrome. Pediatr Res 2000;48:821–8.
18. Mahoney BS, Petty CN, Nyberg DA, et al. The "stuck twin" phenomenon: ultrasonographic findings, pregnancy outcome, and management with serial amniocentesis. Am J Obstet Gynecol 1990;163:1513–22.
19. Quintero RA, Bornick PW, Morales WJ. Selective photocoagulation of communicating vessels of monochorionic twins with selective growth retardation. Am J Obstet Gynecol 2001;185:689–96.
20. Rand L, Feldstein VA, Lee H, et al. RUNT: relatively undergrown with normal twin [abstract]. In: Programs and Abstracts of the Annual Conference of the American Institute of Ultrasound Medicine (AIUM). New York, April 2–5, 2009.
21. Wong AE, Sepulveda W. Acardiac anomaly: current issues in prenatal assessment and treatment. Prenat Diagn 2005;25:796–806.
22. Moore TR, Gale S, Benirschke K. Perinatal outcome of 49 pregnancies complicated by acardiac twinning. Am J Obstet Gynecol 1990;163:907–12.
23. Lee H, Wagner AJ, Sy E, et al. Efficacy of radiofrequency ablation for twin-reversed arterial perfusion sequence. Am J Obstet Gynecol 2007;196:459 e1–e4.

24. Rand L, Eddleman KA, Stone JL. Long-term outcomes in multiple gestations. Clin Perinatol 2005;32:495–513.

25. Jelin AC, Norton ME, Bartha AI, et al. Intracranial magnetic resonance imaging findings in the surviving fetus after spontaneous monochorionic cotwin demise. Am J Obstet Gynecol 2008;199:398 e1–e5.

26. Jelin AC, Rand L, Glenn O, et al. Intracranial abnormalities visualized on fetal imaging in surviving monochorionic co-twins following fetal ablation procedures [abstract]. In: Programs and Abstracts of the Annual Conference of the American Institute of Ultrasound Medicine (AIUM). New York, April 2–5, 2009.

Fetal Surgery for Myelomeningocele

Shinjiro Hirose, MD*, Diana L. Farmer, MD

KEYWORDS

- Fetal surgery • Myelomeningocele • Hydrocephalus • Shunt

Myelomeningocele (MMC), a nonlethal neural tube defect, occurs in approximately 1 in 2000 live births in the United States. Developmentally, it arises early in gestation at about the third week and results in an open spinal canal with exposed neural elements in the form of a flat neural placode. The neural placode can undergo further injury in utero, and thus gives rise to the "two-hit" hypothesis of neurologic injury in MMC, with the first "hit" being the original defect and the second one being additional injury to the exposed neural elements of the spinal cord. Fetal intervention and repair would potentially ameliorate this second injury. This concept is the foundation for the rationale for prenatal repair of these neural tube defects.

Although the exact cause of MMC is unknown, its origin is believed to be multifactorial. Folate deficiency in mothers is associated with an increased incidence of MMC. Folate supplements in pregnant women have decreased the rate of MMC by as much as 70% and are now considered a standard regimen for expectant mothers. In addition, environmental exposure to toxins and drugs has been implicated in the development of MMC. Finally, genetic abnormalities, such as mutations in the PAX3 gene, may have a role in the development of MMC, as seen in Waardenburg's syndrome.

Patients who have MMC have significant clinical findings and morbidity. Most infants who have MMC are born alive and healthy; however, up to 30% of patients die before adulthood because of respiratory, urinary, or central nervous system complications. Virtually all newborns who have MMC have the Chiari hindbrain malformation and most develop hydrocephalus, requiring ventriculoperitoneal (VP) shunting. The spinal level of the defect determines the degree of motor and somatosensory deficit. In addition, these patients often have dysfunction of bladder and bowel control and loss of sexual function.

FETAL SURGERY
Rationale

As stated previously, the main rationale behind fetal surgery for MMC is based on the two-hit hypothesis. The first hit is the original developmental defect that causes the

Division of Pediatric Surgery, Department of Surgery, Fetal Treatment Center, University of California, San Francisco, 513 Parnassus Avenue, HSW-1601, San Francisco, CA 94143–0570, USA
* Corresponding author.
E-mail address: hiroses@surgery.ucsf.edu (S. Hirose).

Clin Perinatol 36 (2009) 431–438
doi:10.1016/j.clp.2009.03.008
0095-5108/09/$ – see front matter. Published by Elsevier Inc.

perinatology.theclinics.com

open neural tube defect. The second hit is postulated to be direct neural injury from exposure to amniotic fluid and by means of direct trauma to the exposed neural elements.[1,2] This theory is supported by several observations. First, early ultrasound examinations of fetuses that have MMC can demonstrate normal hind limb movement, suggesting a later loss of function, correlating with in utero injury to the spinal cord.[3] Second, postmortem analysis of stillborn and aborted fetuses that have MMC demonstrates significant recent injury to the exposed neural placode.[1] Finally, patients who have milder forms of neural tube defects in which the abnormal neural elements remain covered with skin or a membrane have more normal neural development than those patients who have MMC.[4] More recently, observations with curly-tailed mice (which develop a primary defect of neural tube formation) have demonstrated normal anatomic and functional correlation with normal mice; however, the mice then develop progressive neurologic degeneration during gestation, also suggesting this second hit.[5]

Animal Models

Before undertaking fetal MMC repair in humans, animal models were developed for the study of MMC and potential fetal interventions. Surgical models in rodents, rabbits, sheep, and nonhuman primates have all shown similar findings as in human disease: paraplegia, extremity deformity, urinary and bowel dysfunction, hydrocephalus, and the Chiari malformation. Prenatal closure of these surgically created defects has shown improvement in motor function, urinary function, and reversal of the Chiari malformation, with normal or near-normal hindbrain development and morphology. Several different animal models have demonstrated that the Chiari malformation occurs with surgically created MMC and that it can be reversed with in utero repair.[6–10] Further animal studies demonstrating improved neurologic function after in utero repair of surgically created MMC have also been published. Julia and colleagues[11] demonstrated improved neurologic function in the rabbit model using somatosensory evoked potentials after birth. Another study examining anal sphincter development after fetal MMC repair in the sheep model was published by Yoshizawa and colleagues.[12,13] In those experiments, rectum and anal sphincter muscles were histologically examined. Findings in unrepaired animals included hypoplastic longitudinal muscles in the sphincter complex and an underdeveloped submucosal nerve plexus. These structures were preserved in animals that underwent in utero repair.

Human Experience

Before MMC, fetal surgery had been reserved for specific situations in which there would be significant perinatal morbidity or mortality. This approach was adopted to minimize maternal risk and morbidity and to maximize potential benefit in the fetus. Previously treated diseases included obstructive uropathy; congenital diaphragmatic hernia; twin-twin transfusion syndrome; and nonimmune hydrops attributable to massive shunting within a mass, as seen in sacrococcygeal teratoma, or mediastinal shift, as seen in cystic adenoid malformation. MMC is the first nonlethal fetal malformation treated with in utero surgery. To minimize maternal morbidity, the first attempts at human fetal MMC repair were done fetoscopically. This technique was independently attempted at the Vanderbilt University Medical Center (VUMC) in Nashville, Tennessee, and at the University of California, San Francisco (UCSF).[14–16]

The VUMC group reported four fetoscopic repairs in which a maternal laparotomy was performed and a three-port access technique was used. The amniotic fluid was replaced with carbon dioxide, and the defects were covered with a maternal skin graft.

Two of the four fetuses survived; at birth, no evidence of the skin graft was found and the patients required reoperation for postnatal repair.[14,15]

The UCSF group reported three cases, but only one was successfully closed fetoscopically. In that patient, the MMC defect was closed with a decellularized dermal matrix patch; however, at birth, the repair was incomplete and required an additional operation to close the MMC, and a VP shunt was also placed. The two other patients were converted to open repairs. There were two deaths in this series: one from a spontaneous abortion and the other from postnatal urosepsis.[16]

Outcomes

Hydrocephalus

After these largely failed attempts at minimally invasive repair, the VUMC group began performing open fetal MMC repair (**Fig. 1**). After 2 years, they reported their results, stating that the open repair method is superior to the fetoscopic method. The VUMC group also found that hindbrain herniation was improved in the patients who had undergone fetal surgical repair of their MMCs and, additionally, that the need for VP shunting was significantly lower in those patients: 59% versus 91% in historic controls.[17] These data were limited in the small number of treated patients, in addition to the lack of standardization of criteria leading to VP shunt placement. Subsequent follow-up data from the VUMC group with subset analysis suggest that repair earlier in gestation, lower lesions, and smaller ventricles before repair are all associated with a lower VP shunt rate.[18,19]

Concurrently, the group at the Children's Hospital of Philadelphia (CHOP) performed open fetal surgical repair of MMC defects and confirmed the findings of

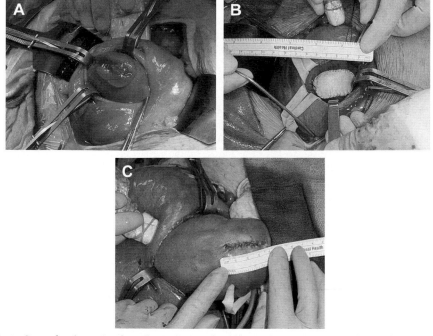

Fig. 1. Open fetal repair of myelomeningocele. (*A*) Myelomeningocele defect before repair. (*B*) Closure of defect with decellularized dermal matrix patch. (*C*) Primary closure of defect.

reversal of hindbrain herniation and improvement in the Arnold-Chiari II malformation in patients who had undergone fetal repair.[20] These findings were also corroborated by studies of head biometry in pre- and postnatal MRI scans in prenatally repaired MMC and postnatal repair.[21] Furthermore, decreased shunt rates and less ventriculomegaly were also noted in the patients who had undergone fetal MMC repair, further mirroring the findings at the VUMC.[22]

Neurologic function

At all three centers, the initial findings after fetal MMC repair did not demonstrate any significant improvement in neurologic function or hind limb movement. Follow-up data have been mixed. At the UCSF, only two of nine survivors had functional improvement greater than two spinal levels above the MMC lesion. The remaining patients' neurologic function correlated well with the level of the spinal lesion.[16] The VUMC group initially compared the neurologic outcomes of the patients who had undergone fetal MMC repair with historical controls and found no improvement.[23] In a later study, the outcomes of those patients were compared with matched controls at the University of Alabama, Birmingham. Again, no improvement in neurologic function was found.[24] In contradistinction, Danzer and colleagues[25] from the CHOP group examined 54 patients who had fetal MMC repair and found that 57% of patients had neurologic function better than what was predicted from the level of their spinal defect. Their median follow-up was 66 months and ranged from 36 to 133 months. Factors that were associated with a lower likelihood of independent ambulation included higher level lesions and presence of a clubfoot deformity.

Maternal morbidity and prematurity

An important finding in the VUMC data was the occurrence of significant maternal morbidity: intraoperative placenta abruption, uterine dehiscence, and small bowel obstruction.[26] Recently, more data have been published regarding outcomes of the mothers and fetuses undergoing fetal interventions for MMC. To date, there have been no specific studies examining maternal outcomes after MMC repair. Two limited studies suggest that maternal morbidity is low and that fertility after fetal surgery is preserved, however.[27,28]

Two reports have been published from the VUMC group regarding prematurity in neonates who underwent fetal repair of MMC. In the first report, Hamdan and colleagues[29] compared whether repair before 25 weeks of gestation affected gestational age at birth. Those data suggested that the degree of prematurity was independent of the gestational age at fetal repair. In a follow-up study, Hamdan and colleagues[30] compared the complication rate of premature infants who had fetal repair of MMC at the VUMC. Using controls matched for gestational age, gender, birth weight, antenatal steroid use, and mode of delivery, they found no significant difference in the incidence of morbidity associated with prematurity.

Urologic function

Studies of urologic outcome in infants who underwent prenatal closure of MMC have uniformly demonstrated no improvement in urologic function. The VUMC group examined 16 patients with a mean age of 6.5 months and compared urodynamic studies with those from historic controls. They found similar results between the two groups.[31] The UCSF group examined 6 patients who had fetal MMC repair and corroborated the findings of the VUMC group.[32]

CLINICAL TRIAL

From the preliminary data discussed previously, it is not clear whether or not prenatal repair of MMC is truly beneficial when compared with standard postnatal therapy. As a result, a prospective, randomized, National Institutes of Health-funded, multicenter trial for fetal surgery for MMC was proposed and is currently underway at the VUMC, UCSF, and CHOP. There are two primary research questions in this trial. First is whether or not fetal surgery for MMC improves outcome as measured by death or the need for a VP shunt within the first year of life as compared with postnatal surgery. The second question is whether or not prenatal repair of MMC improves neurologic function at 30 months of age as predicted by the spinal level of the lesion. Secondary research objectives include whether the Chiari II malformation is improved, whether neuromotor outcome is improved at 12 and 30 months of age, and what are the long-term psychological and reproductive consequences for the parents. Inclusion and exclusion criteria for the trial are listed in **Box 1**. Operative procedures are

---

Box 1

Inclusion and exclusion criteria for the ongoing myelomeningocele clinical trial in the United States

Inclusion criteria

1. MMC at level T1 through S1 with hindbrain herniation

2. Maternal age of 18 years or older

3. Gestational age at randomization of 19 weeks to 25 weeks and 6 days

4. Normal karyotype

Exclusion criteria

1. Nonresident of the United States

2. Nonsingleton pregnancy

3. Insulin-dependent pregestational diabetes

4. Fetal anomaly not related to MMC

5. Kyphosis in the fetus of 30° or greater

6. Current or planned cerclage or documented history of incompetent cervix

7. Short cervix (<20 mm)

8. Placenta previa or placental abruption

9. Body mass index of 35 or greater

10. Previous spontaneous delivery before 37 weeks of gestation

11. Maternal-fetal Rh isoimmunization, Kell sensitization, or neonatal alloimmune thrombocytopenia

12. Maternal HIV- or hepatitis B-positive status

13. Known hepatitis C positivity

14. Uterine anomaly, such as large or multiple fibroids or müllerian duct abnormality

15. Other maternal medical condition that is a contraindication to surgery or general anesthesia

16. Patient does not have a support person

17. Inability to comply with travel and follow-up requirements

standardized in this trial, in addition to follow-up. A team neurosurgeon as part of the trial is designated to help guide the physicians caring for the infant to ensure uniformity in the decision to place a VP shunt. This prospective randomized trial is in its sixth year, and as of February 1, 2009, it has enrolled 150 of a planned 200 patients.

NEW DIRECTIONS

In an attempt to improve on nerve repair and regeneration in MMC, Fauza and colleagues[33] recently published a study in a sheep model in which murine neural stem cells were applied to the defect during fetal repair. Neurologic outcomes in the animals treated with stem cells were comparable to those in animals that underwent standard fetal repair. There were qualitative improvements in hind limb movement in the animals that received stem cells, however. In addition, after histologic analysis, the neural stem cells showed survival and engraftment and seemed to be more concentrated at areas of greatest damage, suggesting that they may "home in" on the most injured areas. Finally, on further histochemical analysis, the engrafted neural stem cells were found to remain in a largely undifferentiated state, possibly suggesting a neurotrophic secretory or chaperone-like role for these stem cells.[33] These data are largely preliminary but may support further study into a multifaceted approach to MMC repair.

Newer less invasive methods of fetal MMC treatment have been investigated in animals as well. Recent surgical experiments in fetal sheep have demonstrated the feasibility of robot-assisted closure of MMC defects.[34] In an attempt to revisit the feasibility for minimally invasive repair, further attempts at refining those techniques have shown promise in the ovine model.[35,36] Furthermore, prenatal steroid treatment in a rabbit model of MMC has been shown to reduce inflammation in the neural placode at delivery. In addition, in that study, preterm delivery was associated with less hindbrain herniation.[37] These findings might suggest that anti-inflammatory medications may be beneficial in protecting the exposed neural elements in MMC from intrauterine injury.

SUMMARY

MMC can be a devastating disease with significant morbidity and mortality within the first few decades of life. Fetal intervention for MMC may improve hydrocephalus and hindbrain herniation associated with the Arnold-Chiari II malformation and may reduce the need for VP shunting. As of now, there is little evidence that prenatal repair of MMC improves neurologic function—sensory, motor, or urologic. MMC is the first nonlethal disease under consideration and study for fetal surgery. As a result, potential improvements in outcome must be balanced with maternal safety and well-being, in addition to that of the unborn patient. The current multicenter trial should provide answers regarding the benefit of fetal surgery for MMC. In addition, other significant insights should be gleaned from the trial regarding optimal treatment of patients who have MMC and maternal safety in open fetal surgery.

REFERENCES

1. Hutchins GM, Meuli M, Meuli-Simmen C, et al. Acquired spinal cord injury in human fetuses with myelomeningocele. Pediatr Pathol Lab Med 1996;16(5): 701–12.

2. Heffez DS, Aryanpur J, Hutchins GM, et al. The paralysis associated with myelo-meningocele: clinical and experimental data implicating a preventable spinal cord injury. Neurosurgery 1990;26(6):987–92.
3. Korenromp MJ, van Gool JD, Bruinese HW, et al. Early fetal leg movements in myelomeningocele. Lancet 1986;1(8486):917–8.
4. Oya N, Suzuki Y, Tanemura M, et al. Detection of skin over cysts with spina bifida may be useful not only for preventing neurological damage during labor but also for predicting fetal prognosis. Fetal Diagn Ther 2000;15(3):156–9.
5. Stiefel D, Copp AJ, Meuli M. Fetal spina bifida in a mouse model: loss of neural function in utero. J Neurosurg 2007;106(Suppl 3):213–21.
6. Pedreira DA, Sanchez e Oliveira Rde C, Valente PR, et al. Validation of the ovine fetus as an experimental model for the human myelomeningocele defect. Acta Cir Bras 2007;22(3):168–73.
7. von Koch CS, Compagnone N, Hirose S, et al. Myelomeningocele: characterization of a surgically induced sheep model and its central nervous system similarities and differences to the human disease. Am J Obstet Gynecol 2005;193(4):1456–62.
8. Weber Guimaraes Barreto M, Ferro MM, Guimaraes Bittencourt D, et al. Arnold-Chiari in a fetal rat model of dysraphism. Fetal Diagn Ther 2005;20(5):437–41.
9. Bouchard S, Davey MG, Rintoul NE, et al. Correction of hindbrain herniation and anatomy of the vermis after in utero repair of myelomeningocele in sheep. J Pediatr Surg 2003;38(3):451–8 [discussion: 451–8].
10. Galvan-Montano A, Cardenas-Lailson E, Hernandez-Godinez B, et al. [Development of an animal model of myelomeningocele and options for prenatal treatment in Macaca mulatta]. Cir Cir 2007;75(5):357–62 [in Spanish].
11. Julia V, Sancho MA, Albert A, et al. Prenatal covering of the spinal cord decreases neurologic sequelae in a myelomeningocele model. J Pediatr Surg 2006;41(6): 1125–9.
12. Yoshizawa J, Sbragia L, Paek BW, et al. Fetal surgery for repair of myelomeningocele allows normal development of the rectum in sheep. Pediatr Surg Int 2003;19(3):162–6.
13. Yoshizawa J, Sbragia L, Paek BW, et al. Fetal surgery for repair of myelomeningocele allows normal development of anal sphincter muscles in sheep. Pediatr Surg Int 2004;20(1):14–8.
14. Bruner JP, Richards WO, Tulipan NB, et al. Endoscopic coverage of fetal myelomeningocele in utero. Am J Obstet Gynecol 1999;180(1 Pt 1):153–8.
15. Bruner JP, Tulipan NB, Richards WO, et al. In utero repair of myelomeningocele: a comparison of endoscopy and hysterotomy. Fetal Diagn Ther 2000;15(2):83–8.
16. Farmer DL, von Koch CS, Peacock WJ, et al. In utero repair of myelomeningocele: experimental pathophysiology, initial clinical experience, and outcomes. Arch Surg 2003;138(8):872–8.
17. Bruner JP, Tulipan N, Paschall RL, et al. Fetal surgery for myelomeningocele and the incidence of shunt-dependent hydrocephalus. JAMA 1999;282(19):1819–25.
18. Tulipan N, Sutton LN, Bruner JP, et al. The effect of intrauterine myelomeningocele repair on the incidence of shunt-dependent hydrocephalus. Pediatr Neurosurg 2003;38(1):27–33.
19. Bruner JP, Tulipan N, Reed G, et al. Intrauterine repair of spina bifida: preoperative predictors of shunt-dependent hydrocephalus. Am J Obstet Gynecol 2004; 190(5):1305–12.
20. Sutton LN, Adzick NS, Bilaniuk LT, et al. Improvement in hindbrain herniation demonstrated by serial fetal magnetic resonance imaging following fetal surgery for myelomeningocele. JAMA 1999;282(19):1826–31.

21. Danzer E, Johnson MP, Bebbington M, et al. Fetal head biometry assessed by fetal magnetic resonance imaging following in utero myelomeningocele repair. Fetal Diagn Ther 2007;22(1):1–6.

22. Johnson MP, Sutton LN, Rintoul N, et al. Fetal myelomeningocele repair: short-term clinical outcomes. Am J Obstet Gynecol 2003;189(2):482–7.

23. Tulipan N, Bruner JP, Hernanz-Schulman M, et al. Effect of intrauterine myelomeningocele repair on central nervous system structure and function. Pediatr Neurosurg 1999;31(4):183–8.

24. Tubbs RS, Chambers MR, Smyth MD, et al. Late gestational intrauterine myelomeningocele repair does not improve lower extremity function. Pediatr Neurosurg 2003;38(3):128–32.

25. Danzer E, Gerdes M, Bebbington MW, et al. Lower extremity neuromotor function and short-term ambulatory potential following in utero myelomeningocele surgery. Fetal Diagn Ther 2009;25(1):47–53.

26. Tulipan N, Bruner JP. Myelomeningocele repair in utero: a report of three cases. Pediatr Neurosurg 1998;28(4):177–80.

27. Farrell JA, Albanese CT, Jennings RW, et al. Maternal fertility is not affected by fetal surgery. Fetal Diagn Ther 1999;14(3):190–2.

28. Longaker MT, Golbus MS, Filly RA, et al. Maternal outcome after open fetal surgery. A review of the first 17 human cases. JAMA 1991;265(6):737–41.

29. Hamdan AH, Walsh W, Heddings A, et al. Gestational age at intrauterine myelomeningocele repair does not influence the risk of prematurity. Fetal Diagn Ther 2002;17(2):66–8.

30. Hamdan AH, Walsh W, Bruner JP, et al. Intrauterine myelomeningocele repair: effect on short-term complications of prematurity. Fetal Diagn Ther 2004;19(1):83–6.

31. Holzbeierlein J, Pope JI, Adams MC, et al. The urodynamic profile of myelodysplasia in childhood with spinal closure during gestation. J Urol 2000;164(4):1336–9.

32. Holmes NM, Nguyen HT, Harrison MR, et al. Fetal intervention for myelomeningocele: effect on postnatal bladder function. J Urol 2001;166(6):2383–6.

33. Fauza DO, Jennings RW, Teng YD, et al. Neural stem cell delivery to the spinal cord in an ovine model of fetal surgery for spina bifida. Surgery 2008;144(3):367–73.

34. Aaronson OS, Hernanz-Schulman M, Bruner JP, et al. Myelomeningocele: prenatal evaluation—comparison between transabdominal US and MR imaging. Radiology 2003;227(3):839–43.

35. Pedreira DA, Oliveira RC, Valente PR, et al. Gasless fetoscopy: a new approach to endoscopic closure of a lumbar skin defect in fetal sheep. Fetal Diagn Ther 2008;23(4):293–8.

36. Kohl T, Hartlage MG, Kiehitz D, et al. Percutaneous fetoscopic patch coverage of experimental lumbosacral full-thickness skin lesions in sheep. Surg Endosc 2003;17(8):1218–23.

37. Fontecha CG, Peiro JL, Aguirre M, et al. The effect of prenatal treatment with steroids and preterm delivery in a model of myelomeningocele on the rabbit foetus. Pediatr Surg Int 2007;23(5):425–9.

Cardiac Anomalies in the Fetus

Christopher G. B. Turner, MD[a], Wayne Tworetzky, MD[b,c],
Louise E. Wilkins-Haug, MD, PhD[d], Russell W. Jennings, MD[e,f,*]

KEYWORDS
- Congenital heart disease • Fetal intervention
- Hypoplastic left heart syndrome • Pulmonary atresia
- Balloon dilatation • Valvuloplasty

As the most frequent congenital anomaly and the leading cause of death among infants in the United States, congenital heart disease (CHD) is an attractive target for fetal therapy. With the development of successful neonatal repair for many types of CHD over the last 20 years, earlier postnatal therapy to restore physiologic anatomy has been encouraged, and fetal therapy has become the next frontier. Concurrent advances in interventional catheterization and fetal imaging provided a foundation for the novel field of fetal cardiac intervention. This article focuses on the current status of in utero catheter interventions for CHD with particular interest in therapy for defects characterized by progressive stenosis or atresia of the semilunar valves, the aortic and pulmonary, with development of subsequent ventricular hypoplasia.

FETAL CIRCULATION

In the normal fetal circulation, oxygenated blood from the umbilical vein is able to stream efficiently through the foramen ovale (FO) to the left heart and up to the brain. The desaturated blood from the superior vena cava is directed through the ductus arteriosus (DA) back to the placenta for reoxygenation (**Fig. 1**). Because pulmonary

[a] Department of Surgery, Children's Hospital Boston, 300 Longwood Avenue, Fegan 3, Boston, MA 02115, USA
[b] Department of Pediatrics, Harvard Medical School, 300 Longwood Avenue, Pavillion 2, Boston, MA 02115, USA
[c] Fetal Cardiology Program, Children's Hospital Boston, 300 Longwood Avenue, Fegan 3, Boston, MA 02115, USA
[d] Department of Maternal Fetal Medicine, Brigham and Women's Hospital, 75 Francis St., Boston, MA 02115, USA
[e] Department of Surgery, Harvard Medical School, 300 Longwood Avenue, Pavillion 2, Boston, MA 02115, USA
[f] Advanced Fetal Care Center, Department of Surgery, Children's Hospital Boston, 300 Longwood Avenue, Fegan 3, Boston, MA 02115, USA
* Corresponding author. Advanced Fetal Care Center, Department of Surgery, Children's Hospital Boston, 300 Longwood Avenue, Fegan 3, Boston, MA 02115.
E-mail address: russell.jennings@childrens.harvard.edu (R.W. Jennings).

Clin Perinatol 36 (2009) 439–449
doi:10.1016/j.clp.2009.03.015
0095-5108/09/$ – see front matter
© 2009 Elsevier Inc. All rights reserved.

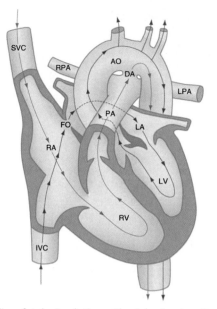

Fig. 1. Normal intracardiac fetal circulation. Physiologic shunting through the patent foramen ovale (FO) and the patent ductus arteriosus (DA). Oxygenated blood from the placenta (*red arrows*) reaches the right atrium (RA) by means of the inferior vena cava (IVC). This well-oxygenated blood is shunted preferentially from the RA across to the left atrium (LA) through the FO and then is ejected out the left ventricle (LV) to the ascending aorta (AO). Deoxygenated blood (*blue arrows*) returning from the superior vena cava (SVC) preferentially travels from RA into the RV, then out through the main pulmonary artery (PA). Because of the high pulmonary vascular resistance in the fetal lungs, this deoxygenated blood bypasses lungs and enters the descending aorta by means of the DA. (*From* Insaba AF. Cardiac disorders. In: Marx JA, editor. Rosen's emergency medicine: concepts and clinical practice. 6th edition. Philadelphia: Elsevier; 2006. p. 2568; with permission.)

vascular resistance is higher than systemic vascular resistance, blood shunts through the DA from the right side to the left, diverting around the lungs. At the moment of birth, however, pulmonary vascular resistance suddenly drops, the shunt reverses, and blood flows through the lungs. As the FO and DA close in the postnatal period, two distinct circuits are formed, the pulmonary and systemic vasculatures.

With severe semilunar valve pathology, however, there is only a single functional ventricular pump, the left ventricle in the case of pulmonary atresia (PA), and the right ventricle in the case of aortic stenosis (AS). In these situations, the DA is essential to continue perfusion to the systemic or pulmonary vasculature, and the FO is essential to allow the mixture of oxygenated and deoxygenated blood in the single ventricle system. As blood flows preferentially through the patent FO rather than the high-pressure ventricle, however, the reduction in flow through the ventricle retards growth, and in part, contributes to eventual hypoplasia.

In addition to semilunar pathology, if the atrial septum is intact (IAS) or severely stenosed, the circuit on the side of the atretic semilunar valve will become obstructed. In the extremely rare case of PA with a stenotic atrial septum, the fetal circulation is impaired and often not compatible with fetal life. In the case of established hypoplastic left heart syndrome (HLHS) with an intact atrial septum, the postnatal circulation is impaired and not compatible with neonatal life.

The most common indication for a fetal cardiac intervention is to attempt to prevent the development of right or left ventricular (LV) hypoplasia. In the approach to fetal cardiac interventions for semilunar valve stenosis, therefore, there are two fundamental conditions:

One must understand the in utero characteristics of the heart defect that would predict progression to ventricular hypoplasia.

One must understand the characteristics of the heart defect that indicate that an in utero intervention might lead to improvement in cardiac growth and function.

Moreover, one needs to understand the features that indicate the heart defect is too far advanced and that fetal intervention would be futile and provide unnecessary risk to the mother and fetus.

DIAGNOSTIC STUDIES

Echocardiography is the preferred modality for screening and determining the severity of semilunar valve stenosis. Color Doppler imaging can identify reduced flow through the aortic valve and retrograde flow in the transverse aortic arch, the hallmark of evolving HLHS in this defect. The pressure gradient across the valve is affected by the degree of stenosis and the competitive retrograde arch flow, as well as the function of the left ventricle. A low gradient therefore may indicate a stenotic valve with poor LV function. Other indicators of LV dysfunction and evolving HLHS include retrograde flow in the aortic arch supplied via the ductus arteriosus, diminished mitral valve diastolic excursion with reduced inflow, left-to-right flow across the FO, or left-to-right bulge of an intact atrial septum.[1-4] Also, although rare, a thrombus can form in the dilated left ventricle.

Thousands of prenatal screening ultrasounds are needed to detect a small number of cardiac defects. Despite increased screening and improved detection rates, most cardiac defects remain undiagnosed prenatally. If CHD is suspected, the mother should be referred to a pediatric cardiologist as soon as possible. This early referral allows for confirmation of the diagnosis, appropriate counseling, and arrangement for delivery and treatment at a center capable of treating complex congenital heart defects.[5,6] Early prenatal diagnosis also allows for the option of palliative or therapeutic in utero interventions for amenable cardiac defects.[7-9] Because these therapies are available at only a few centers, early prenatal detection is critical. Increased overall screening rates, improved detection, and earlier referral will allow for more patients to potentially benefit from in utero interventions.

CONGENITAL HEART DEFECTS APPROPRIATE FOR FETAL INTERVENTION

Fetal intervention offers the tantalizing possibility to reverse the pathologic process before significant cardiac structural and functional deterioration has occurred. Early relief of semilunar valve stenosis in utero may reverse the progression toward ventricular hypoplasia.[10-12] This section discusses the specific defect on the left and right side.

Defects on the Left Side

Aortic valve defects in the fetus range from mild stenosis with an adequately sized ventricle to severe stenosis with evolving HLHS, a term that implies that the left ventricle is unable to sustain systemic circulation. With a patent FO, blood in the left atrium flows preferentially to the low-pressure right atrium rather than the high-pressure left ventricle. The resultant diminished flow through the left heart causes arrest of LV growth and HLHS. Occasionally the left ventricle can be of normal size, but the myocardium becomes damaged and fibrotic with significantly reduced filling and poor systolic function. In fetuses with aortic stenosis and an intact or restrictive atrial septum, there is no low-pressure outlet for blood entering the left heart, so the left atrium and ventricle may become severely dilated. This may lead to severe mitral regurgitation from mitral annular dilation, with the resultant elevated pressure and compression of the right heart causing right heart failure and hydrops fetalis. Patients with HLHS, one of the most serious CHDs, require palliative surgery at birth to make the right ventricle the systemically functioning ventricle, or occasionally primary neonatal heart transplantation. Therefore severe aortic valve stenosis with evolving HLHS is the defect for which fetal intervention is most likely to be considered.[1–3,7–9,13–15]

Several centers have offered in utero aortic valvuloplasty as an alternative treatment for midgestation fetal AS, with a high probability of progression of HLHS.[7,9,14,16] The objective of fetal aortic valvuloplasty is to relieve the obstruction to LV ejection, thereby reducing LV work and damage, increasing flow through the left heart, and slowing or preventing the progression to HLHS. Recent studies from the authors' center demonstrate that fetal aortic valvuloplasty may increase blood flow through the left heart and improve left heart growth.[14,16] An oversized balloon was associated with moderate or severe aortic regurgitation that was tolerated by the fetus and improved through the gestation.[16]

To achieve maximal benefit from the procedure, it must be performed before the occurrence of irreversible pathology. Much remains unknown with respect to the evolution of this CHD.[17,18] Early attempts at fetal aortic valvuloplasties performed in the third trimester were too late in gestation to reverse the disease, demonstrating that the window for intervention must occur as early as possible during the second trimester.

Based on the current understanding of the risk–benefit ratio of fetal intervention, fetal aortic valvuloplasty should not be performed in fetuses with AS that will not otherwise progress to HLHS. Anatomic dimensions of left heart structures at the time of diagnosis alone do not predict progression to HLHS. Instead, physiologic aberrations such as reversed blood flow in the transverse aortic arch, left-to-right flow across the FO, monophasic mitral valve inflow, and moderate-to-severe LV dysfunction in midgestation are important signs of evolving HLHS.[19] These findings may be useful for identifying appropriate candidates for fetal aortic valvuloplasty.

The presence of an intact or highly restrictive atrial septum (I/HRAS) is a predictor of poor outcome among patients with HLHS.[20–23] Maintenance of a postnatal circulation depends on an atrial septal defect (ASD) to allow the left atrium to decompress into the right heart. Without an adequate ASD, left atrial hypertension prevents adequate pulmonary flow, and these infants die shortly after birth without immediate intervention. Anatomic studies have described an intact atrial septum in approximately 6% of patients with HLHS, and clinically deleterious restriction to flow at the level of the atrial septum occurring in as many as 22%.[24,25] In a recent series at a major referral center with aggressive management involving prenatal diagnosis and planned delivery, survival was only 28%.[26] At the authors' institution, a series of 24 fetuses that underwent attempted ASD creation in utero revealed that the procedure can be performed with a high rate of technical success. Of 21 attempted procedures, 19 were technically successful. Creation of a defect greater than or equal to 3 mm was associated with better postnatal oxygenation and less frequent need for emergent postnatal intervention, but it was not shown to improve survival.[27]

Defects on the Right Side

In a similar fashion to aortic valve disease, pulmonary valve disease occupies a spectrum from mild stenosis to severe atresia. Pulmonary atresia with an intact ventricular septum (PA/IVS) produces hypoplastic right heart syndrome (HRHS). Some fetuses with severe tricuspid regurgitations may develop high central venous pressures and resultant fetal hydrops. The size and rate of growth of the fetal tricuspid valve accurately predicts postnatal outcomes and may be used for selecting patients for fetal therapy.[28] In addition, a right ventricular (RV)-dependant coronary artery supply results in increased mortality after birth and is considered the most severe form. These infants will require a palliative circulation or transplantation. If the fetus is likely to require single ventricle palliation after birth, some fetuses with PA/IVS are appropriate candidates for fetal intervention.

Unlike the left ventricle, the right ventricle has some capacity to grow postnatally, and RV decompression in infancy allows the potential for RV growth. RV decompression in utero presumably also should lead to RV growth. Several attempts have been made at treating this defect in utero, but there have been no reports in which the infant did not require postnatal surgery also.[29–31] Further evolution in the technique for right-sided heart interventions is needed, which may also benefit additional defects such as tetralogy of Fallot with pulmonary atresia and hypoplastic pulmonary arteries.

PROCEDURE
Technique

Several techniques have been attempted for fetal balloon valvuloplasty. The least invasive involves maternal sedation with percutaneous access to the fetus, as originally described by Allan.[7–9] A more invasive technique involves a laparotomy to

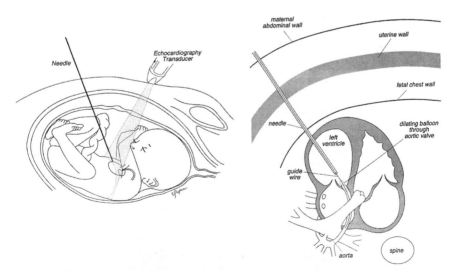

Fig. 2. Ideal fetal position and cannula course for aortic valvuloplasty. Course of cannula corresponds to unobstructed pathway from maternal abdomen to left ventricle apex to aortic valve. (*From* Tworetzky W, Wilkins-Haug L, Jennings RW, et al. Balloon dilation of severe aortic stenosis in the fetus: potential for prevention of hypoplastic left heart syndrome: candidate selection, technique, and results of successful intervention. Circulation 2004;110(15):2127; with permission.)

expose the uterus, which allows for easier manipulation of the fetus, improved ultra-sound image quality, and shorter distance to the fetal heart. The most invasive tech-nique involves a uterine incision and fetal exposure, which allows for femoral and carotid artery access.[32] The more invasive techniques offer direct contact and the

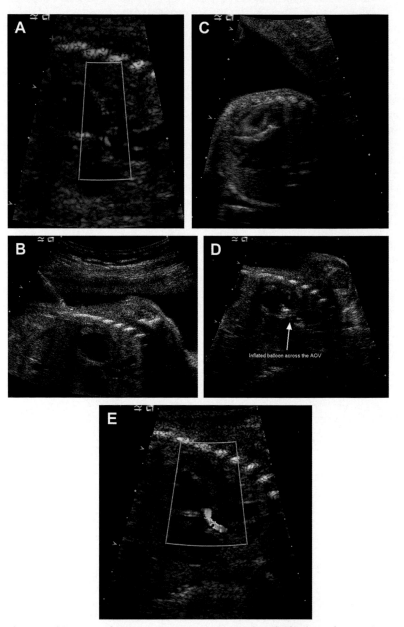

Fig. 3. Ultrasound images of percutaneous in utero aortic valvuloplasty for aortic stenosis. (*A*) Aortic valve flow before intervention. (*B*) Alignment of needle. (*C*) Guide wire across aortic valve in ascending aorta. (*D*) Inflated balloon across the aortic valve. (*E*) Aortic valve flow after intervention.

possibility of improved technical success, but these benefits occur at the cost of increased maternal morbidity and premature delivery. Therefore, less-invasive percutaneous techniques when possible are preferable.

Techniques at Children's Hospital Boston and Brigham and Women's Hospital have evolved with the collaboration of many departments. Percutaneous transthoracic cardiac puncture has been most effective, with minimal maternal risk. The access point to the fetal heart depends on the type of procedure. All procedures are performed under two-dimensional ultrasound guidance. The needle used to access the fetal heart is preferably as small as possible, such as a 19G cannula. A minilaparotomy is performed to expose the uterus only if certain factors require it, such as fetal position, anterior placenta, and maternal body habitus.

For aortic balloon valvuloplasty, the large dilated left ventricle is the most easily accessed structure with proximity to the aortic valve. The cannula and stylet needle are advanced through the maternal abdomen, uterine wall, and fetal chest wall (**Fig. 2**). The cannula, guide wires, and balloon shafts are premeasured and marked, allowing positioning within the fetal heart by both external measurements and ultrasound imaging. Correct fetal positioning is critical; the left ventricle is entered only when:

The left chest is anterior.
There are no limbs between the uterine wall and apex.
The apex is within 9 cm of the abdominal wall.
The outflow track is parallel to the cannula course.

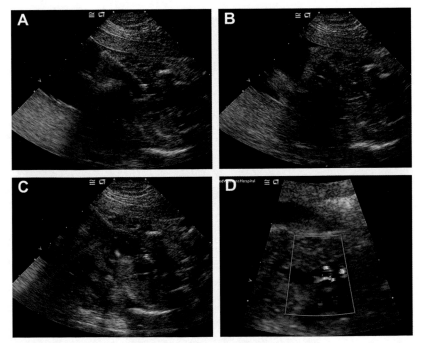

Fig. 4. Ultrasound images of percutaneous in utero pulmonary valvuloplasty for pulmonary atresia with intact ventricular septum. (*A*) Needle aimed at pulmonary valve. (*B*) Guide wire across pulmonary valve in pulmonary artery. (*C*) Inflated balloon across the pulmonary valve. (*D*) Pulmonary valve flow after intervention.

The balloon valvuloplasty itself is performed with a small coronary artery balloon over a thin, floppy-tipped guide wire. The balloon is inflated with pressure gauges to precise inflation diameters. Flow across the dilated aortic valve is confirmed with echocardiography (**Fig. 3**).

For pulmonary balloon valvuloplasty, the right ventricle is accessed, although it makes a more difficult target than the left because of small size, complex geometry, and valvular atresia. The same principles of measurement and position are used. Flow across the dilated pulmonary valve is confirmed with echocardiography (**Fig. 4**).

For atrial septoplasty, the right atrium is accessed through the right chest wall. An unobstructed line is identified from the fetal right atrium, through the left atrium, and into a left pulmonary vein. An 18G or 19G introducer cannula on a sharp metal obturator is advanced into the right atrium and against the atrial septum. The septum is punctured by the tip of the introducer or, more commonly, with a 22G Chiba needle (Cook Incorporated, Bloomington, IN). A wire then is introduced into the left atrium or a pulmonary vein, and the Chiba needle is exchanged for a balloon angioplasty catheter. The balloon is inflated fully several times before the cannula is removed. Flow across the new atrial septal defect is confirmed with echocardiography (**Fig. 5**).

Anesthesia

Anesthesia is a necessary element of any of these procedures. Although maternal sedation is possible, inhaled anesthetic allows for maximal uterine relaxation and easy conversion to an open procedure if necessary. Additional fetal anesthesia is

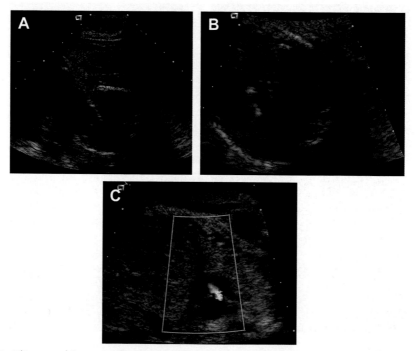

Fig. 5. Ultrasound images of percutaneous in utero atrial septoplasty for hypoplastic left heart syndrome. (*A*) Needle penetrating left atrium from right atrium. (*B*) Balloon across atrial septum. (*C*) Atrial septum flow after intervention.

administered through an intramuscular injection, which allows for fetal manipulation and optimal positioning. At Children's Hospital Boston, a combination of fentanyl, pancuronium, and atropine are used. Atropine counteracts the bradycardia that can occur with fetal and uterine manipulation.

COMPLICATIONS

Fetal complications are usually treatable. Bradycardia is common with needle access to the ventricle, occurring in about 50% of cases, and uncommon with needle access to the atrium. The arrhythmia resolves by stopping manipulations or with intracardiac administration of epinephrine, either into the muscle or by direct injection. Pericardial effusions are also common and, if moderate to large, they can be drained successfully.

Low maternal complication rates also have been possible with in utero catheter interventions. Despite well-executed procedures and extensive preprocedure evaluation to exclude maternal contraindications, complications from the anesthesia, laparotomy, and uterine manipulation do occur. A sick fetus can cause premature labor or the maternal mirror syndrome, which resembles preeclampsia and requires delivery of the fetus.

SUMMARY

On the frontier of pediatric cardiology, fetal cardiac interventions for CHD offer a promising therapeutic option for those conditions with significant morbidity and mortality from current palliative operations. Early detection and referral of all fetuses with suspected CHD would increase the number of patients that may benefit. Concurrent multidisciplinary collaboration between perinatologists, cardiologists, fetal surgeons, and anesthesiologists will improve patient selection criteria, techniques for safe access to the fetus, the performance of the procedure, and perioperative care.

REFERENCES

1. Sharland GK, Chita SK, Fagg NL, et al. Left ventricular dysfunction in the fetus: relation to aortic valve anomalies and endocardial fibroelastosis. Br Heart J 1991;66(6):419–24.
2. McCaffrey FM, Sherman FS. Prenatal diagnosis of severe aortic stenosis. Pediatr Cardiol 1997;18(4):276–81.
3. Simpson JM, Sharland GK. Natural history and outcome of aortic stenosis diagnosed prenatally. Heart 1997;77(3):205–10.
4. Berning RA, Silverman NH, Villegas M, et al. Reversed shunting across the ductus arteriosus or atrial septum in utero heralds severe congenital heart disease. J Am Coll Cardiol 1996;27(2):481–6.
5. Tworetzky W, McElhinney DB, Reddy VM, et al. Improved surgical outcome after fetal diagnosis of hypoplastic left heart syndrome. Circulation 2001;103(9): 1269–73.
6. Bonnet D, Coltri A, Butera G, et al. Detection of transposition of the great arteries in fetuses reduces neonatal morbidity and mortality. Circulation 1999;99(7):916–8.
7. Maxwell D, Allan L, Tynan MJ. Balloon dilatation of the aortic valve in the fetus: a report of two cases. Br Heart J 1991;65(5):256–8.
8. Allan LD, Maxwell DJ, Carminati M, et al. Survival after fetal aortic balloon valvoplasty. Ultrasound Obstet Gynecol 1995;5(2):90–1.

9. Kohl T, Sharland G, Allan LD, et al. World experience of percutaneous ultrasound-guided balloon valvuloplasty in human fetuses with severe aortic valve obstruction. Am J Cardiol 2000;85(10):1230–3.

10. Tweddell JS, Hoffman GM, Mussatto KA, et al. Improved survival of patients undergoing palliation of hypoplastic left heart syndrome: lessons learned from 115 consecutive patients. Circulation 2002;106(12 Suppl 1):I82–9.

11. Fishman NH, Hof RB, Rudolph AM, et al. Models of congenital heart disease in fetal lambs. Circulation 1978;58(2):354–64.

12. Hornberger LK, Sanders SP, Rein AJ, et al. Left heart obstructive lesions and left ventricular growth in the midtrimester fetus. A longitudinal study. Circulation 1995; 92(6):1531–8.

13. Daubeney PE, Sharland GK, Cook AC, et al. Pulmonary atresia with intact ventricular septum: impact of fetal echocardiography on incidence at birth and postnatal outcome. UK and Eire Collaborative Study of Pulmonary Atresia with Intact Ventricular Septum. Circulation 1998;98(6):562–6.

14. Tworetzky W, Wilkins-Haug L, Jennings RW, et al. Balloon dilation of severe aortic stenosis in the fetus: potential for prevention of hypoplastic left heart syndrome: candidate selection, technique, and results of successful intervention. Circulation 2004;110(15):2125–31.

15. Vida VL, Bacha EA, Larrazabal A, et al. Hypoplastic left heart syndrome with intact or highly restrictive atrial septum: surgical experience from a single center. Ann Thorac Surg 2007;84(2):581–5 [discussion: 586].

16. Marshall AC, Tworetzky W, Bergersen L, et al. Aortic valvuloplasty in the fetus: technical characteristics of successful balloon dilation. J Pediatr 2005;147(4): 535–9.

17. Sinclair BG, Sandor GG, Farquharson DF. Effectiveness of primary level antenatal screening for severe congenital heart disease: a population-based assessment. J Perinatol 1996;16(5):336–40.

18. Carvalho JS, Mavrides E, Shinebourne EA, et al. Improving the effectiveness of routine prenatal screening for major congenital heart defects. Heart 2002;88(4): 387–91.

19. Makikallio K, McElhinney DB, Levine JC, et al. Fetal aortic valve stenosis and the evolution of hypoplastic left heart syndrome: patient selection for fetal intervention. Circulation 2006;113(11):1401–5.

20. Photiadis J, Urban AE, Sinzobahamvya N, et al. Restrictive left atrial outflow adversely affects outcome after the modified Norwood procedure. Eur J Cardiothorac Surg 2005;27(6):962–7.

21. Stasik CN, Gelehrter S, Goldberg CS, et al. Current outcomes and risk factors for the Norwood procedure. J Thorac Cardiovasc Surg 2006;131(2):412–7.

22. Daebritz SH, Nollert GD, Zurakowski D, et al. Results of Norwood stage I operation: comparison of hypoplastic left heart syndrome with other malformations. J Thorac Cardiovasc Surg 2000;119(2):358–67.

23. Canter CE, Moorehead S, Huddleston CB, et al. Restrictive atrial septal communication as a determinant of outcome of cardiac transplantation for hypoplastic left heart syndrome. Circulation 1993;88(5 Pt 2):II456–60.

24. Forbess JM, Cook N, Roth SJ, et al. Ten-year institutional experience with palliative surgery for hypoplastic left heart syndrome. Risk factors related to stage I mortality. Circulation 1995;92(Suppl 9):II262–6.

25. Rychik J, Rome JJ, Collins MH, et al. The hypoplastic left heart syndrome with intact atrial septum: atrial morphology, pulmonary vascular histopathology, and outcome. J Am Coll Cardiol 1999;34(2):554–60.

26. Glatz JA, Tabbutt S, Gaynor JW, et al. Hypoplastic left heart syndrome with atrial level restriction in the era of prenatal diagnosis. Ann Thorac Surg 2007;84(5): 1633–8.
27. Marshall AC, Levine J, Morash D, et al. Results of in utero atrial septoplasty in fetuses with hypoplastic left heart syndrome. Prenat Diagn 2008;28(11):1023–8.
28. Salvin JW, McElhinney DB, Colan SD, et al. Fetal tricuspid valve size and growth as predictors of outcome in pulmonary atresia with intact ventricular septum. Pediatrics 2006;118(2):e415–20.
29. Arzt W, Tulzer G, Aigner M, et al. Invasive intrauterine treatment of pulmonary atresia/intact ventricular septum with heart failure. Ultrasound Obstet Gynecol 2003;21(2):186–8.
30. Tulzer G, Arzt W, Franklin RC, et al. Fetal pulmonary valvuloplasty for critical pulmonary stenosis or atresia with intact septum. Lancet 2002;360(9345):1567–8.
31. Galindo A, Gutierrez-Larraya F, Velasco JM, et al. Pulmonary balloon valvuloplasty in a fetus with critical pulmonary stenosis/atresia with intact ventricular septum and heart failure. Fetal Diagn Ther 2006;21(1):100–4.
32. Adzick NS, Harrison MR. Fetal surgical therapy. Lancet 1994;343(8902):897–902.

Prenatal Stem Cell Transplantation and Gene Therapy

Matthew T. Santore, MD[a], Jessica L. Roybal, MD[a], Alan W. Flake, MD[b],*

KEYWORDS

- Prenatal treatment • Fetal therapy • Gene therapy
- Hematopoietic stem cell transplantation
- Immunologic tolerance

Advances in prenatal diagnosis have led to the prenatal management and treatment of various congenital diseases. Whereas surgical treatment has been applied successfully to specific anatomic defects that place the fetus at risk of death or life-long disability, the indications for fetal surgical intervention have remained relatively limited. In contrast, prenatal stem cell and gene therapy await clinical application, but have tremendous potential to treat a range of genetic disorders. If there are biologic advantages unique to fetal development that favor fetal stem cell or gene therapy over postnatal treatment, prenatal therapy may become the preferred approach to treating any disease that can be prenatally diagnosed and cured by stem cell or gene therapy. The conceptual leap, from prenatal treatment of only life-threatening fetal disease to the prenatal treatment of anticipated pediatric and adult disease could expand the future application of fetal therapy dramatically.

PRENATAL STEM CELL THERAPY

A working definition of a stem cell is: "a cell that can self-replicate and can give rise to more than one type of mature daughter cell." Thus, the term stem cell incorporates a range of cells with different capacities for proliferation and differentiation. Terminology used to classify stem cells includes:

Totipotent—stem cells capable of giving rise to an intact organism including germinal tissues

[a] Department of Surgery, Children's Center for Fetal Research, Children's Hospital of Philadelphia, University of Pennsylvania School of Medicine, Abramson Research Building, Room 1114, 3615 Civic Center Boulevard, Philadelphia, PA, 19104-4318, USA
[b] Department of Surgery, Children's Center for Fetal Research, Children's Hospital of Philadelphia, University of Pennsylvania School of Medicine, Abramson Research Building, Room 1116B, 3615 Civic Center Boulevard, Philadelphia, PA, 19104-4318, USA
* Corresponding author.
E-mail address: flake@email.chop.edu (A.W. Flake).

Clin Perinatol 36 (2009) 451–471
doi:10.1016/j.clp.2009.03.006
0095-5108/09/$ – see front matter © 2009 Elsevier Inc. All rights reserved.

Pluripotent—stem cells capable of giving rise to cells derived from all three germ layers, but not capable of independently forming an organism

Multipotent or organ-specific—stem cells capable of giving rise to the cells comprising a single organ system or tissue.

Although all of these types of stem cells might have future therapeutic application in the fetus, a complete discussion of all foreseeable stem cell applications in the fetus is beyond the scope of this article. Suffice it to say that if the biologic advantages for cellular transplantation in the fetus are validated, one could imagine that any postnatal application of stem cells to a prenatally detectable disease might be more effectively and safely performed in the fetus. At the present time, the most likely and eminent application of stem cell therapy to the fetus is in utero hematopoietic stem cell transplantation (IUHCT), and the authors will confine their discussion to this stem cell type as a paradigm for all prenatal stem cell therapy.

The hematopoietic stem cell (HSC) is a multipotent stem cell that maintains functional hematopoiesis by generation of all hematopoietic lineages throughout fetal and adult life.[1] It is the most extensively characterized stem cell and the only adult-derived stem cell that has been prospectively isolated to purity. Although HSC derived from embryonic or fetal sources may have many biologic advantages, there are significant practical and ethical barriers to using the embryo or fetus as an HSC source.[2] Thus, the authors feel that the most likely initial application of IUHCT will use adult HSC derived from bone marrow (BM) or peripheral blood (PB), and will focus this article on this specific approach.

The Rationale for In Utero Hematopoietic Stem Cell Transplantation

There are a few disorders that have a compelling rationale for IUHCT based on the prevention of irreversible damage to the fetus before birth (ie, glycogen storage diseases with neurologic involvement). The rationale for IUHCT in most instances, however, is based on unique opportunities related to normal developmental events that may facilitate cellular engraftment and avoid complications associated with postnatal BM transplantation.[3] Perhaps the most important of these is normal immunologic development, which provides the opportunity for induction of fetal tolerance.[4] Early in gestation, the immune system undergoes a process of self-education. This occurs primarily in the fetal thymus and consists of two components, the positive selection of prelymphocytes for recognition of self-major histocompatibility complex antigen (MHC) and a negative selection (deletion) of prelymphocytes that have high-affinity recognition of self-antigen in association with self-MHC. This leaves a repertoire of lymphocytes that recognize foreign antigen in association with self-MHC.[5,6] Thus, introduction of foreign cells that are capable of appropriate antigen presentation in the thymus before completion of this process should result in donor-specific immune tolerance. This makes possible strategies of allogeneic tolerance induction to maintain hematopoietic engraftment after IUHCT, or perhaps of more immediate clinical application, to facilitate further cellular or organ transplantation in a tolerant recipient after birth.[7–9] The most compelling evidence for the efficacy of fetal tolerance comes from experiments of nature where dizygotic twins share placental circulation resulting in intrauterine exchange of circulating HSC with resultant life-long hematopoietic chimerism and donor-specific tolerance for the sibling twin.[10–12] Of relevance to clinical application, the existence of chimerism in human[13–15] and nonhuman primate[16,17] twins is documented well. In the case of dizygotic human twins, the frequency of chimerism is relatively high (8% for twins and 21% for triplets), and levels of chimerism in some cases have been at a level that would be therapeutic for most hematologic diseases. These findings have long provided proof in principle for the therapeutic potential of IUHCT. Because natural chimeras result from the mixing of hematopoietic cells by means of placental vascular anastomoses, however, the exposure to allogeneic blood components occurs continuously and begins very early in gestation, which is difficult to replicate experimentally. This article reviews the experimental data that support the capacity of IUHCT to induce donor-specific tolerance.

Another perceived advantage of IUHCT is the normal process of HSC migration and engraftment in hematopoietic tissues. Fetal life is the only time that large-scale migration of stem cells occurs to seed tissue compartments. Definitive hematopoiesis begins in the yolk sac or aorto-gonadal-mesonephric (AGM) region, migrates to the fetal liver, and finally to the bone marrow.[18,19] It is conceivable that these migrations could provide opportunities to selectively engraft donor HSC without the need for myeloablation, a primary cause of morbidity and mortality in postnatal BM transplantation. It also is recognized, however, that the fetal hematopoietic system represents a highly competitive environment because of the excess of circulating HSCs and their relatively high proliferative and competitive capacity.[20–22] Taking full advantage of this opportunity will require a better understanding of the regulatory signals controlling the migration and engraftment of HSC to fetal hematopoietic compartments so that they can be manipulated to provide a competitive advantage for donor HSC.[23] Finally, the fetus is extremely small, weighing less than 35 g at 12 weeks gestation, allowing the transplantation of much larger cell doses on a per kilogram basis than can be achieved after birth. Taken together, the normal biology of the fetus allows the potential for a therapeutic recapitulation of ontogeny, with engraftment, migration, differentiation, and expansion of HSC to reconstitute the defective hematopoietic compartment or induce donor-specific tolerance for facilitation of minimally toxic postnatal transplantation.

Experimental support for in utero hematopoietic stem cell transplantation

Great progress has been made toward IUHCT in animal models over the past 30 years, representing an essential foundation for any future clinical application of IUHCT. The first experimental studies of IUHCT by Fleischman and Mintz remain some of the most informative. They used transplacental injection of donor BM cells at E11 into fetal mice with a stem cell deficiency based on the absence of c-kit.[24] In these studies, the degree of erythroid replacement correlated with the degree of underlying anemia, with complete early replacement by donor erythroid cells in lethally anemic homozygous mice. Mintz subsequently noted that hematopoietic reconstitution could be achieved by engraftment of a single HSC in this noncompetitive model.[25] These early studies were directed toward questions in stem cell biology rather than IUHCT as a potential therapeutic approach. Nevertheless, they demonstrate the importance of host cell competition as a barrier to engraftment after IUHCT. Later studies by Blazar and colleagues[26] confirmed the ability to achieve multilineage chimerism after IUHCT in stem cell-deficient recipients, and the ability to achieve only lymphoid reconstitution (split chimerism) in the mouse severe combined immunodeficiency (SCID) model, which has a T-cell proliferation and survival defect.[27,28] Thus, in the presence of a lineage deficiency, IUHCT was able to reconstitute the defective lineage. It appeared, however, that competitive pressure from the normal host lineages prevented multilineage donor cell expression. These studies reaffirm the importance of host cell competition, whether at the level of the stem cell, or lineage progenitor in limiting engraftment after IUHCT. One therefore would expect that achieving donor cell engraftment after IUHCT in normal animal models with a competitive hematopoietic compartment would be much more difficult.

In general, most studies of IUHCT in normal animal models including the goat,[29,30] dog,[31,32] primate,[33–36] and mouse[37–40] have confirmed this expectation and demonstrated minimal or no detectable engraftment. The exception is the ovine model. Early data in the ovine model appeared promising with achievement of potentially therapeutic levels of allogeneic engraftment (up to 30%) after a single injection of fetal liver-derived donor cells.[41] In fact, the ovine model has even been permissive for xenogeneic engraftment with stable engraftment of human HSC from various sources.[42–45] The reason for the relative success of IUHCT in the sheep remains unclear. Although subsequent results using adult BM-derived cells have not been as favorable, it remains the easiest of large animal models to engraft. Nevertheless, the sheep studies, while not directly clinically applicable, have confirmed the potential of IUHCT by demonstrating the achievement of long-term stable multilineage allogeneic chimerism.

With increasing experimental and clinical experience, it became clear that there were significant barriers to successful engraftment after IUHCT, and that the fetal hematopoietic environment posed very different challenges than encountered in postnatal BM transplantation.[3] To systematically examine the relative importance of these barriers and develop strategies to overcome them, the development of the normal allogeneic murine model was critical. The available inbred and transgenic strains, defined immunology, large litter size, minimal cost, and short gestation of the mouse allow studies to be performed that simply were not possible in other species. In addition, the mouse is stage-for-stage, very similar to people with respect to hematopoietic and immunologic ontogeny. In utero HSC transplants can be performed early in gestation (11 to 15 days) during a time when hematopoiesis is confined to the fetal liver, and before completion of thymic processing and the appearance of mature lymphocytes in the peripheral circulation. Finally, the normal mouse initially proved very difficult to engraft, making it a legitimate model for investigation of barriers to engraftment. The authors and other, only were able to achieve polymerase chain reaction (PCR)-detectable microchimerism for several years in hematopoietically normal mouse strains.[26,37,38,40,46,47]

With improvements in the murine model, the authors were able to deliver higher doses of cells, raising levels of donor chimerism in some recipients into the range measurable by flow cytometry. With generation of macrochimeric mice, it became evident that levels of chimerism of greater than 1% to 2% resulted in the consistent association of donor-specific tolerance across full MHC barriers as evidenced by nonreactivity to donor in mixed lymphocyte reaction and acceptance of donor skin grafts for more than 8 weeks. Mechanistic analysis of tolerance in chimeric mice supported a primary mechanism of deletion of donor reactive lymphocytes, although deletion was not complete, implicating the presence of peripheral tolerance mechanisms also.[8,9,46,48,49] Thus IUHCT appeared to result in normal immunologic processing of donor cells with high level deletion of donor reactive lymphocytes in the thymus and presumably generation of donor-specific T-regulatory cells to control donor-reactive cells that escape thymic deletion. The next step was to demonstrate proof in principle for the potentially important clinical strategy of using IUHCT for tolerance induction, followed by postnatal nontoxic bone marrow transplantation to enhance levels of chimerism to therapeutic levels. Three different nontoxic postnatal strategies were demonstrated to work:

Preparative low-dose total body irradiation followed by T-cell depleted BMT[9]
Donor-specific lymphocyte infusion without BMT[8]
Low-dose busulfan as a single agent preparative regimen, followed by BMT.[7]

In each study, complete or near complete replacement of host hematopoiesis by donor cells was achieved essentially without toxicity or graft versus host disease

(GVHD). These studies form the basis for what the authors believe will be the first successful strategy for application of IUHCT to competitive hematologic disorders.[50]

Despite this success in the murine model, however, there are unexplained observations that suggested an additional barrier to engraftment beyond host cell competition. First, despite what appeared to be consistent delivery of donor cells, the authors observed long-term donor chimerism in only approximately one third of recipients. Second, engraftment differed significantly between strain combinations. These issues suggested immunologic barriers, either innate or adaptive, that limited engraftment. The authors therefore decided to re-examine the question of an immunologic barrier to engraftment using a modification of their previous model, i.e., intravenous injection by means of the vitelline vein rather than intra-peritoneal (IP) injection.[51,52] This technique overcomes the volume limitation of IP injection and allows delivery of much larger doses of cells. There is the additional advantage that the success of the injection can be monitored visually, removing the uncertainty of cell delivery that exists with the IP approach. By performing early tracking of donor cells and long-term assessment of donor chimerism, the authors were able to document that 100% of allogeneic and congenic recipients maintained high levels of engraftment up to 3 weeks after IUHCT. Between 3 and 5 weeks, however, 70% of allogeneic animals lost their engraftment, whereas 100% of congenic animals remained chimeric. Thus the higher cell doses and consistent delivery in this study unmasked a previously unrecognized, very clear difference in the incidence of chimerism between congenic and allogeneic donors, supporting the presence of an adaptive immune barrier to engraftment after IUHCT.[53] The authors since have confirmed the presence of an adaptive cellular and humoral alloresponse that is quantitatively higher in nonchimeric versus chimeric animals. This finding was incongruous with the authors' previous demonstration of long-term chimerism in some animals and the presence of deletional tolerance, prompting additional studies into the mechanism of this response. The authors now have demonstrated that the immune response is in reality a maternal immune response that is transferred to the neonate by means of maternal breast milk.[54] If pups are fostered on a surrogate mother who has not been exposed to donor antigen, the frequency of chimerism remains 100%. The mechanism of this transfer of adaptive immunity is under investigation. These data confirm the validity of fetal tolerance, as all of the transplanted animals are tolerant of donor and appear to maintain chimerism indefinitely. Obviously murine placentation, maternal fetal trafficking of antibodies and cells, and the time course of events after IUHCT are dramatically different in mice compared with large animal models or during human pregnancy. Nevertheless, it raises the question of whether maternal immunization is an issue in large animal models and clinical circumstances, and whether it is a limitation to engraftment after IUHCT. This is a critical question to answer before clinical application, and it only can be addressed in relevant large animal models. In addition, recent evidence supports a possible role for the innate immune system (natural killer [NK] cells) in ablating engraftment in circumstances of minimal levels of chimerism after IUHCT.[55] Further studies are needed to understand the relative importance of NK cells as a barrier to engraftment.

As mentioned previously, there has been very limited success after IUHCT in large animal models, although recently that has begun to change. Successful achievement of measurable multilineage chimerism after IUHCT with associated donor-specific tolerance for swine leukocyte antigen (SLA)-matched kidney transplants has been demonstrated in the SLA inbred pig model.[56,57] With their success in the murine model, the authors recently began translational studies in the canine model using dogs that have the canine analog of human leukocyte adhesion deficiency (canine leukocyte adhesion deficiency or CLAD). CLAD-affected dogs have a severe immunodeficiency that results in death before 6 months of age, whereas the CLAD carrier is phenotypically normal. Neither the affected, nor carrier dogs have a significant competitive defect in the HSC compartment or in any of the lineages. Therefore, the CLAD model should be representative of the degree of host cell competition expected for most target diseases. This is supported by prior experience in the canine model by Blakemore and others in which minimal levels of engraftment have been achieved after IUHCT.[31,32] In addition, the canine model has been used extensively for BMT experiments and has been validated as a preclinical model from the perspective of GVHD, the most concerning potential complication of IUHCT.[58,59] In their first study in the canine model, the authors demonstrated that low-level chimerism can be achieved by IUHCT, and that these levels of chimerism can:

Ameliorate or cure the clinical phenotype of CLAD

Result in associated donor-specific tolerance in some animals that is adequate to facilitate postnatal enhancement of chimerism to potentially therapeutic levels using the single-agent, low-dose busulfan conditioning regimen, followed by transplantation of T-cell depleted BM from the same donor.[60]

In this study, the authors saw no significant toxicity and no GVHD. They are encouraged that the results of IUHCT in the canine model appear remarkably similar to their results in the murine model, suggesting that results in the murine model can be translated to clinical application.

Clinical application of in utero hematopoietic stem cell transplantation

The early success of IUHCT in the sheep model was followed by many attempts around the world to perform IUHCT for various hematologic disorders during the late 1980s and 1990s. The international clinical experience with IUHCT has been reviewed previously. It can be summarized as discouraging with the exception of severe combined immunodeficiency (SCID), which has been treated successfully by IUHCT in several centers.[61–64] SCID, however, is a unique disorder that provides a survival and proliferative advantage for donor T-cells, and the engraftment achieved has been documented only to reconstitute the T-cell lineage (split chimerism). Thus it can be stated that IUHCT has not been clinically successful in establishing engraftment in a hematopoietically competitive recipient. As most of the anticipated target disorders such as the hemoglobinopathies, other types of immunodeficiencies, and the lysosomal storage diseases are competitively normal, methods must be developed to overcome host cell competition before further attempts at clinical application. The strategy of prenatal tolerance induction to facilitate nontoxic postnatal BMT lowers the threshold of chimerism required for clinical application of IUHCT. Methods to selectively enhance donor cell competition and thereby further enhance donor chimerism achieved by IUHCT have been and are being developed in animal models[23] and need translational application in appropriate preclinical large animal models. The authors feel that if adequate engraftment can be achieved to consistently induce donor-specific tolerance without GVHD in a preclinical model, then clinical trials of IUHCT for treating genetic disorders that can be prenatally diagnosed and treated by mixed hematopoietic chimerism, such as the hemoglobinopathies and selected immunodeficiency disorders should be initiated.

PRENATAL GENE THERAPY

Gene therapy generally can be defined as gene transfer to an individual's cells for therapeutic benefit. Methods to achieve gene transfer to mammalian cells have been available for decades, but human application of gene therapy has been limited by several obstacles, some of which may be addressed by prenatal application. The most compelling rationale for prenatal gene therapy is to prevent disease onset in circumstances where a disease has devastating manifestations before birth. In most circumstances, however, as in cellular therapy, the rational for prenatal gene therapy relates to opportunities presented for gene transfer by normal events during development. In adult life, stem cells are extremely low-frequency populations that may be difficult to access because of tissue distribution and anatomic barriers. During specific developmental periods, however, stem cell and progenitor cell populations exist at high relative frequencies, and may be accessible to gene transfer, providing a unique window of opportunity for gene transfer to all of the nascent stem cells of a tissue compartment. As in cellular transplantation, the immature immune system of the fetus may allow tolerance to immunogenic transgenes or viral products that would be rejected by the intact immune system in the postnatal patient. The lack of a fetal immune response against the viral vector and transgene makes stable, long-term transduction possible and theoretically would allow postnatal treatment with the same vector and transgene. Finally, in utero gene transfer to the extremely small fetus allows much higher vector-to-cell ratios to be delivered, a major advantage for efficiency of transduction, and in circumstances where large-scale production of vector is difficult. These advantages obviate many of the most important obstacles to postnatal gene therapy.

Methods of Gene Transfer

There are several gene transfer methods to choose from depending upon one's goals and the circumstances that apply. Nonviral DNA delivery methods including naked DNA combined with microbubble-enhanced ultrasound, the gene gun, and electroporation have been proposed as safer alternatives to viral vectors.[65–68] These methods, however, generally have been too inefficient or impractical for most in vivo applications. In contrast to nonviral methods, gene transfer by viral vectors is a relatively efficient and extremely versatile approach. Viruses are highly evolved biologic machines that efficiently penetrate hostile host cells and exploit the host's cellular machinery to facilitate their replication. Ideally, viral vectors harness the viral infection pathway but avoid the subsequent replicative expression of viral genes that causes toxicity. This traditionally is achieved by deleting some, or all, of the coding regions from the viral genome, but leaving intact those sequences that are needed for the vector function, such as elements required for the packaging of viral DNA into virus capsid, or the integration of vector DNA into host chromatin. The chosen expression cassette then is cloned into the viral backbone in place of those sequences that were deleted. The deleted genes encoding proteins involved in replication or capsid/envelope proteins are included in a separate packaging construct. The vector genome and packaging construct then are cotransfected into packaging cells to produce recombinant vector particles. Because the vector is ultimately responsible for the transfer of genes to the fetus, the choice of vector is of utmost importance in fetal gene therapy. Although a complete discussion of viral vector technology is beyond the scope of this article, a specific vector type usually is chosen based on several considerations such as tissue tropism, packaging capacity, the ability to integrate into host genomic DNA, immunogenicity, and the ability of the investigator to obtain or manufacture the vector. The primary viral vector groups and their advantages and disadvantages are shown in **Table 1**.

Table 1
Primary viral vector groups and their properties

Vector Type	Coding Material	Packaging Capacity	Tissue Tropism	Vector Genome	Advantages	Disadvantages
Retrovirus	RNA	8 kb	Only dividing cells	Integrated	Prolonged gene transfer in dividing cells	Requires cell division, oncogenesis
Lentivirus	RNA	8 kb	Broad, including stem cells	Integrated	Integrates into nondividing cells	Potential for oncogenesis
HSV-1	ds DNA	40 kb	Neural	Episomal	Large packaging capacity, strong tropism for neurons	Inflammatory response, limited tropism
AAV	ss DNA	<5 kb	Broad	Episomal >90% Integrated <10%	Noninflammatory Nonpathogenic	Small packaging capacity, complex production
Adenovirus	ds DNA	8 kb 30kb[a]	Broad	Episomal	Extremely efficient gene transfer in most tissues	Capsid-mediated potent immune response, transient expression in dividing cells

Abbreviations: AAV, adeno-associated virus; ds DNA, double-stranded DNA; HSV-1, herpes simplex virus-1; ss DNA, single stranded DNA.
[a] Helper-dependent.

Rationale for Specific Vector Application to In Utero Hematopoietic Stem Cell Transplantation

The use of a specific vector for fetal gene transfer is evolving toward newer-generation vectors that provide both relative safety and efficacy. Whereas first-generation adeno-viral vectors were highly efficient with broad tropism, they did not integrate into the host genome, and they are highly immunogenic. This resulted in short duration of expression in rapidly dividing fetal cells, and significant inflammatory responses when administered after the onset of immunocompetence.[69–72] Given these disadvantages, there are few clinical applications where adenoviral vectors would be optimal except those where only a short duration of expression is required very early in gestation. Experimental applications for adenoviral vector include any circumstance where only short-term gene expression is desirable, or when transgene expression is required within 12 to 24 hours after transduction.[73] Adeno-associated virus vectors (AAV) are single-stranded DNA viruses that are gaining in application because of their safety and low immunogenicity.[74] Although they integrate into the genome at low frequency, most AAV expression is episomal; therefore the expression is limited in rapidly dividing fetal tissues. Tropism can be influenced by viral serotype, however, and the vectors can be targeted to tissues with low turnover such as skeletal muscle, liver, and the central nervous system (CNS) to achieve relatively durable expression. Limitations of AAV are their limited packaging capacity and slow expression profile, which can take up to 2 or more weeks for peak expression of transgene. This can be a major limitation in fetal mouse models because of short gestation but less of an issue clinically. Permanent expression of transgene after IUGT in most tissues requires gene transfer to the stem cell population that generates and maintains that tissue with an integrating viral vector. Retroviral vectors were the first integrating vectors to be used. Retroviruses, however, require cell division for transduction, a major limitation for transduction of relatively quiescent stem cell populations. More recently, lentiviral vectors, including those derived from a replication-incompetent HIV, have been introduced and are highly efficient at infecting dividing and nondividing cells with low immunogenicity.[75,76] Pseudotyping the lentivirus with a specific viral envelope, such as vesicular stomatitis virus protein G (VSVG), improves lentivirus stability and helps target the transgene to specific tissues.[77,78]

Modes and Timing of Prenatal Gene Transfer

In addition to the type and titer of vector used, the developing fetus offers a multitude of variables that profoundly influence the distribution and efficiency of transduction. The primary variables relate to the mode and timing of vector administration and once again are integrally related to normal developmental anatomy and events. A prime example is the amniotic cavity. This space forms at the earliest stages of embryogenesis and is theoretically accessible for gene transfer from the developmental stage of formation of the bilaminar embryonic disk throughout the remainder of gestation. Injection of vector into the amniotic space would be predicted to have an efficiency of transduction that depends upon the ability of the vector to contact the cell, and the tropism and titer of the vector used. For each stem cell population or tissue that comes in contact with the amniotic fluid, however, there is a developmental window of accessibility for specific cell populations.[79,80] For the example of the amniotic cavity, there are three obvious explanations for major changes in stem cell accessibility over time. First, macroscopic changes of embryonic body shape, like folding and closure, may determine the period of direct contact with the amniotic fluid.[79–84] Second, differentiation of epithelium, such as formation of the periderm and epithelial stratification in skin, or placode formation and invagination, may obscure access to the expanding stem cell or progenitor cell population.[81,85–88] Third, fetal physiologic movements, like breathing and swallowing, help to extend the distribution of amniotic fluid to internal spaces exposing additional cell populations.[89,90] In this context, it is not surprising that major differences in distribution of transduction are observed with intra-amniotic injection at different developmental stages. For instance, skin stem cells that give rise to all of the skin and skin appendages can be transduced easily and efficiently between E8 and E10 (**Fig. 1**A), but formation of the periderm makes them inaccessible thereafter.[91] Similarly, neural ectoderm, which gives rise to the CNS, peripheral nervous system, neural crest derived cells, and retina only

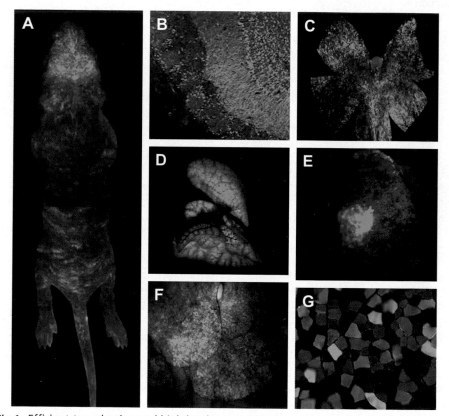

Fig. 1. Efficient transduction and high-level expression of transgene in organs after in utero gene transfer. The figure demonstrates extensive transduction of various organs after various modes of prenatal gene transfer using a GFP marker gene. (*A*) Extensive skin expression at 1 year of age after intra-amniotic gene transfer (IAGT) at E8 using lentiviral vector. (*B*) Section of hippocampal brain tissue 1 year after IAGT at E8 with lentiviral vector. Extensive Green Fluorescence Protein (GFP) expression is seen in all layers of the hippocampus. (*C*) Flat mount image of the retina showing extensive and widespread GFP expression 1 year after IAGT with lentiviral vector at E8. (*D*) Whole lung expression of GFP from lung epithelium after IAGT at E16 with adenoviral vector. (*E*) GFP expression from the lung interstitium in a localized area of the lung after direct injection of adenoviral vector into the lung bud at E15.5. (*F*) Extensive GFP expression from the liver 1 month after E10 intracardiac injection of lentiviral vector. (*G*) GFP expression from hind limb muscle groups 1 year after IAGT with lentiviral vector at E8.

can be transduced by means of the amniotic cavity before E9 in the mouse when the neural tube closes (**Fig. 1**B and **1**C).[92] Finally, murine lung epithelium can be transduced during a narrow window of gestation (E16 to 17), which corresponds to the onset of fetal breathing movements and is before significant lung fluid production (**Fig. 1**D).[89]

Although gestational age-dependent changes in the pattern of transduction with intra-amniotic gene transfer represents an extreme example, similar observations can be made throughout gestation with vector administration to different compartments or organs. What can be stated generally is that the dependence of stem cell accessibility on developmental stage is greater for all modes of administration at earlier gestational time points than later, and likewise the efficiency of stem cell transduction is, in general, greater earlier than later in development. In addition, advantages of prenatal gene transfer such as immunologic tolerance and the vector particle-to-cell number ratio are favored by gene transfer during early developmental stages. The authors therefore believe that the most impressive results of prenatal gene transfer will be seen when it is applied earlier, rather than later.

A primary determinant of the distribution of transduction is the developmental compartment that the vector is delivered into. For instance, the distribution of transduction after intra-amniotic administration (ectodermal, neuroectodermal) is dramatically different than administration of vector to the extracoelomic cavity (heart, kidney, pancreas) at the same time in gestation. Similarly, intravascular administration by means of an intracardiac injection at E10 results in a completely different distribution of transduction (hematopoietic, endothelial, osteogenic, liver, cardiac) than intra-amniotic or extracoelomic. This can be particularly relevant to targeting specific organs and providing some specificity of transduction by the presence of anatomic barriers or to targeting specific types of stem cells like the hemangioblast (capable of both blood and endothelial differentiation).

Experimental Progress in Prenatal Gene Therapy

Thus far, prenatal gene therapy has been limited to proof in principle studies in animal models; however, as in all gene therapy, significant progress has been made. Although a complete review of all of the prenatal gene transfer studies performed thus far is beyond the scope of this article, the authors will mention studies relevant to a few of the most promising target disorders.

Hemophilia disorders

The hemophilias are attractive targets for prenatal gene therapy, because they are relatively common inherited disorders that may have initial manifestations early in life or in some cases prenatally. They can be cured by a low percentage of normal secreted protein activity, and the secreted protein does not need to be regulated tightly for cure of disease or to avoid toxicity. The protein does not need to be produced by a specific cell type, avoiding issues of vector specificity. Finally, a primary limitation to postnatal administration of clotting factors or to postnatal approaches to gene therapy thus far has been the immunologic response.[93,94]

There have been several prenatal murine gene transfer studies directed toward hemophilia. The first significant study used adenoviral vector encoding factor 8 delivered by intraperitoneal injection at E15 and achieved therapeutic but transient levels of factor expression.[95] Schneider and colleagues injected either adenoviral vector or AAV encoding factor 9 by various routes (intramuscularly, IP, or intravenously) into fetal mice. The highest sustained levels were achieved with intramuscular adenoviral vector, but the levels declined over time.[96] No immunologic response was noted to either the vector or the human factor 9 transgene product. The first study using an integrating vector came from Waddington and colleagues,[97] who injected a lentiviral vector encoding human factor 9 into the vitelline vein of immunocompetent hemophilia mice and observed therapeutic levels of factor 9 expression (9% to 16%) for the full 14-month duration of the study. Blood coagulability improved in hemophilia mice, and no humoral or cellular immune response against the protein was detected. Recently, Sabatino and colleagues examined tolerance after pre- or neonatal intramuscular administration of AAV serotypes 1 and 2. Although low levels of factor 9 were achieved, the interesting finding in this study was the observation of tolerance after AAV-1 but not AAV-2 administration in the pre- or neonatal period. This was attributed to the relative delay in expression of the AAV-2 serotype, presumably to a point when immune recognition could occur.[98]

The data from these studies support the promise of prenatal gene therapy strategies for treating hemophilias. Other clotting disorders related to deficiency of secreted proteins also might be candidates for prenatal gene therapy. For example, deficiency of A disintegrin and metalloprotease with thrombospondin 13 (ADAMTS13) results in thrombotic thrombocytopenic purpura (TTP). Niiya and colleagues[99] recently demonstrated sustained correction of ADAMTS13 deficiency in the murine model after either E8 intra-amniotic or E14 intravascular injection of lentiviral vector (**Fig. 1F**).

Muscular dystrophy

Duchenne's and other forms of muscular dystrophy (MD) are also appealing target disorders for prenatal gene therapy. Although the disease does not manifest during fetal life, there may be tremendous biologic advantages afforded by developmental events such as formation of the skeletal muscle compartment by migrating myogenic progenitors, transduction of the relative high frequency of myogenic stem cells after formation of this compartment, immunologic tolerance to dystrophin and vector products, and advantages afforded by the relatively small size of the fetal muscle compartment relative to the adult.[100–102] In addition, one would anticipate that normal myofibers would have a survival advantage in this disease and that progressive replacement of the abnormal muscle fibers would occur given an adequate number of corrected myogenic stem cells.

Prenatal studies in the murine model have demonstrated that viral vectors can transduce muscle in the fetus, with the efficiency of transduction depending upon may factors. Modifications of the vectors such as specific serotypes of AAV or the origin or pseudotype of lentiviral vectors may effect tropism of the vector for muscle fibers or myogenic progenitors. Timing and mode of administration can have major influence on the distribution and efficacy of muscle transduction. Intramuscular administration provides the highest level of expression in the injected muscle but only in a limited area, and achieving correction of all effected muscle groups would require multiple injections.[96,103,104] Systemic administration by means of the peritoneal or intravascular routes at E14 to 15 has shown variable efficacy, but high dose intravenous administration appears promising, with relatively high-0level transduction of both skeletal and cardiac muscle groups, particularly with favorable serotype AAV vectors. A less clinically applicable but highly efficient method of transduction of the muscle compartment is very early intra-amniotic gene transfer with lentiviral vector at a time before completion of gastrulation. At this time, myogenic precursors line the primitive streak and can be accessed before its closure with remarkable levels of ultimate gene expression in the caudad muscle compartments (**Fig. 1G**). Of course, one of the limitations in any gene therapy strategy for the treatment of MD is the size of the dystrophin molecule, which exceeds the packaging capacity of any of the vectors discussed. Minidystrophin molecules have been engineered that appear to at least approximate dystrophin function and can be packaged easily into a lentiviral vector and even into an AAV vector. The efficacy of these molecules to fully correct severe MD has not been tested fully, however. Recently, full-length dystrophin was packaged in a fully deleted adenoviral vector and tested by prenatal intramuscular injection in the dystrophin deficient mouse model. Unfortunately, levels of gene transfer were not high enough to fully correct the dystrophic muscle.[105] Much more work needs to be done to fully explore the potential of prenatal gene therapy for MD.

Central nervous system disorders

One of the most compelling rationales for prenatal gene therapy applies to the lysosomal stage diseases where deposition of substrate in the CNS and associated neurologic damage can occur before birth. The results of postnatal BMT in these disorders have been disappointing because of the limited ability of donor cells to cross the blood–brain barrier, suggesting that direct treatment of the CNS will be necessary to address the CNS disease. Although there was early speculation that systemically administered vector in the fetus could cross the immature blood–brain barrier and achieve efficient CNS transduction, that has not proven to be the case.[106] More direct strategies such as intraventricular or intraparenchymal injections have been much more promising. Specifically recent studies by Wolfe and colleagues demonstrated that intraventricular injection of AAV-1 in fetal mucopolysaccharidosis type 8 mice resulted in efficient transduction of both CNS and spinal cord and complete reversal of pathology in all areas of the brain for at least 1 year.[107] The authors recently observed very impressive transduction of CNS progenitors and ultimately parenchyma after early intra-amniotic gene transfer before closure of the neural canal using lentiviral vectors (**Fig. 1**B). This level of gene transfer would provide correction of many CNS disorders, although it would require very early prenatal diagnosis, well before current capabilities.

Cystic fibrosis and other lung disorders

The lung has proven to be one of the more challenging organs to treat by either prenatal or postnatal gene therapy strategies. Prenatal strategies include intratracheal injection with or without simultaneous tracheal occlusion, direct intraparenchymal injection, and intra-amniotic injection. The least invasive and most frequently attempted is intra-amniotic injection. Although there were early studies suggesting efficacy of this approach despite low levels of pulmonary transduction,[108] subsequent studies have not replicated that success.[109,110] As discussed previously, the window for gene transfer to the pulmonary epithelium with this approach is limited to the period immediately after onset of fetal breathing movements in mice (around E16) and diminishes thereafter as production of lung liquid creates a net egress of fluid out of the lung. At that time, near complete distribution of vector can be achieved throughout the developing airways, and with vectors such as adenovirus (**Fig. 1**D) and specific serotypes of AAV, with high tropism for pulmonary epithelium, extensive gene transfer can be achieved. Adenoviral use is limited to the preimmune period because of inflammatory response.[70–72] Unfortunately, integrating viruses demonstrate much less efficient transduction, and expression thus far with all vectors has been transient. Treatment of cystic fibrosis likely would require transduction of the stem cell compartment of the lung with an integrating vector, and that has not been demonstrated. In addition, the window for efficient intra-amniotic gene transfer to lung has not been defined in other species or people, and clinical application may require concomitant tracheal occlusion for practical or technical reasons.[70–72,111,112]

The direct approach of intraparenchymal injection has demonstrated success proportionate to the efficiency of the vector used, but gene expression is limited to a small area of the lung (**Fig. 1**E), and has also been transient.[113,114] This technique may be very valuable, however, in experimental applications examining the effects of localized gene expression on development or disease biology.[73]

Adverse Effects and Safety Concerns

Before in utero gene therapy can be applied to people, several safety concerns must be addressed. Although the risks of postnatal gene therapy have been recognized and extensively discussed, there are specific risks that may be higher for the fetus than the postnatal subject. The most concerning of these are insertional mutagenesis, disruption of normal organ development, and germline transmission.[115]

Insertional mutagenesis is a major concern with integrating viral vectors and is the subject of intense investigation. The clinical observation of four cases of T-cell leukemia, diagnosed 31 to 68 months after retroviral-mediated gene therapy for X-linked SCID (SCID-XI) led to a temporary halt of gene therapy trials using retroviral vector. Lymphocyte analysis revealed that insertional mutagenesis had occurred in all four of the cases.[116,117] In the only study documenting oncogenesis after prenatal gene transfer, Themis and colleagues[118] reported a high incidence of postnatal liver tumors in mice after prenatal injection with an early form of third-generation equine infectious anemia virus (EAIV) vectors with self-inactivating (SIN) configuration, but not when using a similar vector with an HIV backbone. It remains unclear whether insertional mutagenesis led to tumor formation, but it demonstrates that the fetus may be particularly sensitive to certain vectors.

The effects of prenatal gene transfer on organ development need to be considered with any prenatal gene transfer strategy. Certainly strategies involving expression of growth factors, transcription factors, or other regulatory molecules have significant potential to alter normal organ development, particularly early in gestation. A dramatic example is the authors' recent finding that interstitial expression of fibroblast growth factor 10 in the developing rat lung results in formation of cystic adenomatous malformations.[73] Also, direct toxicity of either the virus or inappropriately regulated transgene would have great potential to impact organ growth.

Germline transmission is a safety concern as well as a bioethical issue. The goal of in utero gene therapy is to modify somatic cells, but undesired gene transfer to germline cells is possible. In the human fetus, the primordial germ cells are compartmentalized in the gonads by 7 weeks gestation.[119] The germline should be accessible only through the vascular system, so targeted gene therapy that is administered after this time period should not affect the germline. Several groups have assessed germline transmission directly after in utero gene transfer. Tran and colleagues[120] performed intraperitoneal injections of retroviral vector into fetal sheep and examined the germ cells by PCR and breeding experiments. Gene transfer to the germline was not detected. Lee and colleagues[121] subsequently investigated germ cell transfer after intraperitoneal, intrapulmonary, and intracardiac administration of HIV-1 derived lentiviral pseudotyped VSV-G vectors in fetal rhesus monkeys. At early postnatal time points, there was no sign of transgene in the germ cells of those monkeys that received intrapulmonary or intracardiac injections. The intraperitoneal approach, however, resulted in gene transfer to a subpopulation of female gonadal cells, but this was not detected in male gonads. Porada and colleagues also investigated germ cell transmission after intraperitoneal retroviral gene transfer in fatal sheep. Breeding studies were negative, but PCR on the purified sperm from injected rams and immunohistochemistry of sectioned testes showed low-level transduction of germ cells.[122] The same group recently determined that germ cell transduction varied depending on the gestational age of the injected fetus. Later gestational vector administration may minimize the risk of germline transmission.[123] These studies suggest that the frequency of germline transduction is low and related to gestational age and mode of vector administration. The question is what level of germline transduction, if any, would be acceptable?

Future Challenges

Although great progress has been made, there are many remaining challenges for prenatal cellular and gene therapy. Challenges for IUHCT primarily are related to overcoming the competitive barriers to engraftment in the fetus, and better defining the innate and adaptive immune limitations to engraftment in large animals and people. Although the strategy of prenatal tolerance induction for facilitation of postnatal BMT is nearing clinical application, a single-step treatment consisting of IUHCT with achievement of therapeutic levels of engraftment would be ideal. In the author's opinion, it is unlikely that high levels of engraftment can be achieved in the fetus without the development of a highly specific, nontoxic method for fetal myeloablation.

Fetal gene therapy has even greater potential to prevent the onset of inherited genetic diseases, but it is still in the early experimental stage. Proof in principle for fetal gene therapy for many disorders already has been demonstrated in rodent and large animal models. Safety concerns involving the risk of insertional mutagenesis, the effect on organ development, and the importance of low-level germ cell transmission need to be investigated extensively in appropriate preclinical animal models before application in people. The ethics of fetal gene therapy and its potential to alter the human genome also need to be considered. Although greater tissue specificity and safety likely can be accomplished by using tissue specific promoters, or regulated transgene expression, safer gene transfer technologies will need to be developed to alleviate these concerns.

REFERENCES

1. Weissman IL, Shizuru JA. The origins of the identification and isolation of hematopoietic stem cells, and their capability to induce donor-specific transplantation tolerance and treat autoimmune diseases. Blood 2008;112:3543–53.
2. Kamm FM. Ethical issues in using and not using embryonic stem cells. Stem Cell Rev 2005;1:325–30.
3. Flake AW, Zanjani ED. In utero hematopoietic stem cell transplantation: Ontogenic opportunities and biologic barriers. Blood 1999;94:2179–91.
4. Billingham R, Brent L, Medawar PB. Actively acquired tolerance of foreign cells. Nature 1953;172:603–7.
5. Takahama Y. Journey through the thymus: stromal guides for T-cell development and selection. Nat Rev Immunol 2006;6:127–35.
6. Palmer E. Negative selection–clearing out the bad apples from the T-cell repertoire. Nat Rev Immunol 2003;3:383–91.
7. Ashizuka S, Peranteau WH, Hayashi S, et al. Busulfan-conditioned bone marrow transplantation results in high-level allogeneic chimerism in mice made tolerant by in utero hematopoietic cell transplantation. Exp Hematol 2006;34:359–68.
8. Hayashi S, Peranteau WH, Shaaban AF, et al. Complete allogeneic hematopoietic chimerism achieved by a combined strategy of in utero hematopoietic stem cell transplantation and postnatal donor lymphocyte infusion. Blood 2002;100:804–12.

9. Peranteau WF, Hayashi S, Hsieh M, et al. High-level allogeneic chimerism achieved by prenatal tolerance induction and postnatal nonmyeloablative bone marrow transplantation. Blood 2002;100:2225–34.

10. Anderson D, Billingham R, Lampkin G, et al. The use of skin grafting to distinguish between monozygotic and dizygotic twins in cattle. Heredity 1951;5:379–97.

11. Cragle R, Stone W. Preliminary results of kidney grafts between cattle chimeric twins. Transplantation 1967;5:328–35.

12. Owen RD. Immunogenetic consequences of vascular anastomoses between bovine cattle twins. Science 1945;102:400–1.

13. Gill T. Chimerism in humans. Transplant Proc 1977;9:1423–31.

14. Hansen HE, Niebuhr E, Lomas C. Chimeric twins. T.S. and M.R. reexamined. Hum Hered 1984;34:127–30.

15. Thomsen M, Hansen HE, Dickmeiss E. MLC and CML studies in the family of a pair of HLA haploidentical chimeric twins. Scand J Immunol 1977;6:523–8.

16. Picus J, Aldrich WR, Letvin NL. A naturally occurring bone-marrow-chimeric primate. I. Integrity of its immune system. Transplantation 1985;39:297–303.

17. Picus J, Holley K, Aldrich WR, et al. A naturally occurring bone marrow-chimeric primate. II. Environment dictates restriction on cytolytic T lymphocyte-target cell interactions. J Exp Med 1985;162:2035–52.

18. Christensen JL, Wright DE, Wagers AJ, et al. Circulation and chemotaxis of fetal hematopoietic stem cells. PLoS Biol 2004;2:0368–77.

19. Medvinsky A, Dzierzak E. Definitive hematopoiesis is autonomously initiated by the AGM region. Cell 1996;86:897–906.

20. Harrison DE, Zhong RK, Jordan CT, et al. Relative to adult marrow, fetal liver repopulates nearly five times more effectively long-term than short-term. Exp Hematol 1997;25:293–7.

21. Rebel VI, Miller CL, Eaves CJ, et al. The repopulating potential of fetal liver hematopoietic stem cells in mice exceeds that of their liver adult bone marrow counterparts. Blood 1996;87:3500–7.

22. Shaaban AF, Kim HB, Milner R, et al. A kinetic model for homing and migration of prenatally transplanted marrow. Blood 1999;94:3251–7.

23. Peranteau WH, Endo M, Adibe OO, et al. CD26 inhibition enhances allogeneic donor-cell homing and engraftment after in utero hematopoietic-cell transplantation. Blood 2006;108:4268–74.

24. Fleischman R, Mintz B. Prevention of genetic anemias in mice by microinjection of normal hematopoietic cells into the fetal placenta. Proc Natl Acad Sci U S A 1979;76:5736–40.

25. Mintz B, Anthony K, Litwin S. Monoclonal derivation of mouse myeloid and lymphoid lineages from totipotent hematopoietic stem cells experimentally engrafted in fetal hosts. Proc Natl Acad Sci U S A 1984;81:7835–9.

26. Blazar BR, Taylor PA, Vallera DA. Adult bone marrow-derived pluripotent hematopoietic stem cells are engraftable when transferred in utero into moderately anemic fetal recipients. Blood 1995;85:833–41.

27. Blazar BR, Taylor PA, Vallera DA. In utero transfer of adult bone marrow cells into recipients with severe combined immunodeficiency disorder yields lymphoid progeny with T- and B-cell functional capabilities. Blood 1995;86:4353–66.

28. Waldschmidt TJ, Panoskaltsis-Mortari A, McElmurry RT, et al. Abnormal T cell-dependent B-cell responses in SCID mice receiving allogeneic bone marrow in utero. Severe combined immune deficiency. Blood 2002;100:4557–64.

29. Lovell KL, Kraemer SA, Leipprandt JR, et al. In utero hematopoietic stem cell transplantation: a caprine model for prenatal therapy in inherited metabolic diseases. Fetal Diagn Ther 2001;16:13–7.

30. Pearce R, Kiehm D, Armstrong D, et al. Induction of hematopoietic chimerism in the caprine fetus by intraperitoneal injection of fetal liver cells. Experientia 1989;45:307–8.

31. Blakemore K, Hattenburg C, Stetten G, et al. In utero hematopoietic stem cell transplantation with haploidentical donor adult bone marrow in a canine model. Am J Obstet Gynecol 2004;190:960–73.

32. Omori F, Lutzko C, Abrams-Ogg A, et al. Adoptive transfer of genetically modified human hematopoietic stem cells into preimmune canine fetuses. Exp Hematol 1999;27:242–9.

33. Harrison MR, Slotnick RN, Crombleholme TM, et al. In utero transplantation of fetal liver haemopoietic stem cells in monkeys. Lancet 1989;2:1425–7.

34. Shields LE, Gaur L, Delio P, et al. The use of CD 34(+) mobilized peripheral blood as a donor cell source does not improve chimerism after in utero hematopoietic stem cell transplantation in non-human primates. J Med Primatol 2005;34:201–8.

35. Shields LE, Gaur LK, Gough M, et al. In utero hematopoietic stem cell transplantation in nonhuman primates: the role of T cells. Stem Cells 2003;21:304–13.

36. Cowan MJ, Tarantal AF, Capper J, et al. Long-term engraftment following in utero T cell-depleted parental marrow transplantation into fetal rhesus monkeys. Bone Marrow Transplant 1996;17:1157–65.

37. Carrier E, Gilpin E, Lee TH, et al. Microchimerism does not induce tolerance after in utero transplantation and may lead to the development of alloreactivity. J Lab Clin Med 2000;136:224–35.

38. Carrier E, Lee TH, Busch MP, et al. Induction of tolerance in nondefective mice after in utero transplantation of major histocompatibility complex-mismatched fetal hematopoietic stem cells. Blood 1995;86:4681–90.

39. Howson-Jan K, Matloub YH, Vallera DA, et al. In utero engraftment of fully H-2-incompatible versus congenic adult bone marrow transferred into nonanemic or anemic murine fetal recipients. Transplantation 1993;56:709–16.

40. Kim HB, Shaaban AF, Yang EY, et al. Microchimerism and tolerance after in utero bone marrow transplantation in mice. J Surg Res 1998;77:1–5.

41. Flake AW, Harrison MR, Adzick NS, et al. Transplantation of fetal hematopoietic stem cells in utero: the creation of hematopoietic chimeras. Science 1986;233:776–8.

42. Srour EF, Zanjani ED, Brandt JE, et al. Sustained human hematopoiesis in sheep transplanted in utero during early gestation with fractionated adult human bone marrow cells. Blood 1992;79:1404–12.

43. Zanjani ED, Flake AW, Rice H, et al. Long-term repopulating ability of xenogeneic transplanted human fetal liver hematopoietic stem cells in sheep. J Clin Invest 1994;93:1051–5.

44. Zanjani ED, Pallavicini MG, Flake AW, et al. Engraftment and long-term expression of human fetal hemopoietic stem cells in sheep following transplantation in utero. J Clin Invest 1992;89:1178–88.

45. Narayan AD, Chase JL, Lewis RL, et al. Human embryonic stem cell-derived hematopoietic cells are capable of engrafting primary as well as secondary fetal sheep recipients. Blood 2006;107:2180–3.

46. Kim HB, Shaaban AF, Milner R, et al. In utero bone marrow transplantation induces tolerance by a combination of clonal deletion and anergy. J Pediatr Surg 1999;34:726–30.

47. Pallavicini MG, Flake AW, Madden D, et al. Hemopoietic chimerism in rodents transplanted in utero with fetal human hemopoietic cells. Transplant Proc 1992;24:542–3.

48. Hayashi S, Abdulmalik O, Peranteau WH, et al. Mixed chimerism following in utero hematopoietic stem cell transplantation in murine models of hemoglobinopathy. Exp Hematol 2003;31:176–84.

49. Hayashi S, Hsieh M, Peranteau WH, et al. Complete allogeneic hematopoietic chimerism achieved by in utero hematopoietic cell transplantation and cotransplantation of LLME-treated, MHC-sensitized donor lymphocytes. Exp Hematol 2004;32:290–9.

50. Merianos DJ, Tiblad E, Laje P, et al. Breast milk transmission of maternal alloantibodies activates a prenatal immune response that limits allogeneic engraftment after in utero hematopoietic stem cell transplantation in the murine model. Blood 2008;112(11):362a.

51. Waddington SN, Mitrophanous KA, Ellard FM, et al. Long-term transgene expression by administration of a lentivirus-based vector to the fetal circulation of immuno-competent mice. Gene Ther 2003;10:1234–40.

52. Javazon EH, Merchant AM, Danzer E, et al. Reconstitution of hematopoiesis following intrauterine transplantation of stem cells. Methods Mol Med 2005; 105:81–94.

53. Peranteau WH, Endo M, Adibe OO, et al. Evidence for an immune barrier after in utero hematopoietic-cell transplantation. Blood 2007;109:1331–3.

54. Merianos D, Heaton T, Flake AW. In utero hematopoietic stem cell transplantation: progress toward clinical application. Biol Blood Marrow Transplant 2008; 14:729–40.

55. Durkin ET, Jones KA, Rajesh D, et al. Early chimerism threshold predicts sustained engraftment and NK-cell tolerance in prenatal allogeneic chimeras. Blood 2008;112:5245–53.

56. Lee PW, Cina RA, Randolph MA, et al. Stable multilineage chimerism across full MHC barriers without graft-versus-host disease following in utero bone marrow transplantation in pigs. Exp Hematol 2005;33:371–9.

57. Lee PW, Cina RA, Randolph MA, et al. In utero bone marrow transplantation induces kidney allograft tolerance across a full major histocompatibility complex barrier in Swine. Transplantation 2005;79:1084–90.

58. Storb R, Deeg HJ, Raff R, et al. Prevention of graft-versus-host disease. Studies in a canine model. Ann N Y Acad Sci 1995;770:149–64.

59. Storb R, Thomas ED. Graft-versus-host disease in dog and man: the Seattle experience. Immunol Rev 1985;88:215–38.

60. Peranteau WH, Heaton TE, Gu Y-C, et al. Haploidentical in utero hematopoietic cell transplantation improves phenotype and can induce tolerance for postnatal same donor transplants in the canine leukocyte adhesion deficiency model. Biology of Blood and Bone Marrow Transplantation 2009;15:293–305.

61. Flake A, Roncarolo M-G, Puck J, et al. Treatment of X-linked severe combined immunodeficiency by in utero transplantation of paternal bone marrow. N Engl J Med 1996;335:1806–10.

62. Touraine JL, Raudrant D, Laplace S. Transplantation of hemopoietic cells from the fetal liver to treat patients with congenital diseases postnatally or prenatally. Transplant Proc 1997;29:712–3.

63. Wengler G, Lanfranchi A, Frusca T, et al. In-utero transplantation of parental CD34 haematopoietic progenitor cells in a patient with X-linked severe combined immunodeficiency (SCIDX1). Lancet 1996;348:1484–7.

64. Westgren M, Ringden O, Bartmann P, et al. Prenatal T-cell reconstitution after in utero transplantation with fetal liver cells in a patient with X-linked severe combined immunodeficiency. Am J Obstet Gynecol 2002;187:475–82.

65. Endoh M, Koibuchi N, Sato M, et al. Fetal gene transfer by intrauterine injection with microbubble-enhanced ultrasound. Mol Ther 2002;5:501–8.

66. Sato M, Tanigawa M, Kikuchi N. Nonviral gene transfer to surface skin of mid-gestational murine embryos by intraamniotic injection and subsequent electro-poration. Mol Reprod Dev 2004;69:268–77.

67. Yoshizawa J, Li XK, Fujino M, et al. Successful in utero gene transfer using a gene gun in midgestational mouse fetuses. J Pediatr Surg 2004;39:81–4.

68. Gubbels SP, Woessner DW, Mitchell JC, et al. Functional auditory hair cells produced in the mammalian cochlea by in utero gene transfer. Nature 2008;455:537–41.

69. David A, Cook T, Waddington S, et al. Ultrasound-guided percutaneous delivery of adenoviral vectors encoding the beta-galactosidase and human factor IX genes to early gestation fetal sheep in utero. Hum Gene Ther 2003;14:353–64.

70. Sylvester KG, Yang EY, Cass DL, et al. Fetoscopic gene therapy for congenital lung disease. J Pediatr Surg 1997;32:964–9.

71. Yang EY, Cass DL, Sylvester KG, et al. BAPS Prize–1997. Fetal gene therapy: efficacy, toxicity, and immunologic effects of early gestation recombinant adeno-virus. British association of paediatric surgeons. J Pediatr Surg 1999;34:235–41.

72. Iwamoto HS, Trapnell BC, McConnell CJ, et al. Pulmonary inflammation associ-ated with repeated, prenatal exposure to an E1, E3-deleted adenoviral vector in sheep. Gene Ther 1999;6:98–106.

73. Gonzaga S, Henriques-Coelho T, Davey M, et al. Cystic adenomatoid malforma-tions are induced by localized FGF10 overexpression in fetal rat lung. Am J Respir Cell Mol Biol 2008;39:346–55.

74. Mueller C, Flotte TR. Clinical gene therapy using recombinant adeno-associated virus vectors. Gene Ther 2008;15:858–63.

75. Olsen JC. Gene transfer vectors derived from equine infectious anemia virus. Gene Ther 1998;5:1481–7.

76. Zufferey R, Nagy D, Mandel RJ, et al. Multiply attenuated lentiviral vector achieves efficient gene delivery in vivo. Nat Biotechnol 1997;15:871–5.

77. Sena-Esteves M, Tebbets JC, Steffens S, et al. Optimized large-scale production of high titer lentivirus vector pseudotypes. J Virol Methods 2004;122:131–9.

78. Steffens S, Tebbets J, Kramm CM, et al. Transduction of human glial and neuronal tumor cells with different lentivirus vector pseudotypes. J Neurooncol 2004;70:281–8.

79. Findlater GS, McDougall RD, Kaufman MH. Eyelid development, fusion and subsequent reopening in the mouse. J Anat 1993;183(Pt 1):121–9.

80. Kaufman MH, Bard J. The anatomical basis of mouse development. San Diego (CA): Academic Press; 1999.

81. Baker CV, Bronner-Fraser M. Vertebrate cranial placodes I. Embryonic induction. Dev Biol 2001;232:1–61.

82. Blackburn CC, Manley NR. Developing a new paradigm for thymus organogen-esis. Nat Rev Immunol 2004;4:278–89.

83. Graw J. The genetic and molecular basis of congenital eye defects. Nat Rev Genet 2003;4:876–88.

84. Pispa J, Thesleff I. Mechanisms of ectodermal organogenesis. Dev Biol 2003; 262:195–205.

85. Hardman MJ, Sisi P, Banbury DN, et al. Patterned acquisition of skin barrier function during development. Development 1998;125:1541–52.

86. M'Boneko V, Merker HJ. Development and morphology of the periderm of mouse embryos (days 9–12 of gestation). Acta Anat (Basel) 1988;133:325–36.

87. Byrne C, Hardman M, Nield K. Covering the limb—formation of the integument. J Anat 2003;202:113–23.

88. Kaufman MH. The atlas of mouse development. San Diego (CA): Academic Press; 1992.

89. Buckley SM, Waddington SN, Jezzard S, et al. Factors influencing adenovirus-mediated airway transduction in fetal mice. Mol Ther 2005;12:484–92.

90. Holzinger A, Trapnell BC, Weaver TE, et al. Intraamniotic administration of an adenoviral vector for gene transfer to fetal sheep and mouse tissues. Pediatr Res 1995;38:844–50.

91. Endo M, Zoltick PW, Peranteau WH, et al. Efficient in vivo targeting of epidermal stem cells by early gestational intraamniotic injection of lentiviral vector driven by the keratin 5 promoter. Mol Ther 2008;16:131–7.

92. Endo M, Zoltick PW, Chung DC, et al. Gene transfer to ocular stem cells by early gestational intraamniotic injection of lentiviral vector. Mol Ther 2007;15:579–87.

93. Hasbrouck NC, High KA. AAV-mediated gene transfer for the treatment of hemophilia B: problems and prospects. Gene Ther 2008;15:870–5.

94. Zaiss AK, Muruve DA. Immunity to adeno-associated virus vectors in animals and humans: a continued challenge. Gene Ther 2008;15:808–16.

95. Lipshutz GS, Sarkar R, Flebbe-Rehwaldt L, et al. Short-term correction of factor VIII deficiency in a murine model of hemophilia A after delivery of adenovirus murine factor VIII in utero. Proc Natl Acad Sci U S A 1999;96:13324–9.

96. Schneider H, Muhle C, Marie Douar A, et al. Sustained delivery of therapeutic concentrations of human clotting factor IX—a comparison of adenoviral and AAV vectors administered in utero. J Gene Med 2002;4:46–53.

97. Waddington SN, Nivsarkar MS, Mistry AR, et al. Permanent phenotypic correction of hemophilia B in immunocompetent mice by prenatal gene therapy. Blood 2004;104:2714–21.

98. Sabatino DE, Mackenzie TC, Peranteau W, et al. Persistent expression of hF.IX After tolerance induction by in utero or neonatal administration of AAV-1-F.IX in hemophilia B mice. Mol Ther 2007;15:1677–85.

99. Niiya M, Endo M, Shang D, et al. Correction of ADAMTS13 Deficiency by in Utero gene transfer of lentiviral vector encoding ADAMTS13 genes. Mol Ther 2009;17: 34–41.

100. Bouchard S, MacKenzie TC, Radu AP, et al. Long-term transgene expression in cardiac and skeletal muscle following fetal administration of adenoviral or adeno-associated viral vectors in mice. J Gene Med 2003;5:941–50.

101. Mackenzie TC, Kobinger GP, Kootstra NA, et al. Efficient transduction of liver and muscle after in utero injection of lentiviral vectors with different pseudotypes. Mol Ther 2002;6:349–58.

102. MacKenzie TC, Kobinger GP, Louboutin JP, et al. Transduction of satellite cells after prenatal intramuscular administration of lentiviral vectors. J Gene Med 2005;7:50–8.

103. Weisz B, David AL, Gregory LG, et al. Targeting the respiratory muscles of fetal sheep for prenatal gene therapy for Duchenne muscular dystrophy. Am J Obstet Gynecol 2005;193:1105–9.

104. Gregory LG, Waddington SN, Holder MV, et al. Highly efficient EIAV-mediated in utero gene transfer and expression in the major muscle groups affected by Duchenne muscular dystrophy. Gene Ther 2004;11:1117–25.

105. Reay DP, Bilbao R, Koppanati BM, et al. Full-length dystrophin gene transfer to the mdx mouse in utero. Gene Ther 2008;15:531–6.
106. Westlake VJ, Jolly RD, Jones BR, et al. Hematopoietic cell transplantation in fetal lambs with ceroid-lipofuscinosis. Am J Med Genet 1995;57:365–8.
107. Karolewski BA, Wolfe JH. Genetic correction of the fetal brain increases the lifespan of mice with the severe multisystemic disease mucopolysaccharidosis type VII. Mol Ther 2006;14:14–24.
108. Larson JE, Morrow SL, Happel L, et al. Reversal of cystic fibrosis phenotype in mice by gene therapy in utero. Lancet 1997;349:619–20.
109. Buckley SM, Waddington SN, Jezzard S, et al. Intra-amniotic delivery of CFTR-expressing adenovirus does not reverse cystic fibrosis phenotype in inbred CFTR-knockout mice. Mol Ther 2008;16:819–24.
110. Davies LA, Varathalingam A, Painter H, et al. Adenovirus-mediated in utero expression of CFTR does not improve survival of CFTR knockout mice. Mol Ther 2008;16:812–8.
111. David AL, Weisz B, Gregory L, et al. Ultrasound-guided injection and occlusion of the trachea in fetal sheep. Ultrasound Obstet Gynecol 2006;28:82–8.
112. Luton D, Oudrhiri N, de Lagausie P, et al. Gene transfection into fetal sheep airways in utero using guanidinium-cholesterol cationic lipids. J Gene Med 2004;6:328.
113. Henriques-Coelho T, Gonzaga S, Endo M, et al. Targeted Gene Transfer to Fetal Rat Lung Interstitium by Ultrasound-guided Intrapulmonary Injection. Mol Ther 2007;15:340–7.
114. Tarantal AF, McDonald RJ, Jimenez DF, et al. Intrapulmonary and intramyocardial gene transfer in rhesus monkeys (Macaca mulatta): safety and efficiency of HIV-1-derived lentiviral vectors for fetal gene delivery. Mol Ther 2005;12:87–98.
115. Prenatal gene tranfer. scientific, medical, and ethical issues: a report of the recombinant DNA advisory committee. Hum Gene Ther 2000;11:1211–29.
116. Hacein-Bey-Abina S, Garrigue A, Wang GP, et al. Insertional oncogenesis in 4 patients after retrovirus-mediated gene therapy of SCID-X1. J Clin Invest 2008;118:3132–42.
117. Uren AG, Kool J, Berns A, et al. Retroviral insertional mutagenesis: past, present and future. Oncogene 2005;24:7656–72.
118. Themis M, Waddington SN, Schmidt M, et al. Oncogenesis following delivery of a nonprimate lentiviral gene therapy vector to fetal and neonatal mice. Mol Ther 2005;12:763–71.
119. David AL, Peebles D. Gene therapy for the fetus: is there a future? Best Pract Res Clin Obstet Gynaecol 2008;22:203–18.
120. Tran ND, Porada CD, Zhao Y, et al. In utero transfer and expression of exogenous genes in sheep. Exp Hematol 2000;28:17–30.
121. Lee CC, Jimenez DF, Kohn DB, et al. Fetal gene transfer using lentiviral vectors and the potential for germ cell transduction in rhesus monkeys (Macaca mulatta). Hum Gene Ther 2005;16:417–25.
122. Porada CD, Park PJ, Tellez J, et al. Male germ-line cells are at risk following direct-injection retroviral-mediated gene transfer in utero. Mol Ther 2005;12:754–62.
123. Park PJ, Colletti E, Ozturk F, et al. Factors determining the risk of inadvertent retroviral transduction of male germ cells following in Utero gene transfer in sheep. Hum Gene Ther 2009;20:201–15.

Fetal Tissue Engineering

Christopher G.B. Turner, MD[a], Dario O. Fauza, MD[a,b,*]

KEYWORDS

- Fetal tissue engineering • Tissue engineering
- Structural anomalies • Congenital anomalies
- Fetal cells • Fetal stem cells

The fetus is, perhaps, the ultimate tissue-engineering subject, both as a donor and a host. The many exclusive characteristics of fetal cells, in conjunction with the developmental and long-term impacts of engineered graft implantations into a fetus, add new dimensions to tissue engineering, which expand its reach to realms unequaled by any other age group.

Attempts at harnessing the prospective benefits of the therapeutic use of fetal cells or tissues date many decades before the modern era of transplantation. The first reported transplantation of human fetal tissue took place in 1922, when a fetal adrenal graft was transplanted into a patient who had Addison's disease.[1] This and a few other similar efforts that followed in the years thereafter, involving different fetal cells and tissues, failed. It was only in the last three decades that fetal tissue transplantation in people has started to lead to favorable outcomes, yet by and large anecdotally.

Fetal cells or tissues also have been used as helpful investigational tools since the 1930s. Cultures of different fetal cell lines, and commercial preparations of human fetal tissue, have been used routinely in viral isolation/culture and to produce vaccines, for example, among other applications. Companies long have employed fetal cells and extraembryonic structures such as placenta, amnion, and the umbilical cord to screen new pharmaceutical, biotechnology, and even cosmetic products for toxicity, teratogenicity, and carcinogenicity. Fetal cell and tissue banks have been operating in the United States and abroad for decades as research sources.

Although such a large body of data has come out of research involving fetal cells or tissues, perhaps surprisingly, comparatively little has been done on the true engineering of fetal tissue, through culture and placement of fetal cells into matrices or membranes, or through other in vitro manipulations before implantation. Human trials of open-systems tissue engineering (ie, constructs consisting of cells seeded onto

a Department of Surgery, Children's Hospital Boston, 300 Longwood Avenue, Fegan 3, Boston, MA 02115, USA
b Harvard Medical School, Department of Surgery, 300 Longwood Avenue, Fegan 3, Boston, MA 02115, USA
* Corresponding author. Children's Hospital Boston, 300 Longwood Avenue, Fegan 3, Boston, MA 02115.
E-mail address: dario.fauza@childrens.harvard.edu (D.O. Fauza).

Clin Perinatol 36 (2009) 473–488
doi:10.1016/j.clp.2009.03.005   perinatology.theclinics.com
0095-5108/09/$ – see front matter © 2009 Elsevier Inc. All rights reserved.

different scaffolds) involving fetal cells have yet to be performed, and a relatively small number of animal experiments have been reported. The use of fetal cells in experimental engineered constructs first was reported by Vacanti and colleagues[2] in the late 1980s, as part of the introductory study on selective cell transplantation using bioabsorbable, synthetic polymers as matrices. This and a subsequent similar experiment from the same group, all using rodents, did not include structural replacement or functional data.[3]

Fetal constructs as a means of structural and functional replacement first were reported experimentally in 1997 in large animal models.[4,5] Those studies introduced a novel therapeutic concept in perinatal surgery, involving the (preferably minimally invasive) procurement of fetal cells, which are used to engineer tissue in vitro in parallel to the remainder of gestation, so that an infant, or a fetus, with a prenatally diagnosed birth defect could benefit from having autologous, expanded tissue readily available for surgical implantation in the perinatal period. This concept has been known as fetal tissue engineering.

This article offers an outlook of the current status of the still immature field of fetal tissue engineering, along with other germane information.

BIOLOGIC CONSIDERATIONS

Perennial complications of tissue engineering include vascularization and growth limitations, differentiation and function restraints, incorporation barriers, immunologic rejection (in nonautologous applications), and cell/tissue delivery hurdles. Most of those problems can be managed better, if not totally prevented, when fetal cells are used. Because of their biologic properties, both in vitro and in vivo, fetal cells are an excellent raw material for tissue engineering.

Fetal Cells

Compared with postnatal cells, most fetal cells multiply significantly more rapidly and more often in culture. Depending on the cell line considered, however, this is more or less pronounced, or, in a few cases, not evident at all. Fetal cells can survive at lower oxygen tensions than those tolerated by mature cells and are therefore more resistant to hypoxia during in vitro manipulations. They also typically lack long extensions and strong intercellular adhesions. Probably because of all those characteristics, fetal cells tend to display better survival after refrigeration and cryopreservation protocols when compared with adult cells.

Because they are very plastic in their differentiation potential, fetal cells respond better than more mature cells to environmental cues. Data from fetal myoblasts, osteoblasts, and mesenchymal amniocytes suggest that focused manipulations in culture or in a bioreactor can be designed so as to steer fetal cells into producing enhanced constructs. Also, at least in part because of their proliferation and differentiation capacities, fetal cells long have been recognized as ideal targets for gene transfers.

Characteristically, fetal mesenchymal stem cells (MSCs) express HLA class 1, but not HLA class 2. Although the presence of interferon gamma in the growth medium could initiate the intracellular synthesis and cell surface expression of HLA class 2 in these cells, normally neither undifferentiated nor differentiated fetal MSCs induce proliferation of allogenic lymphocytes in mixed cultures. This indicates that fetal MSCs may not elicit much alloreactive lymphocyte proliferation. These characteristics suggest that engineered constructs made with fetal cells should be less susceptible to rejection in heterologous applications. Even xenologous implantations eventually may become viable, as studies suggest that fetal cells also are tolerated better in cross-species transplantations, including in people.[6] At the same time, however, the expression of major histocompatibility complex antigens in the fetus and, hence, fetal allograft survival in immunocompetent recipients, is age- and tissue-specific.

Fetal cells often produce high levels of angiogenic and trophic factors, which enhance their ability to engraft and grow in vivo. Interestingly, those factors also can facilitate regeneration of surrounding host tissues. For example, significant clinical and hematological improvement has been described following fetal liver stem cell transplantation in people, even when there is no clear evidence of engraftment. These improvements have been attributed to regeneration of autologous hematopoiesis and inhibition of tumor cell growth promoted by the infused cells, through mechanisms that have yet to be determined fully.

Fetal Cell Sources

Fetal cells obtainable in amounts compatible with tissue engineering processing can be procured from various sites, in addition to the fetus itself. So far, proven viable sources have included the amniotic fluid, placenta, and umbilical cord blood. Of all these, the amniotic fluid and placenta are the least invasive ones, to a good extent because amniocentesis and chorionic villus sampling are widely accepted routine forms of prenatal diagnostic screening, which also obviates any ethical objection to the procurement from these sources.[7] This is particularly true for the amniotic fluid, in that an amniocentesis typically is offered to any mother with a fetus in whom a structural anomaly has been diagnosed by prenatal imaging, after such diagnosis. Further, an amniocentesis is the safest of any invasive prenatal diagnostic method, having long been associated with a less than 0.5% spontaneous abortion rate.[8] A small extra aliquot of amniotic fluid could be obtained at that time for tissue engineering purposes without any additional risk to the mother or fetus (**Fig. 1**).

Amniotic fluid

The cellular profile of the amniotic fluid varies throughout gestation. The mechanisms responsible for the production and turnover of the fluid itself are thought to also play a role in determining the cell types present in the amniotic cavity. In the first half of gestation, most of the amniotic fluid derives from active sodium and chloride transport across the amniotic membrane and fetal skin, with concomitant passive movement of water. In the second half, most of the fluid comes from fetal micturition. An additional substantial source of amniotic fluid is secretion from the respiratory tract. Fetal swallowing and gastrointestinal (GI) tract excretions, while not voluminous, also impact the composition of the amniotic fluid. As a result of such fluid dynamics, cells present in the urinary, respiratory, and GI tracts are shed into the amniotic cavity, in addition to skin cells. More importantly, however, embryonic and fetal cells from all three germ layers long have been identified therein.[9–12] Finally, select fetal pathologic states, such as neural tube and body wall defects for example, may lead to the presence of cells that are not normally found in the amniotic fluid in healthy pregnancies, which also could be clinically useful.

The fact that certain progenitor cells can be found in the amniotic fluid first was reported in 1993, when cells identified as hematopoietic progenitor cells were found there before the 12th week of gestation, possibly coming from the yolk sac.[13] A study from 1996 was the first to suggest the possibility of mutilineage potential of nonhematopoietic cells present in the amniotic fluid.[14] The presence of MSCs in the amniotic fluid, also referred to as mesenchymal amniocytes, has been proposed for many years. The differentiation potential of amniotic MSCs, however, has started to be determined only quite recently.[15–17] These cells can be differentiated into not only

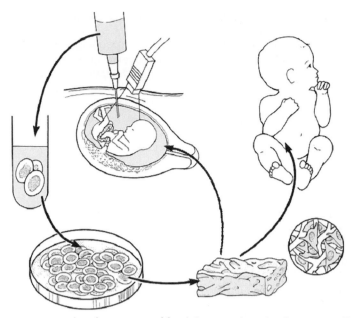

Fig. 1. Diagram representing the concept of fetal tissue engineering from naturally occurring amniotic fluid cells for the treatment of birth defects. A small aliquot of amniotic fluid is obtained from a diagnostic amniocentesis, which is performed regularly when a structural anomaly is diagnosed by prenatal imaging screening. Fetal tissue then is engineered in vitro from select amniotic progenitor cells while pregnancy continues, so that the newborn, or a fetus, can benefit from having autologous, expanded tissue promptly available for surgical reconstruction, either at birth or in utero.

mesodermal, but also ectodermal and endodermal cell lineages, rendering them particularly suitable for tissue engineering.[16–22] To date, there has been no conclusive evidence that cKit-positive stem cells recently reported in the amniotic fluid are different from amniotic MSCs.[21–23]

The authors have described a very simple protocol for isolation of mesenchymal amniocytes, based on mechanical separation and natural selection by the culture medium.[18,24] Other protocols for isolation of these cells also have been described.[16,25] Animal data have shown that amniotic fluid-derived MSCs proliferate significantly faster in culture than immunocytochemically comparable cells derived from fetal or adult subcutaneous connective tissue, neonatal bone marrow, and umbilical cord blood.[24,26,27] In people, the expansion potential of mesenchymal amniocytes exceeds that of bone marrow MSCs.[16,18] The phenotype of human mesenchymal amniocytes expanded in vitro is comparable to that reported for MSCs derived from second trimester fetal tissue and adult bone marrow.[19,28,29]

Maternal blood

Fetal cells can be found in the maternal circulation in most human pregnancies. Indeed, fetal progenitor cells have been found to persist in the circulation of women decades after child birth.[30] Interestingly, a novel population of fetal cells, the so-called pregnancy-associated progenitor cells (PAPCs), appears to differentiate in diseased/ injured maternal tissue, seemingly providing some measure of local repair. The precise phenotypical identity of these cells remains unknown. They are thought to be either a hematopoietic stem cell, a mesenchymal stem cell, or possibly a novel cell type. At this time, peripheral maternal blood has yet to be proven as a viable source of fetal cells in enough numbers for tissue engineering applications. Still, this perspective certainly deserves continued scrutiny.

The Fetus as a Host

Several advantages of a fetus receiving an engineered construct in utero could be envisioned, not only from a theoretical perspective, but also from clinical and experimental evidence derived from simple intrauterine cellular transplantation studies previously reported. Prospective advantages encompass

Induction of graft tolerance in the fetus due to its relative immunologic immaturity at early gestational ages

Induction of donor-specific tolerance in the fetus by concurrent or previous intra-uterine transplantation of hematopoietic progenitor cells

A completely sterile environment

The presence of hormones, cytokines, and other intercellular signaling factors that may enhance graft survival and development

The unique wound-healing properties of the fetus

Early prevention of clinical manifestations of disease, before they can cause irre-versible damage

Most of those advantages should be more or less evident, depending on the timing of prenatal transplantation.

CURRENT APPLICATIONS

Major congenital anomalies are present in approximately 3% of all newborns. Those diseases are responsible for nearly 20% of deaths occurring in the neonatal period and virtually immeasurable morbidity rates throughout childhood and later in life. Treatment of many congenital anomalies is hindered regularly by the scarce availability of normal tissues or organs, either in autologous or allologous fashion, especially at birth. Autologous grafting often is not an option in newborns because of donor site size limitations, and the ever-present severe donor shortage hindering practically all forms of transplantation is even more critical during the neonatal period. Fetal tissue engineering has emerged as a viable option to overcome these hurdles and offers a new alternative for treating these anomalies.

Although yet to be fully explored, several studies using fetal tissue engineering as a means to treat congenital anomalies have been reported in large animal models.[4,15,17,18,24,31–42] So far, these studies have involved models of relatively few congenital anomalies. Nonetheless, given the results reported to date, many other birth defects are likely candidates to eventually benefit from this therapeutic principle. The following section contains remarks on select experimental developments.

Diaphragmatic Hernia

According to the Congenital Diaphragmatic Hernia (CDH) Study Group, most infants who have CDH cannot have their diaphragmatic defect closed primarily.[43] Most of these patients end up receiving a prosthetic diaphragmatic patch. The dramatic improvement in survival of patients who had CDH experienced over the last two decades also has included patients who had prosthetic diaphragmatic repair, a well-known risk factor for recurrence of the hernia, which can occur in up to half of these patients.[44–47] Hernia recurrence is believed to derive from normal growth, which leads to traction and eventual detachment of the prosthesis. In addition to recurrence, repair of CDH with artificial prosthetic patches also has been linked with higher rates of infection, adhesions, and both thoracic and spinal column deformities, when compared with primary repair.[48,49] The use of a patch made of living autologous tissue conceivably could overcome much of the morbidity associated with prosthetic diaphragmatic repair. Given the timing of CDH repair in the neonatal period, an autologous construct would have to be made with fetal cells.

The first experimental report of engineered diaphragmatic replacement dates to 2000, when the authors used the concept of fetal tissue engineering with myoblast-based constructs to that end in an ovine model.[31] The authors' subsequent efforts have focused on the engineering of a diaphragmatic tendon, rather than a muscle patch, for various reasons. Except for the rare cases of complete diaphragmatic agenesis, the native residual diaphragmatic muscle seems to develop and function normally in most children who have CDH. Also, a sizeable portion of the normal diaphragm is comprised of a tendon. Besides, meaningful muscular function driven by substantial nerve ingrowth from the host has yet to be shown in engineered skeletal muscle grafts in large animal models. In a comparison between tendon-based and muscle-based constructs, the authors observed improved structural and biomechanical outcomes in vivo in the former, with eventual loss of myogenic identity of the donor cells in the latter.[40]

Amniotic MSCs have proven particularly effective and practical for diaphragmatic tendon engineering (**Fig. 2**).[35,40] By default, these cells tend to assume a fibroblastic/myofibroblastic phenotype, which is consistent with their intended function as living, engineered tendons. All these previous studies also have pointed to the fact that scaffold composition and architecture are determining factors of outcome, even when a preferable cell source is used.

Although much still can be pursued in optimizing different variables of diaphragmatic patch graft engineering, the currently prevalent high recurrence rates, combined with what has been achieved experimentally, arguably warrant initial clinical experience with fetal tissue engineering as a means to repair a CDH that cannot be closed primarily. This is expected for the not too distant future, pending regulatory approval, presently under review.

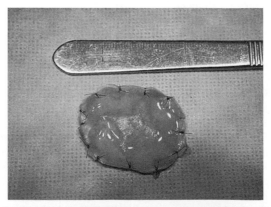

Fig. 2. Gross view of a diaphragmatic tendon patch engineered from ovine amniotic mesenchymal stem cells before surgical implantation.

Airway Anomalies

The treatment of the more severe forms of congenital tracheal anomalies, such as long-segment stenosis, atresia, and agenesis, remains fundamentally unsolved in pediatric surgery.[50] As is customary when an optimal procedure for a given disease has yet to be described, numerous surgical techniques and a plethora of either natural or artificial prostheses have been described, all of which have been fraught with complications such as stenosis, infection, implant extrusion, poor growth, and inconsistent functional outcomes.[51–56] A relatively recent development, cadaveric tracheal transplantation, has not improved this scenario.[57] Not surprisingly, overall mortality remains high.[55,56,58]

Primary anastomosis after resection is the treatment of choice for congenital tracheal defects and usually can be performed successfully for defects spanning up to 30% of the expected tracheal length. Unfortunately, however, over 50% of the cases involve more than 50% of the trachea, making primary reconstruction impossible without excessive anastomotic tension. Correction of long-length tracheal deformities would require a conduit that is rigid enough to prevent collapse on inspiration while remaining flexible enough to bend with the neck. A tissue-engineered conduit could offer these features, and have the potential for growth with the child. The authors have applied the principle of fetal tissue engineering in different experimental models of airway repair. They have shown that cartilage engineered from either fetal auricular chondrocytes or bone marrow-derived MSCs can be used to successfully repair tracheal defects in utero[32,33] The authors also have shown that cartilage can be engineered from fetal umbilical cord blood MSCs.[36] A considerable limitation of these early studies, however, is the fact all these cell sources are not easily accessible and carry a substantial risk for fetal and maternal morbidity or prolonged intervals between cell procurement and airway repair.

More recently, the authors have shown that cartilaginous grafts engineered from amniotic MSCs have a unique extracellular matrix composition, when compared with cartilage engineered from other perinatal MSCs, and when compared with native hyaline and elastic cartilage (**Fig. 3**).[27] Such composition proved particularly suitable for surgical implantation. Indeed, the authors have shown, in a large animal model, that cartilaginous grafts from amniotic MSCs could be a means for tracheal reconstruction.[41] Interestingly, although the grafts were engineered devoid of respiratory epithelium, they all became lined with pseudostratified columnar epithelium in vivo, and the animals were able to breathe spontaneously postoperatively. Stridor, however, eventually ensued in most subjects, likely because portions of the grafts remodeled into fibrous cartilage, leading to variable degrees of stenosis over time. Still, given the potential impact of fetal tissue engineering on the currently dismal prognosis of fetuses with major airway disease, further studies are warranted.

Another possible application of fetal tissue engineering is in the treatment of congenital cervical tumors. The prenatal detection of a cervical mass raises the prospect of clinically relevant airway compromise and respiratory distress at birth, often associated with significant airway damage, either from the disease process itself, or as a consequence of therapeutic measures such as emergency intubations or tracheostomies or the resection of the mass.[59–61] The planned availability of autologous engineered fetal cartilage could help minimize some of these complications.

Cardiovascular Anomalies

Congenital heart disease is the most frequent form of congenital anomaly and the leading cause of death among infants in the United States. Most congenital cardiac

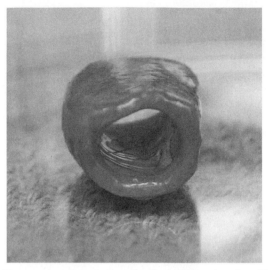

Fig. 3. A representative, cross-sectional view of a three-dimensional cartilaginous tube engineered from amniotic mesenchymal stem cells seeded onto a polyglycolic acid matrix, previously maintained in a bioreactor under chondrogenic conditions.

anomalies involve variable degrees of myocardial, valvar, or vascular deformities. Although primary repairs are often possible, implantation of different types of prosthesis may be necessary in more complex cases. Complications of prosthetic cardiac repair include thrombogenesis, absent contractility, lack of growth, material-related failures, and suture line ruptures, all of which contribute to significant morbidity and mortality.[62] Myocardial, valvar, and vascular tissue engineering are potentially improved alternatives to current methods of cardiac reconstruction, some of which already have been shown to be viable when fetal cells are employed.

A contractile autologous engineered patch could be valuable for repairing a severe septal defect, or as a means to replace myocardium in select cases of cardiac hypoplasia. Several investigators are working on this concept using two basic approaches. One, cellular cardiomyoplasty, involves simple direct injection of select cell suspensions, such as MSCs, into the myocardium, so as to possibly overcome the heart's inability to regenerate, as it has no known stem cells, and the mature cardiomyocyte is a terminally differentiated cell that does not enter the cell cycle to a significant degree.[63] Yet, the notion of differentiating MSCs, including some of fetal origin, into cardiomyocytes has met with conflicting results.[20,64,65] The other approach involves creating a three-dimensional implantable graft by seeding cells onto a scaffold. These constructs have a defined structure and may lead to more meaningful myocardial augmentation when transplanted. The authors have shown experimentally that an autologous fetal myoblast-based engineered muscle patch implanted onto the myocardium can display prolonged donor cell survival and engraftment, with eventual expression of proteins typical of a cardiomyocyte-like lineage on the donor cells. Conclusive documentation of myocardial transdifferentiation of these cells, along with functional analyses, remains to be described, however.

The engineering of heart valves normally involves two different layers, so as to mimic native valve architecture. An inner myofibroblast/fibroblast-based layer could produce the extracellular matrix profile typically responsible for the unique biomechanical properties found in heart valves, while an endothelial cell-based layer would produce an antithrombogenic and blood-compatible surface. The fabrication of such heart valves from both umbilical cord-derived and amniotic fluid-derived progenitor cells has been described in vitro.[66,67] Conclusive in vivo data on the ability of these structures to function as valve replacements remain to be described, however.

Deformities of the large vessels of the base of the heart are frequently a major component of congenital cardiac disease. In recent years, a Japanese group has accumulated considerable clinical experience with the use of conduits engineered from endothelial cells obtained from a peripheral vein as vascular replacements in low-pressure systems, in children with varying forms of complex congenital cardiovascular anomalies.[68,69] Current methods are focusing on the use of autologous bone marrow progenitor cells for seeding scaffold tubes based on special composite copolymers.[70,71] Thus far, the midterm outcome of engineered vascular grafts in children has shown continued patency, with balloon angioplasty having been required in some cases to treat tissue overgrowth at anastomotic sites. The long-term growth, remodeling, and biomechanical profile of these grafts remain unknown. Perhaps most importantly, prospective human trials comparing tissue-engineered conduits with those consisting solely of synthetic materials remain to be conducted. Still, the use of fetal cells in this setting, which has yet to be reported, could lead to improved results and deserves investigation.

Bone Defects

Several congenital defects involve some degree of bone loss, such as craniofacial, chest wall, and limb defects. Tissue engineering has proven viable in bone replacement ever since the late 1990s.[72] Both osteoblasts obtained from periosteal biopsies and bone marrow-derived MSCs have been described as viable cell sources in different, essentially anecdotal clinical applications.[72–75] Prenatal delivery of MSCs, for example, from first trimester peripheral fetal blood, also has been shown to ameliorate genetic bone disorders, such as osteogenesis imperfecta, both experimentally and clinically.[76–78] More recently, the authors have demonstrated that bone grafts can be engineered from amniotic MSCs and electrospun nanofibers (**Fig. 4**). These grafts have been used in the postnatal repair of full-thickness sternal defects, in a leporine model.[42] In light of these previous experimental and clinical data, the perspective of employing fetal tissue engineering for structural bone replacement seems to be another realistic prospect for the future.

Neural Tube Defects

Failure of the neural tube to close by the end of the fourth week of gestation leads to different forms of a midline vertebral defect (spina bifida), most often in the dorsal portion of the lumbosacral vertebrae. Spina bifida leads to injury/loss of spinal cord tissue at and below the lesion. Common manifestations include paraplegia, urinary and fecal incontinence, sexual dysfunction, and secondary musculoskeletal deformities. Overall mortality and morbidity rates remain high.[79]

Classical treatment of spina bifida consists of surgical closure of the spinal canal soon after birth, with lifelong support and rehabilitation usually necessary. Given that the neural damage associated with this disease is thought to be, at least in part, secondary to the exposure of the spinal cord to the amniotic fluid and local trauma, prenatal surgical closure of the defect has been performed at a few centers in an attempt to improve outcome. Although a large multicenter clinical trial of fetal repair (the Management of Myelomeningocele Study) is ongoing, clinical experience suggests that prenatal closure of spina bifida has had a limited impact on spinal cord function.[80–82]

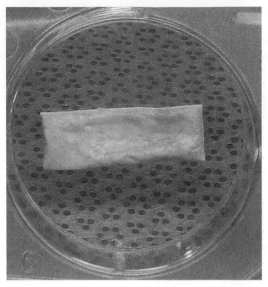

Fig. 4. Gross view of engineered bone made with human amniotic mesenchymal stem cells and electrospun nanofibers.

Neural stem cells (NSCs) have been shown to mediate repair in various postnatal central nervous system impairments, including in the spinal cord.[83–86] The authors have started to explore experimentally the notion of prenatal delivery of (fetal) NSCs as a potential means of promoting spinal cord repair and enhancing prenatal surgical coverage of spina bifida.[87] A pilot study has shown that donor NSCs selectively engrafted within the most damaged areas of the spinal cord and retained an undifferentiated state in vivo, producing neurotrophic factors locally. These early findings, taken together with the large body of data on the use of NSCs in other forms of spinal cord injury, support further investigation into this multifaceted prenatal therapy, combining local NSC delivery to the cord with mechanical/surgical repair aimed at inducing local protective or regenerative processes.

TRANSLATIONAL CONSIDERATIONS

In The United States, the Food and Drug Administration (FDA) has mandatory jurisdiction over cell-based therapies, such as tissue engineering. An elaborate and costly infrastructure is necessary for the development and manufacture of engineered tissue suitable for FDA validation. Such regulatory clearance demands cell and construct manufacturing at so-called good manufacturing practice (GMP) facilities, which not only must fulfill strict physical and operational requirements, but also be controlled by a critical mass of highly trained personnel. Another practical intricacy is the fact that certain tissues require preconditioning in intricate bioreactors, which may not be readily compatible with large-scale manufacturing or shipping.[88] All of these underlying hurdles translate into chronic difficulties in establishing clinical trials, particularly multicenter ones.

Regulatory constraints have hampered clinical translation of many tissue engineering therapies significantly.[89] The FDA often has been criticized for slow approval processes, which include both justifiable and questionable requirements. This predicament has been attributed, at least to some extent, to the lack of clear, predictable regulatory frameworks and to doubts concerning the proper classification of different tissue-engineered products. This is particularly evident when stem cells (including fetal) are to be used, in that, besides eventual ethical concerns, they typically trigger regulatory demands for unique safety data sets, more notably on genomic stability and tumorigenesis.

These constraints often have contributed, among other factors, to rendering tissue engineering products commercially unsustainable in the long run.[90,91] Indeed, many firms driven by an initial substantial interest in tissue engineering have exited the market over the last 5 to 10 years. Still, dozens of companies continue to invest in the development of new products.[92,93] It seems that a healthy partnership between academia and industry should be the best option to further expand tissue engineering into clinical reality, a principle that appears to be particularly relevant to fetal tissue engineering, given its sources purely in academia and its sizeable target market, not to mention the perspective of prolonged fetal cell banking.

Regulatory clearance of tissue engineering-based therapies typically involves three sets of requirements: cell manufacturing, scaffold manufacturing, and animal safety data. As it pertains to fetal tissue engineering, the authors recently showed that amniotic MSC manufacturing is feasible within regulatory guidelines, in a GMP-type facility, which has given further impetus to the prospect of timely clinical trials of at least some of the applications discussed previously.[94,95]

ETHICAL CONSIDERATIONS

Any use of fetal cells or tissue expectedly incites intense ethical debate and heavy regulation. Philosophically and theologically, there is no single authoritative position on the independent moral status of the fetus. Tissue sourced from induced abortion conflicts with fetal rights, while tissue sourced from spontaneous abortion is frequently compromised by chromosomal abnormalities, infections, and anoxia. Routine prenatal diagnostic procedures such as amniocentesis or chorionic villus sampling offer viable sources of fetal cells that do not challenge the rights of the unborn child, or place the mother at any additional risk. Used in autologous fashion, no ethical objections to fetal tissue engineering can be justified, as long as the procedure is a valid therapeutic choice for a given perinatal condition. Eventual heterologous applications should fall into the same moral and regulatory frameworks already governing the use of fetal cells, such as from umbilical cord banks.

SUMMARY

Considering the data reported thus far, it is reasonable to speculate that fetal tissue engineering may become an alternative for the perinatal treatment of several congenital anomalies. Moreover, given the feasibility of minimally invasive fetal cell sources, such as amniotic fluid, placenta, and umbilical cord blood, the promise of fetal tissue engineering should apply to both life-threatening and non life-threatening anomalies. Different fetal progenitor cells progressively are becoming relevant, if not indispensable tools in research related to stem cells, tissue engineering, gene therapy, and maternal–fetal medicine. Still, much remains to be learned, and various evolutionary paths, including unsuspected ones, are to be pursued in this relatively new branch of tissue engineering. Fetal tissue engineering also shall benefit from the progress expected for tissue engineering in general. Fertile experimental work from an ever-increasing number of groups has introduced promising novel therapeutic concepts employing fetal cells or the fetus as a host. The reach of fetal tissue engineering, nonetheless, likely will go beyond the perinatal period, offering unique therapeutic perspectives for different age groups.

REFERENCES

1. Hurst AF, Tanner WE, Osman AA. Addison's disease with severe anemia treated by suprarenal grafting. Proc R Soc Med 1922;15:19.
2. Vacanti JP, Morse MA, Saltzman WM, et al. Selective cell transplantation using bioabsorbable artificial polymers as matrices. J Pediatr Surg 1988;23:3–9.
3. Cusick RA, Sano K, Lee H, et al. Heterotopic fetal rat hepatocyte transplantation on biodegradable polymers. Surg Forum 1995;XLVI:658–61.
4. Fauza DO, Fishman SJ, Mehegan K, et al. Videofetoscopically assisted fetal tissue engineering: bladder augmentation. J Pediatr Surg 1998;33:7–12.
5. Fauza DO, Fishman SJ, Mehegan K, et al. Videofetoscopically assisted fetal tissue engineering: skin replacement. J Pediatr Surg 1998;33:357–61.
6. Liechty KW, MacKenzie TC, Shaaban AF, et al. Human mesenchymal stem cells engraft and demonstrate site-specific differentiation after in utero transplantation in sheep. Nat Med 2000;6:1282–6.
7. Fauza D. Amniotic fluid and placental stem cells. Best Pract Res Clin Obstet Gynaecol 2004;18:877–91.
8. Jauniaux E, Rodeck C. Use, risks and complications of amniocentesis and chorionic villous sampling for prenatal diagnosis in early pregnancy. Early Pregnancy 1995;1:245–52.
9. Milunsky A. Amniotic fluid cell culture. In: Milunsky A, editor. Genetic disorder of the fetus. New York: Plenum Press; 1979. p. 75–84.
10. Hoehn H, Salk D. Morphological and biochemical heterogeneity of amniotic fluid cells in culture. Methods Cell Biol 1982;26:11–34.
11. Gosden CM. Amniotic fluid cell types and culture. Br Med Bull 1983;39:348–54.
12. Prusa AR, Marton E, Rosner M, et al. Stem cell marker expression in human trisomy 21 amniotic fluid cells and trophoblasts. J Neural Transm Suppl 2003;67:235–42.
13. Torricelli F, Brizzi L, Bernabei PA, et al. Identification of hematopoietic progenitor cells in human amniotic fluid before the 12th week of gestation. Ital J Anat Embryol 1993;98:119–26.
14. Streubel B, Martucci-Ivessa G, Fleck T, et al. [In vitro transformation of amniotic cells to muscle cells–background and outlook]. Wien Med Wochenschr 1996; 146:216–7.
15. Kaviani A, Jennings RW, Fauza DO. Amniotic fluid-derived fetal mesenchymal cells differentiate into myogenic precursors in vitro [abstract]. J Am Coll Surg 2002;195:S29.
16. In't Anker PS, Scherjon SA, Kleijburg-van der Keur C, et al. Amniotic fluid as a novel source of mesenchymal stem cells for therapeutic transplantation. Blood 2003;102:1548–9.
17. Kunisaki SM, Jennings RW, Fauza DO. Fetal cartilage engineering from amniotic mesenchymal progenitor cells. Stem Cells Dev 2006;15:245–53.
18. Kaviani A, Guleserian K, Perry TE, et al. Fetal tissue engineering from amniotic fluid. J Am Coll Surg 2003;196:592–7.
19. Noort WA, Kruisselbrink AB, In't Anker PS, et al. Mesenchymal stem cells promote engraftment of human umbilical cord blood-derived CD34(+) cells in NOD/SCID mice. Exp Hematol 2002;30:870–8.
20. Zhao P, Ise H, Hongo M, et al. Human amniotic mesenchymal cells have some characteristics of cardiomyocytes. Transplantation 2005;79:528–35.

21. Holden C. Stem cells. Versatile stem cells without the ethical baggage? Science 2007;315:170.
22. Tsai MS, Hwang SM, Tsai YL, et al. Clonal amniotic fluid-derived stem cells express characteristics of both mesenchymal and neural stem cells. Biol Reprod 2006;74:545–51.
23. De Coppi P, Bartsch G Jr, Siddiqui MM, et al. Isolation of amniotic stem cell lines with potential for therapy. Nat Biotechnol 2007;25:100–6.
24. Kaviani A, Perry TE, Dzakovic A, et al. The amniotic fluid as a source of cells for fetal tissue engineering. J Pediatr Surg 2001;36:1662–5.
25. Hurych J, Macek M, Beniac F, et al. Biochemical characteristics of collagen produced by long term cultivated amniotic fluid cells. Hum Genet 1976;31:335–40.
26. Kunisaki SM, Fuchs JR, Azpurua H, et al. A comparison of different perinatal sources of mesenchymal progenitor cells: implications for tissue engineering. In: Hilton Head (SC): Thirty-seventh Annual Meeting of the American Pediatric Surgical Association.
27. Kunisaki SM, Fuchs JR, Steigman SA, et al. A comparative analysis of cartilage engineered from different perinatal mesenchymal progenitor cells. Tissue Eng 2007;13:2633–44.
28. Pittenger MF, Mackay AM, Beck SC, et al. Multilineage potential of adult human mesenchymal stem cells. Science 1999;284:143–7.
29. In't Anker PS, Noort WA, Scherjon SA, et al. Mesenchymal stem cells in human second-trimester bone marrow, liver, lung, and spleen exhibit a similar immunophenotype but a heterogeneous multilineage differentiation potential. Haematologica 2003;88:845–52.
30. Bianchi DW, Johnson KL, Salem D. Chimerism of the transplanted heart. N Engl J Med 2002;346:1410–2.
31. Fauza DO, Marler JJ, Koka R, et al. Fetal tissue engineering: diaphragmatic replacement. J Pediatr Surg 2001;36:146–51.
32. Fuchs JR, Terada S, Ochoa ER, et al. Fetal tissue engineering: In utero tracheal augmentation in an ovine model. J Pediatr Surg 2002;37:1000–6.
33. Fuchs JR, Hannouche D, Terada S, et al. Fetal tracheal augmentation with cartilage engineered from bone marrow-derived mesenchymal progenitor cells. J Pediatr Surg 2003;38:984–7.
34. Fuchs JR, Terada S, Hannouche D, et al. Fetal tissue engineering: chest wall reconstruction. J Pediatr Surg 2003;38:1188–93.
35. Fuchs JR, Kaviani A, Oh JT, et al. Diaphragmatic reconstruction with autologous tendon engineered from mesenchymal amniocytes. J Pediatr Surg 2004;39:834–8.
36. Fuchs JR, Hannouche D, Terada S, et al. Cartilage engineering from ovine umbilical cord blood mesenchymal progenitor cells. Stem Cells 2005;23:958–64.
37. Fuchs JR, Nasseri BA, Vacanti JP, et al. Postnatal myocardial augmentation with skeletal myoblast-based fetal tissue engineering. Surgery 2006;140:100–7.
38. Kaviani A, Perry TE, Barnes CM, et al. The placenta as a cell source in fetal tissue engineering. J Pediatr Surg 2002;37:995–9.
39. Krupnick AS, Balsara KR, Kreisel D, et al. Fetal liver as a source of autologous progenitor cells for perinatal tissue engineering. Tissue Eng 2004;10:723–35.
40. Kunisaki SM, Fuchs JR, Kaviani A, et al. Diaphragmatic repair through fetal tissue engineering: a comparison between mesenchymal amniocyte- and myoblast-based constructs. J Pediatr Surg 2006;41:34–9.
41. Kunisaki SM, Freedman DA, Fauza DO. Fetal tracheal reconstruction with cartilaginous grafts engineered from mesenchymal amniocytes. J Pediatr Surg 2006;41:675–82.

42. Steigman SA, Ahmed A, Shanti RM, et al. Sternal repair with bone grafts engineered from amniotic mesenchymal stem cells. J Pediatr Surg 2009, in press.
43. Clark RH, Hardin WD Jr, Hirschl RB, et al. Current surgical management of congenital diaphragmatic hernia: a report from the Congenital Diaphragmatic Hernia Study Group. J Pediatr Surg 1998;33:1004–9.
44. Atkinson JB, Poon MW. ECMO and the management of congenital diaphragmatic hernia with large diaphragmatic defects requiring a prosthetic patch. J Pediatr Surg 1992;27:754–6.
45. Moss RL, Chen CM, Harrison MR. Prosthetic patch durability in congenital diaphragmatic hernia: a long-term follow-up study. J Pediatr Surg 2001;36:152–4.
46. Lund DP, Mitchell J, Kharasch V, et al. Congenital diaphragmatic hernia: the hidden morbidity. J Pediatr Surg 1994;29:258–62.
47. Kimber CP, Dunkley MP, Haddock G, et al. Patch incorporation in diaphragmatic hernia. J Pediatr Surg 2000;35:120–3.
48. Cullen ML. Congenital diaphragmatic hernia: operative considerations. Semin Pediatr Surg 1996;5:243–8.
49. Greenholz SK. Congenital diaphragmatic hernia: an overview. Semin Pediatr Surg 1996;5:216–23.
50. Airway Reconstruction Team. Recent challenges in the management of congenital tracheal stenosis: an individualized approach. J Pediatr Surg 2005;40:774–80.
51. Hill SA, Milam M, Manaligod JM. Tracheal agenesis: diagnosis and management. Int J Pediatr Otorhinolaryngol 2001;59:63–8.
52. Backer CL, Mavroudis C, Dunham ME, et al. Intermediate-term results of the free tracheal autograft for long segment congenital tracheal stenosis. J Pediatr Surg 2000;35:813–8.
53. Bando K, Turrentine MW, Sun K, et al. Anterior pericardial tracheoplasty for congenital tracheal stenosis: intermediate to long-term outcomes. Ann Thorac Surg 1996;62:981–9.
54. Jacobs JR. Investigations into tracheal prosthetic reconstruction. Laryngoscope 1988;98:1239–45.
55. Wright CD, Graham BB, Grillo HC, et al. Pediatric tracheal surgery. Ann Thorac Surg 2002;74:308–13.
56. Backer CL, Mavroudis C, Gerber ME, et al. Tracheal surgery in children: an 18-year review of four techniques. Eur J Cardiothorac Surg 2001;19:777–84.
57. Jacobs JP, Quintessenza JA, Andrews T, et al. Tracheal allograft reconstruction: the total North American and worldwide pediatric experiences. Ann Thorac Surg 1999;68:1043–51.
58. Chiu PP, Kim PC. Prognostic factors in the surgical treatment of congenital tracheal stenosis: a multicenter analysis of the literature. J Pediatr Surg 2006;41:221–5.
59. Hirose S, Farmer DL, Lee H, et al. The ex utero intrapartum treatment procedure: looking back at the EXIT. J Pediatr Surg 2004;39:375–80.
60. Hirose S, Sydorak RM, Tsao K, et al. Spectrum of intrapartum management strategies for giant fetal cervical teratoma. J Pediatr Surg 2003;38:446–50.
61. Steigman SA, Nemes L, Barnewolt CE, et al. Differential risk for neonatal surgical airway intervention in prenatally diagnosed neck masses. J Pediatr Surg 2009;44:76–9.
62. Li RK, Yau TM, Weisel RD, et al. Construction of a bioengineered cardiac graft. J Thorac Cardiovasc Surg 2000;119:368–75.
63. Taylor DA, Atkins BZ, Hungspreugs P, et al. Regenerating functional myocardium: improved performance after skeletal myoblast transplantation. Nat Med 1998;4:929–33.

64. Sartore S, Lenzi M, Angelini A, et al. Amniotic mesenchymal cells autotransplanted in a porcine model of cardiac ischemia do not differentiate to cardiogenic phenotypes. Eur J Cardiothorac Surg 2005;28:677–84.
65. Iop L, Chiavegato A, Callegari A, et al. Different cardiovascular potential of adult- and fetal-type mesenchymal stem cells in a rat model of heart cryoinjury. Cell Transplant 2008;17:679–94.
66. Schmidt D, Mol A, Breymann C, et al. Living autologous heart valves engineered from human prenatally harvested progenitors. Circulation 2006;114:I125–131.
67. Schmidt D, Achermann J, Odermatt B, et al. Prenatally fabricated autologous human living heart valves based on amniotic fluid derived progenitor cells as single cell source. Circulation 2007;116:I64–70.
68. Shin'oka T, Imai Y, Ikada Y. Transplantation of a tissue-engineered pulmonary artery. N Engl J Med 2001;344:532–3.
69. Matsumura G, Hibino N, Ikada Y, et al. Successful application of tissue engineered vascular autografts: clinical experience. Biomaterials 2003;24:2303–8.
70. Hibino N, Shin'oka T, Matsumura G, et al. The tissue-engineered vascular graft using bone marrow without culture. J Thorac Cardiovasc Surg 2005;129: 1064–70.
71. Shin'oka T, Matsumura G, Hibino N, et al. Midterm clinical result of tissue-engineered vascular autografts seeded with autologous bone marrow cells. J Thorac Cardiovasc Surg 2005;129:1330–8.
72. Vacanti CA, Bonassar LJ, Vacanti MP, et al. Replacement of an avulsed phalanx with tissue-engineered bone. N Engl J Med 2001;344:1511–4.
73. Quarto R, Mastrogiacomo M, Cancedda R, et al. Repair of large bone defects with the use of autologous bone marrow stromal cells. N Engl J Med 2001;344: 385–6.
74. Warnke PH, Springer IN, Wiltfang J, et al. Growth and transplantation of a custom vascularised bone graft in a man. Lancet 2004;364:766–70.
75. Marcacci M, Kon E, Moukhachev V, et al. Stem cells associated with macroporous bioceramics for long bone repair: 6- to 7-year outcome of a pilot clinical study. Tissue Eng 2007;13:947–55.
76. Horwitz EM, Prockop DJ, Fitzpatrick LA, et al. Transplantability and therapeutic effects of bone marrow-derived mesenchymal cells in children with osteogenesis imperfecta. Nat Med 1999;5:309–13.
77. Horwitz EM, Prockop DJ, Gordon PL, et al. Clinical responses to bone marrow transplantation in children with severe osteogenesis imperfecta. Blood 2001;97: 1227–31.
78. Guillot PV, Abass O, Bassett JH, et al. Intrauterine transplantation of human fetal mesenchymal stem cells from first-trimester blood repairs bone and reduces fractures in osteogenesis imperfecta mice. Blood 2008;111:1717–25.
79. Worley G, Schuster JM, Oakes WJ. Survival at 5 years of a cohort of newborn infants with myelomeningocele. Dev Med Child Neurol 1996;38:816–22.
80. Bruner JP, Tulipan N, Paschall RL, et al. Fetal surgery for myelomeningocele and the incidence of shunt-dependent hydrocephalus. JAMA 1999;282:1819–25.
81. Sutton LN, Adzick NS. Fetal surgery for myelomeningocele. Clin Neurosurg 2004; 51:155–62.
82. Sutton LN, Adzick NS, Bilaniuk LT, et al. Improvement in hindbrain herniation demonstrated by serial fetal magnetic resonance imaging following fetal surgery for myelomeningocele. JAMA 1999;282:1826–31.
83. Snyder EY, Deitcher DL, Walsh C, et al. Multipotent neural cell lines can engraft and participate in development of mouse cerebellum. Cell 1992;68:33–51.

84. Whittemore SR, Snyder EY. Physiological relevance and functional potential of central nervous system-derived cell lines. Mol Neurobiol 1996;12:13–38.
85. Teng YD, Lavik EB, Qu X, et al. Functional recovery following traumatic spinal cord injury mediated by a unique polymer scaffold seeded with neural stem cells. Proc Natl Acad Sci USA 2002;99:3024–9.
86. Lu P, Jones LL, Snyder EY, et al. Neural stem cells constitutively secrete neurotrophic factors and promote extensive host axonal growth after spinal cord injury. Exp Neurol 2003;181:115–29.
87. Fauza DO, Jennings RW, Teng YD, et al. Neural stem cell delivery to the spinal cord in an ovine model of fetal surgery for spina bifida. Surgery 2008;144:367–73.
88. Griffith LG, Naughton G. Tissue engineering—current challenges and expanding opportunities. Science 2002;295:1009–14.
89. Ahsan T, Nerem RM. Bioengineered tissues: the science, the technology, and the industry. Orthod Craniofac Res 2005;8:134–40.
90. Bouchie A. Tissue engineering firms go under. Nat Biotechnol 2002;20:1178–9.
91. Fauza DO. Tissue engineering: current state of clinical application. Curr Opin Pediatr 2003;15:267–71.
92. Lysaght MJ, Reyes J. The growth of tissue engineering. Tissue Eng 2001;7:485–93.
93. Vacanti JP. Tissue engineering: from bench to bedside via commercialization. Surgery 2008;143:181–3.
94. Kunisaki SM, Armant M, Kao GS, et al. Tissue engineering from human mesenchymal amniocytes: a prelude to clinical trials. J Pediatr Surg 2007;42:974–80.
95. Steigman SA, Armant M, Bayer-Zwirello L, et al. Preclinical regulatory validation of a 3-stage amniotic mesenchymal stem cell manufacturing protocol. J Pediatr Surg 2008;43:1164–9.

Index

Note: Page numbers of article titles are in **boldface** type.

A

Abdominal masses, MRI in, 290–291
Abortion preference, in clinical trials, 242–243
Acardiac twin. *See* Twin-reversed arterial perfusion sequence/acardiac twin.
Acetaminophen, for NICU, 219, 221
Adeno-associated virus, for gene transfer, 458–459, 462
Adenoviruses, for gene transfer, 458–459
Agenesis, corpus callosal, 280–283
Airway
    anomalies of, tissue engineering for, 479
    obstruction of
        EXIT procedure for, 267–268
        MRI in, 287
Alfentanil, for NICU, 217
Amniocentesis, in defect detection, 231
Amnioreduction, for twin-twin transfusion syndrome, 250–251, 400–401, 408–409
Amniotic fluid, fetal cells in, for tissue engineering, 475–476
Anastomosis, in monochorionic twin pregnancy, 419–421
Anesthesia
    for fetal valvuloplasty, 446–447
    topical, for NICU, 219
Angiogenesis factors, in twin-twin transfusion syndrome, 394
Aortic stenosis, 441–442
    echocardiography in, 303–304, 306–309
    ultrasonography in, 269–270
Aortic valvuloplasty, 303–304, 306–309, 445–446
Atrial natriuretic peptide, in twin-twin transfusion syndrome, 393–394
Atrial septoplasty, 310–311, 442, 446
Atrioventicular block, echocardiography in, 302–303

B

Balloon occlusion, tracheal. *See* Tracheal occlusion.
Barbiturates, for NICU, 218
Benzodiazepines, for NICU, 217–218, 220–221
Biopsy, fetal, 231
Bladder
    histology of, in urinary tract obstruction, 380
    outlet obstruction of, shunt for, 269
Blood, maternal, fetal cells in, for tissue engineering, 476–477
Bone defects, tissue engineering for, 481

Clin Perinatol 36 (2009) 489–501
doi:10.1016/S0095-5108(09)00036-0   perinatology.theclinics.com
0095-5108/09/$ – see front matter © 2009 Elsevier Inc. All rights reserved.

Moving?

Make sure your subscription moves with you!

To notify us of your new address, find your **Clinics Account Number** (located on your mailing label above your name), and contact customer service at:

E-mail: elspcs@elsevier.com

800-654-2452 (subscribers in the U.S. & Canada)
314-453-7041 (subscribers outside of the U.S. & Canada)

Fax number: 314-523-5170

Elsevier Periodicals Customer Service
11830 Westline Industrial Drive
St. Louis, MO 63146

*To ensure uninterrupted delivery of your subscription, please notify us at least 4 weeks in advance of move.